"It All Depends on the Dose"

This is the first volume to take a broad historical sweep of the close relation between medicines and poisons in the Western tradition, and their interconnectedness. They are like two ends of a spectrum, for the same natural material can be medicine or poison, depending on the dose, and poisons can be transformed into medicines, while medicines can turn out to be poisons. The book looks at important moments in the history of the relationship between poisons and medicines in European history, from Roman times, with the Greek physician Galen, through the Renaissance and the maverick physician Paracelsus, to the present, when poisons are actively being turned into beneficial medicines.

Ole Peter Grell is Professor in Early Modern History at The Open University, U.K.

Andrew Cunningham was formerly Senior Research Fellow at the Department of History and Philosophy of Science, University of Cambridge, U.K.

Jon Arrizabalaga is Research Professor in History of Science at the Spanish National Research Council (CSIC), Institución Milà i Fontanals, Barcelona, Spain.

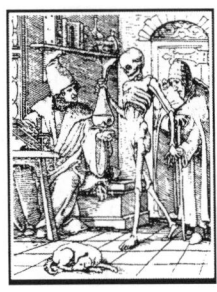

Poison bottle, cobalt blue skull. Wheaton Arts and Cultural Center, Museum of American Glass, Millville, NJ.

The History of Medicine in Context

Series Editors: Andrew Cunningham
Department of History and Philosophy of Science,
University of Cambridge
Ole Peter Grell
Department of History, The Open University

Titles in the series include

Medicine, Trade and Empire
Garcia de Orta's Colloquies on the Simples and Drugs of India (1563)
in Context
Palmira Fontes da Costa

**The Political and Social Dynamics of Poverty, Poor Relief and
Health Care in Early-Modern Portugal**
Laurinda Abreu

The World of Plants in Renaissance Tuscany
Medicine and Botany
Cristina Bellorini

Plague, Print, and the Reformation
The German Reform of Healing, 1473–1573
Erik A. Heinrichs

Pathology in Practice
Diseases and Dissections in Early Modern Europe
Edited by Silvia De Renzi, Marco Bresadola and Maria Conforti

"It All Depends on the Dose"
Poisons and Medicines in European History
Edited by Ole Peter Grell, Andrew Cunningham and Jon Arrizabalaga

For more information about this series, please visit: https://www.routledge.
com/The-History-of-Medicine-in-Context/book-series/HMC

"It All Depends on the Dose"
Poisons and Medicines in European History

Edited by Ole Peter Grell,
Andrew Cunningham and
Jon Arrizabalaga

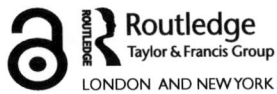
Routledge
Taylor & Francis Group
LONDON AND NEW YORK

First published 2018
by Routledge
2 Park Square, Milton Park, Abingdon, Oxon OX14 4RN

and by Routledge
605 Third Avenue, New York, NY 10017

First issued in paperback 2022

Routledge is an imprint of the Taylor & Francis Group, an informa business

British Library Cataloguing-in-Publication Data
A catalogue record for this book is available from the British Library

Library of Congress Cataloging-in-Publication Data
Names: Grell, Ole Peter, editor.
Title: "It all depends on the dose": poisons and medicines in European history / edited by Ole Peter Grell, Andrew Cunningham and Jon Arrizabalaga.
Description: New York: Routledge, 2018. | Series: The history of medicine in context | Includes bibliographical references and index.
Identifiers: LCCN 2017057421 (print) | LCCN 2017059064 (ebook) | ISBN 9781315521091 (ebook) | ISBN 9781138697614 (hbk: alk. paper) | ISBN 9781315521091 (ebk)
Subjects: LCSH: Drugs—Toxicology—History—Europe. | Poisons—History—Europe. | Drugs—Dose-response relationship.
Classification: LCC RA1238 (ebook) | LCC RA1238 .I83 2018 (print) | DDC 615.9094—dc23
LC record available at https://lccn.loc.gov/2017057421

ISBN 13: 978-1-03-240191-1 (pbk)
ISBN 13: 978-1-138-69761-4 (hbk)
ISBN 13: 978-1-315-52109-1 (ebk)

DOI: 10.4324/9781315521091

Typeset in Sabon
by codeMantra

Contents

Figures

Tables

Contributors

Jeffrey Aronson is Honorary Consultant Physician and Clinical Pharmacologist at the Centre for Evidence Based Medicine, Nuffield Department of Primary Care Health Sciences, Oxford, U.K.

Jon Arrizabalaga is Research Professor in History of Science at the Spanish National Research Council (CSIC), Institución Milà i Fontanals, Barcelona, Spain.

José Ramón Bertomeu-Sánchez is Senior Lecturer in History of Science at the University of Valencia, Spain, and Director of the Institute for the History of Medicine and Science "López Piñero" at the University of Valencia.

Montserrat Cabré is Associate Professor of the History of Science at the Universidad de Cantabria, Spain.

Andrew Cunningham was formerly Senior Research Fellow at the Department of History and Philosophy of Science, University of Cambridge, U.K.

Robin E. Ferner is Director at the West Midlands Centre for Adverse Drug Reactions, City Hospital, Birmingham and Honorary Professor of Clinical Pharmacology, School of Medicine, University of Birmingham.

Ole Peter Grell is Professor in Early Modern History at The Open University, U.K.

Anne Hardy is Honorary Professor at the Centre for History in Public Health at The London School of Hygiene and Tropical Medicine, U.K.

Georgiana Hedesan is Wellcome Trust Fellow at the University of Oxford, U.K.

Helen King is Professor Emerita of Classical Studies at The Open University, U.K.

Alessandro Pastore is Professor Emeritus of Early Modern History at the University of Verona, Italy.

Toine Pieters is Professor in the History of Pharmacy and Allied Sciences at the Descartes Centre for the History and The Philosophy of the Sciences and the Humanities, Utrecht University, The Netherlands.

Alisha Rankin is Associate Professor of History at Tufts University, U.S.A.

Fernando Salmón is Professor of the History of Science at the Universidad de Cantabria, Spain.

Acknowledgements

Most of the contributions in this volume were first given at a conference on the theme, organised by the editors and held in the Institución Milà i Fontanals, Barcelona Division of the Spanish National Research Council, the Consejo Superior de Investigaciones Científicas. We thank the Residència d'Investigadors, where the sessions were held.

We thank the Wellcome Trust and the Research Committee of the Arts Faculty of The Open University for their financial assistance for the conference. We also thank Ashgate Publishing for the reception.

We thank William Bynum and Helen Bynum for their papers given at the conference, on poison in the hospital, and on poison on the stage, respectively, and regret that neither of them felt able to offer final versions for this book. We particularly thank Jeffrey Aronson and Robin E. Ferner for their paper, specially written for this volume, and we also thank John Gabbay for acting as intermediary.

Introduction
Deadly medicine

Andrew Cunningham

Medicines and poisons have been closely related in the Western tradition since at least the time of Hippocrates. Yet historical coverage of the relation between medicines and poisons has been very patchy, and while the history of Greek herbals and their Renaissance counterparts has received substantial study, the most recent novel interest – stemming from the 1960s – has been on the role of narcotics and other addictive drugs.[1] There has been some recent work on the deliberate use of poisons and antidotes in the Middle Ages and in the sixteenth and seventeenth centuries, looking at the issue both in material and metaphorical terms, using literary works to explore both murderous intentions and symbolic significations in the use of poisons and antidotes.[2] By contrast, what we are presenting here is a volume that takes a broad historical sweep of the close relation between medicines and poisons in the Western tradition and of their interconnectedness.[3] They are like two ends of a single spectrum.

The title of our book is a quotation from the writings of the sixteenth-century medical maverick, Paracelsus. It comes from the third of his *Seven Defensiones (Septem Defensiones)*, first published in Cologne in 1564, some twenty-three years after his death. It will be discussed several times by contributors to the present volume, and in several formulations. Paracelsus is here defending himself against other physicians who say that 'the prescriptions I write are poison, corrosive, and an extraction of all that is evil and poisonous in nature'. But in making these accusations, Paracelsus says, his opponents

> are lacking in understanding and ignorant of natural forces. For what has God created that is not blessed with a great gift for the good of man? Why then should poison be rejected and despised, if not the poison but nature be sought?

What matters, Paracelsus argues, is the dose: 'it is not too much, nor too little. He who strikes the middle, receives no poison'.

> If you wish justly to explain each poison, what is there that is not poison? All things are poison, and nothing is without poison: the *Dosis* alone makes a thing not poison.[4]

Or, as we have chosen to render it, 'It all depends on the dose'. It will be seen in the course of this volume that Paracelsus was neither the first nor the last medical man to express this sentiment, though perhaps he did so most pithily.

As Brockliss and Jones have recently written, 'Paracelsus had urged the use of a number of poisonous minerals such as antimony, mercury, and arsenic on the grounds that diseases were poisons which needed to be treated with antidotes',[5] that is to say, with other poisons suitably prepared. As we shall see, for varying reasons, different practitioners over time have frequently used poisons as medicines or as antidotes against other poisons.

At first glance, it might seem that the whole Western tradition of medicine is based on poison, since Asclepius, the Greek god of medicine, is traditionally portrayed with a snake twisting around his staff. However, it appears that this was a non-poisonous species of snake and was there to represent the symbolic value of medicine, though what that symbolism was is still unresolved among historians. These snakes also slithered constantly around the healing temples of the god, interacting with the patients.

The earliest-known surviving works on poisons and antidotes in the Western tradition were two works in Greek, written by Nicander of Colophon around 150 BC, the *Theriaca* and the *Alexipharmaca*.[6] In the first of these, Nicander announces that he 'will expound the forms of savage creatures and their deadly injuries which smite one unforeseen, and countering remedy for the harm'.[7] Spiders, snakes, asps and vipers all have deadly venom, which can be countered in various ways. Best of all is this counter-remedy: 'If however you can cast snakes coupled at a crossroads, alive and just mating, into a pot, and the following medicaments besides, you have a preventive against deadly disasters'.[8] The antidotes are taken from plant leaves and roots, and from animals such as birds and the sea turtles. Spiders, wasps, scorpions, centipedes, salamanders and stingrays are similarly dealt with. The *Alexipharmaca* deals in poetic fashion with other poisons such as aconite, white lead, coriander, hemlock, arrow poison, toads, fungi and other vegetable and mineral substances, with the effects of them in poisoning humans and with an array of antidotes.[9]

In the present volume, Toine Pieters begins the discussion of medicines as poisons and vice versa. He gives an overview of how the highly significant developments in the sciences in the nineteenth century, especially in chemistry, physiology and pharmacology, 'opened new avenues for mass poisoning' (as he puts it) in many fields, including in hospitals. He focuses in particular on the important role of arsenic – the 'king of poisons', as John Parascandola has called it – in the deliberate poisoning of people. He investigates the story of a famous arsenic poisoner active in late-nineteenth-century Leiden, the Jekyll-and-Hyde character, 'Good Mie' and her alternate personality as 'Murderous Mie'. Over the course of the nineteenth century, what had been seen as habituation to a strong drug gradually came to be seen as addiction and abuse. The pharmaceutical developments of the period have come to produce many more medicines that were quickly seen to be poisons.

In the Western tradition of learned medicine, it is Galen who looms largest as model medical thinker and authority. His works were in use into the seventeenth century, so what he had to say about poisons was crucial. In our second chapter, Helen King shows that Galen had extensive experience of poisons and antidotes and wrote about them both at length. She also shows that among ruling families and elsewhere in Roman imperial times, poisons and suspected poisons were widely used against one's enemies. Antidotes were used to accustom the body in advance to poisonous substances, especially the famous mithridatium (mithridate), in order to evade the attempts of poisoners. Dosage was all important. Epidemics, the much-feared appearances of a deadly disease across a whole community, were particularly difficult to account for and to treat in a medical system like that of Galen, based as it was on the individual person and his or her particular humoral balance. King explores how Galen effectively adopted the theory of how poisons work in order to explain also how the whole humoral body works, beginning (as King puts it), 'to think about poison as a model for disease and, indeed, for healing'.

The chapter by Montserrat Cabré and Fernando Salmón takes us into the heart of Christianised Europe and the world of miracles and devotion to the Virgin. They analyse the story of the apparent poisoning of a young girl who had been fasting intensely – but not poisoned by a human agent, nor by a poison introduced from outside her body. She was devoted to the cult of Mary and signalled that her heart was the locus of her illness. Her mother appears to have called for her heart to be anatomised. When the heart was dissected, the onlookers found 'a likeness of the Glorious one, which She [Holy Mary] had graven there'. The finding leads the onlookers to praise Mary. It looks like a case of self-poisoning, the possibility of which had been expounded in the writings of Avicenna, the great Persian writer who developed the Greek tradition from Galen. Cabré and Salmón take us into some of the different ways in which poisoning could be believed to happen, even 'through a glance, a sound or a smell'.

Epidemics, where a whole population suffers from a sudden and usually fatal illness, were difficult to understand in medieval Christian Europe. On the one hand, to believers, epidemics were clearly the action of God, warning or punishing society. On the other, the dominant theoretical medical teaching, derived from Galen, dealt with individuals, not people in the mass. But suffering societies were not passive: they frequently sought out scapegoats such as lepers, Jews or simply foreigners, believing them to have deliberately poisoned the water supply. Jon Arrizabalaga explores these issues in fourteenth-century southern Europe in our fourth chapter, focussing on the so-called 'Black Death' of 1348–49. He shows that the fear caused by epidemics in turn led to the belief that the poison of epidemics could not only be spread deliberately by evil persons, but also be man-made often in the form of powders. Belief in man-made poisons even reached the academic arena of Montpellier University's medical faculty.

Georgiana D. Hedesan's chapter brings us right to Paracelsus himself, the celebrated rejecter of the classical tradition in medicine that had stemmed from Hippocrates and Galen. She concentrates on seven writings by Paracelsus in order to try and find how consistent his teachings on poison were, and on what principles they were based. Paracelsus's basic position is that all diseases are caused by poison of one sort or another, and Hedesan deals with his views on the origin of such poisons in *ens astrale*, a heavenly infection. Paracelsus is not an easy author, and careful analysis is needed to understand his theories, and Hedesan's title indicates the range of fields to which Paracelsus turned: alchemy, potency and imagination. She concludes her analysis by reaffirming the centrality of Christianity to Paracelsus's thinking about poison.

We have seen from the contribution of Cabré and Salmón that the concept of self-poisoning could be legitimately applied in a deeply religious Christian context and, at the same time, be justified from the Greek–Arabic medical tradition. In more recent centuries, there have been a number of celebrated instances of investigators deliberately self-poisoning, but on these occasions simply in order to see what would happen. For instance, John Hunter in 1767 inoculated himself with the poison – the *virus* – of gonorrhoea in an attempt to prove that gonorrhoea and syphilis were the same disease.[10] Ole Grell now takes us on an unexpected journey to the heart of the Protestant Reformation, showing how Martin Luther, himself a former friar and therefore sworn to celibacy, promoted the view that sexual abstinence – that is, the unnatural retention of semen, both male and female – was itself a form of self-poisoning. Its antidote, Luther claimed, was marriage. Again, as Grell shows, this position could find support in classical medical texts by Galen, one of which may have been Luther's source.

Though they may never have experienced them themselves, the people of early modern Western Europe were very familiar with the motifs of poisons and antidotes. They suspended their disbelief when watching many of the plays written for the stage in early modern Europe, in which playwrights frequently resorted to potions, poisons and antidotes as very handy dramatic devices. They distinguish the bad guys who administer the poisons from the good guys who bring the antidotes. The great thing about poisons on the stage is that a stage poison can work as quickly, or slowly, as the dramatist wants or needs, while similarly the antidote can bring a character back to life and resolve the drama at whatever pace is required. Shakespeare adopts such dramatic devices frequently. The tragedy of Romeo and Juliet depends entirely on potions, poisons and antidotes: a wise friar, skilled in the virtues of herbs, gives Juliet a sleeping draught (a potion) to feign death and thus avoid an impending marriage. This seeming death on Juliet's part Romeo mistakes for self-poisoning, leading him to immediately poison himself using poison acquired from an apothecary. In another play revolving around poison, Shakespeare could for the sake of the drama even introduce new anatomical pathways for the poison to travel: Hamlet's sleeping father is poisoned by 'juice of cursed hebenon' poured into his ear, which swiftly 'courses through the natural gates and alleys of the body' and curdles the blood and kills the king. Other characters in *Hamlet* are killed by a poisoned sword or a poisoned drink.

But poison on the stage may not merely be a convenient dramatic device: it can be a metaphor to represent the evil in the society being portrayed, or it can be the trigger for psychological changes or a symbol of such changes. 'In poison there is physic', the Earl of Northumberland says, grieving over the news of the death of his son Percy, known as Hotspur; throwing away his crutch, he resolves on 'bloody courses' to be avenged (*King Henry IV*, Part Two, I, i, 137). He is cured from his own ailment by the poison of the news of his son's death.

These obsessions with the role of poison and antidote in the theatre have been widely adopted for the opera stage as well, especially in scenarios where the poison or drug is false or the wrong one. In Donizetti's comic opera *L'elisir d'amore*, the shy young man is sold a love potion that isn't a love potion – yet it works. In Wagner's *Tristan und Isolde*, by contrast, where the text is full of potions, poisons and antidotes, both actual and psychological, a love drug is administered accidentally instead of a deadly poisonous potion, with extraordinary rapturous results and for which the only antidote is death.

The courts of the Italian Renaissance states have long been notorious for the deployment of poison by those wishing to take over power. This image comes to us from writers such as Stendhal and historians such as Burckhardt. Alessandro Pastore in our seventh chapter, dealing with 'poisoning as politics', confirms, from a wide range of sources, that poisoning was indeed a political weapon in Renaissance Italy, in the courts of local rulers and of the papacy. He shows that diplomatic correspondence of the time had as many rumours of poisoning as valid reports on poisoning. Doctors and political theorists were concerned with how rulers should keep away from harm and familiarise themselves with antidotes, and some rulers such as Cosimo I de' Medici had a ready supply of condemned men on whom to experiment. The papal court was far from immune to poisoners and plotters.

The role or roles of women in making and administering poisons in the early modern period have been widely studied in recent years. Alisha Rankin, by contrast, in Chapter 8 offers a study of the role of women in preparing or procuring antidotes, a possible further skill in their role as healers. She explores whether or how far antidotes to poisons were gendered. She finds much new material in manuscripts, which indicates women's interest in poison antidotes.

Mateu Orfila, who came from the island of Minorca and went on to fame in Paris, is generally credited with creating the science and practice of toxicology; the investigation of poisons, their nature, effects and their detection.

His (1815) *Traité des poisons* became Europe's textbook on the subject. But it was a science in the making, and everything about it was controversial. José Bertomeu-Sánchez explores Orfila's use of live animals for testing poisons and antidotes, and his employment in legal trials as a toxicologist, especially for the detection of arsenic in cases of alleged poisoning. Orfila was a showman as well as an investigative scientist, and Bertomeu-Sánchez highlights Orfila's public performances in front of students, fellow medical men, and in the law courts, as well as his extensive chemical experiments. The developing situation was in no way clear-cut, as is shown by the continued controversy over the existence of 'normal arsenic' in the human body.

Of all the naturally occurring poisons, mercury has perhaps been the most actively employed in civilised life. It was – and still is – everywhere we look, in measuring instruments such as thermometers and barometers, in electric apparatus and lighting, in our mended teeth and in mirrors. It will be a long time before we can live in a mercury-free world. And it was also very actively employed for centuries in attempting to cure syphilis or the pox. The treatment was often more painful than the illness, and it remained questionable whether the use of mercury created a disease rather than cured it. This continued almost to the mid-twentieth century. In Chapter 10, Andrew Cunningham explores this persistent reliance on, and faith in, the restorative properties of mercury: a known poison used against another poison, the *virus* of the pox.

Our final two chapters bring us full circle in this exploration of the relation between poisons and medicines in Western history, for here our contributors deal with current practice in eliciting new medicines from notorious poisons and with new ways of assessing dosage – and hence toxicity – in administering medicines. Louis Pasteur, in seeking a remedy for someone bitten by a rabid dog (rabies), in 1885, discovered that by manipulation of the poison – the *virus* – in the laboratory, he could create an antidote in the form of a vaccine. Pasteur's method was to culture the virus in the laboratory, but solely in living animals. By trial-and-error experimenting, he found that the virus could be made either more virulent or more attenuated, if passed through guinea pigs or rabbits. It was all a matter of timing in the laboratory. And then, increasingly virulent injections of the vaccine could actually cure the patient, as he famously demonstrated with the young Joseph Meister. As he said, the disease – that is, the *virus*, the poison – becomes its own preventive.

In her chapter on food poisoning in the Britain of the 1880s and onwards to the present day, Anne Hardy shows how certain agents most poisonous to man have been turned, through laboratory manipulation, into therapeutic agents. It is a very interesting turn on the Paracelsian view of the relation of poisons and medicines. Drug companies, themselves a new kind of business in the nineteenth century, took up much of this investigative role in their laboratories in the case of ergot – 'a veritable treasure house for drugs' as one of the main investigators called it – and naturally enough, given their commercial interests, they were very interested in dosage. She also shows that interest in using the botulinum toxin was shown by the US military developing bacteriological warfare, though its most widespread use has been as the cosmetic Botox.

Jeffrey K. Aronson and Robin E. Ferner are the authors of our final chapter, which brings the whole discussion of dosage up to date. These authors are both practitioners of clinical pharmacology today, and their contribution here reflects their own present-day research on reactions to medicines and thus on questions of dosage. They draw our attention to the Law of Mass Action propounded by two Norwegian scientists in 1864, which was the foundation of quantitative treatment of pharmacological phenomena and which 'dictates that the magnitude of a pharmacological reaction increases with increasing dose'. Aronson and Ferner trace much subsequent experimental research subsequent to the establishment of that Law, including the introduction of the concept of receptors, and concentration-effect and dose-response lines of inquiry, bringing the whole discussion up to the present day. It seems that it *does* indeed all depend on the dose, though many other factors are involved.

Notes

1 For instance, Roy Porter and Mikuláš Teich, eds., *Drugs and narcotics in history*, Cambridge: Cambridge University Press, 1995.
2 See Sarah Voinier and Guillaume Winter, eds., *Poison et antidote dans l'Europe des XVI et XVII siècles*, Arras: Artois presses université, 2011. Franck Collard, *The crime of poison in the Middle Ages*, Westport, Conn.: Praeger, 2008 (first publ. in French 2003).
3 On poisons and their histories, see, for instance, Lloyd G. Stevenson, *The meaning of poison*, Logan Clendening Lectures on the History and Philosophy of Medicine, Seventh Series, Lawrence: University of Kansas Press, 1959; John Timbrell, *The poison paradox: chemicals as friends and foes*, Oxford: Oxford University Press, 2005; Joel Levy, *Poison: a social history*, Stroud, UK: The History Press, 2011; John Elmsley, *The elements of murder: a history of poison*, Oxford: Oxford University Press, 2005.
4 *Four treatises of Theophrastus von Hohenheim called Paracelsus*. Translated from the original German, with Introductory essays by C. Lillian Temkin, George Rosen, Gregory Zilboorg, and Henry E. Sigerist. Edited with a preface by Henry E. Sigerist. The quotations are from pages 20, 21 and 22, and the translation is by C. Lilian Temkin. The German original is as follows:

> Die da sagen, das meine Recept, so ich schreib, ein Gifft, Corusium, und *Extraction* sein aller bóßheit und gifftigfeit der Natur ... Dann im selbigen puncten sind sie unverstendig, und unwissend in den natürlichen krefften. Dann was ist das Gotterschaffen hat, das nie mit einer grossen gaben begnadet sei, dem Menschen zu guten? Warumb soll dann Gifft verworffen und veracht werden, so doch nicht das Gifft, sonder die Natur gesucht werde? ... Was ist das nit Gifft ist? alle ding sind Gifft, und nichts ohn Gifft, allein die Dosis macht, das ein ding Gifft ist.
> Paracelsus, *Septem Defensiones Die Selbstverteidigung eines Aussenseiters*; reprint of the 1589 edition, pp. 169–170 (60, 62)

5 Laurence Brockliss and Colin Jones, *The medical world of early modern France*, Oxford: Clarendon Press, 1997, p. 122, no direct reference given to the writings of Paracelsus.

6   Scholars still dispute about whether the content of these poems is original with Nicander, or whether it was taken from one Apollodorus, whose writings are cited by Pliny in the *Natural History*.

7   A.S.F. Gow and A.F. Scholfield, eds., *Nicander: the poems and poetical fragments*, Cambridge: Cambridge University Press, 1953, p. 29, the first verse.

8   Gow and Scholfield, p. 35.

9   Peter K. Knoefel and Madeline C. Covi, eds., *A Hellenistic treatise on poisonous animals (the "Theriaca" of Nicander of Colophon): a contribution to the history of toxicology*, Lewiston, NY: The Edwin Mellen Press, 1991.

10 See Wendy Moore, *The knife man*, London: Bantam Press, 2005, pp. 188–197, who concludes that this was an instance of self-experimentation, not carried out on a third party.

1   Poisons in the historic medicine cabinet

Toine Pieters

Suppose that you are stricken with bad luck and you are diagnosed with cancer.[1] About half of all men and a third of all women will be diagnosed with cancer at some point in their lives. In the process, your doctor will tell you about your cancer: the name, size, location, origin, whether it has spread and if it is slow-growing or aggressive. You will certainly ask your doctor about the available treatment options, the success rates and the expected side effects. You will learn that the benefits associated with cancer treatments in terms of survival rates do not come without risk. Most cancer treatments are fraught with iatrogenic harm. High risk/benefit ratios have been integral to the culture of cancer treatment for more than a century.[2] Severe side effects from drugs that are considered poisonous outside of the hospital ward have become an accepted part of life in most cancer treatment centres. The treatment-related morbidity and mortality rates due to cardio- or nephrotoxicity are rather high.[3] Your cancer specialist, trained in healing but frequently frustrated by being unable to deliver a cure, will be prepared to go to any extreme (overdosing and over-drugging) if you allow it. At the same time, you, like most other patients, in a desperate effort to avert a presumed 'death sentence', will be willing to try almost anything hoping for a cure or at least postponing death, thus placing treatment side effects and iatrogenic harm second to potential benefits. Suppose that the doctor and you decide in favour of chemotherapy, you might experience a highly toxic fluid being injected into your veins. The nurse administering it will be wearing protective gloves because the drug could burn his/her skin if even a tiny drop is spilled. You can't help asking yourself, 'If such precautions are needed to be taken on the outside, what is this drug doing to me on the inside?' During your treatment, you might lose your hair by the handful, appetite, weight, skin colour and zest for life.

The aforementioned drastic 21st-century interventionist therapy is practised on a regular basis in cancer clinics around the globe and is as much part of the history of pharmacology and toxicology as the heroic medicine practised in the 18th and 19th centuries. This also applies to early modern last-ditch efforts to save the lives of patients suffering from venereal and other infectious diseases. Historically, European and North American pharmacopoeias included a considerable number of drugs that we now consider poisons. For example, mercury in ointments for the treatment of syphilis or in calomel for intestinal purging, strychnine and arsenic salts as ingredients for tonic medicines, opium to relieve severe pains and tartar emetic for vomiting. Most of these substances were (re)introduced into Western medicine by the renowned 16th-century physician and alchemist Theophrastus Bombastus von Hohenheim (1493–1541), who took the name Paracelsus. In his writings, Paracelsus persistently addressed the question: What is a poison?

The word poison, as we know it, refers to a substance that is harmful or lethal to a living organism.[4] Generally, it is associated with something that harms a person or thing. However, informally, it can be used to signify a drink such as 'What is your poison?' In that sense, poison is etymologically linked to the Latin words *potio* and *poto* (to drink). In Roman and Greek culture, poisons were often prepared in the form of a drinkable concoction that could be used for a state-ordered suicide as for instance in the case of the Greek philosopher Socrates (469–399 BC). It is worth mentioning that in modern Greek, the word *farmaki* is used informally to refer to a poisonous substance. This brings us to the ambiguous and complex ancient Greek word '*pharmakon*', meaning sacrament, spell-giving potion, remedy, poison, talisman, perfume, cosmetic or intoxicant.[5] Thus, the word poison was used to signify both the healing and useful effects as well as the damaging effects of a pharmacon. Paracelsus skilfully exploited this ambiguity by developing the following astute concept of what constitutes the difference between a poisonous and a non-poisonous substance:[6]

> What is there that is not a poison, all things are poison and nothing (is) without poison. Solely the dose determines that a thing is not a poison.

The famous English physician, toxicologist and 'father' of British forensic medicine, Alfred Swaine Taylor (1806–1880), pragmatically paraphrased Paracelsus by arguing that 'a poison in a small dose is a medicine, and a medicine in a larger dose is a poison'.[7] Whether indeed the dose should be considered the single determinant of the poisonous or therapeutic quality of a substance will be up for discussion in this chapter.

The 'Paracelsus principle' of dose and response may be an important conceptual legacy, but in terms of a material and poisonous legacy, Paracelsus had a far greater impact on the history of medicine and toxicology. Inspired by Rhazes' *Liber Secretorum*, Paracelsus reintroduced a number of potent substances to the *materia medica*. Mercury, antimony and arsenic would develop into major commodities with a far-reaching impact on medicine, society and environment. For those historians who love to literally dig into the history of poisons, the riverbeds are a historical treasure and can be read as a cross section of poisonous compounds from arsenic and mercury compounds up to barbiturates and modern-day cytotoxic drugs.[8] In this chapter, I will historically analyse the multidimensional and dynamic role of drugs as poisons and vice versa, shedding light on prototypical trajectories of medical, criminal and social poisoning from the early modern period (15th century) to the current era of modern scientific medicine.

The history of the 'king of poisons' with a Dutch touch

John Parascandola, a historian of pharmacy, crowned arsenic as the 'king of poisons'.[9] And indeed, there is hardly any other poison with a longer, darker, more pervasive historical trajectory than arsenic. From the 15th century onwards, arsenical poisons, publicly known as *poudres de succession*, would become increasingly popular as a method of political assassination and homicide. The most notorious families associated with historical arsenic poisonings are the Borgias and the Medici, but they should really be considered as pioneers who prepared the way, along with Paracelsus, for exponentially growing silent crowds of criminal, iatrogenic and environmental arsenic poisonings.

Efforts to control the availability of arsenic date back to the late 15th century when city authorities across Europe began worrying about the growing and unrestricted sale of poisonous drugs and their focus was on arsenic. The 'king of poisons' became widely regarded as a social poison with the potential to undermine social cohesion in towns and kingdoms. Over time, tighter poison control regimes were put in place. The professional boundaries in the medical marketplace were still fluid with overlap between physic, surgery and pharmacy. Physicians, surgeons and apothecaries were all involved in the testing, preparation and assessment of drugs, poisons and antidotes to some degree.[10] Antidotes such as *antidotum arcenici* or *hydrargyrosus* in the form of a chelating agent were widely used. Dating back to the days of Pedanius Dioscorides (40–90), it was also standard practice to use emetics to treat poisoning. It was assumed that clearing the stomach would eliminate any ingested poison from the body. But, medical history shows that the heroic emesis therapy was far from harmless and frequently induced iatrogenic damage.

From the 16th century onwards, apothecaries were regarded as the most trustful gatekeepers for the sale of toxic medicinal substances. For example, in 1687, the city council of the Dutch city of Leiden curbed the free sale of arsenic powder or what was known as 'rats herb' and passed legislation restricting sales to only those by the town's official pharmacist.[11] Rotterdam, Amsterdam and Haarlem soon followed suit.[12] Although there is little reason to suppose that these town-restricted arsenic acts exerted a significant influence on the overall incidence of poisoning, with druggists still selling significant quantities of rat herb, nevertheless it gradually paved the way for the establishment of pharmacy-centred poison legislation across Europe.

According to Parascandola, arsenic poisoning reached a peak in the 1850s when the use of arsenic compounds exploded in the home, on the farm and in various industries.[13] A wide array of goods contained arsenic including clothes, soap, books, paint, wallpaper, glass and glassware, and popular patent medicines like the tonic Fowler's solution. It is not surprising that given arsenic's routine presence in everyday life and environmental accumulation, a rapidly growing number of people suffered from unintentional poisoning at the end of the 19th and early 20th centuries. Fatalities due to chronic arsenic exposure were most likely far higher than the numbers involved in homicides and the new wave of mariticidal poisonings in attempts to cash in on life-insurance policies. In widely published French criminal records, statistics from 1835 to 1885 for arsenic poisonings figure prominently as 836 out of 1,759 cases.[14] The number of poisoning cases reported was no doubt lower than the actual number of cases, but the introduction of chemical tests made it harder for murderers to get away with their crimes. The development of analytical methods to detect and quantify poisonous chemicals like arsenic (e.g. the Marsh and the Reinsch tests) set the stage for a new field of science, forensics, that would be called upon in court trials and for legally enforced national restrictions on the sale of arsenic and other poisons.[15] Inquests and trials involving suspected and subsequently scientifically confirmed arsenic poisoning had high public visibility throughout the 19th century and well into the 20th century. One example is the Dutch trial of Maria Catharina van der Linden-Swanenburg (1839–1915), known as the 'Leiden poisoner Mie'. Her serial murder cases using arsenic can be found in the *Guinness Book of Records*.[16]

In approximately 1879, murderous Mie began the systematic poisoning of poor local residents in the town of Leiden. Because of her great helpfulness, she was nicknamed 'Good Mie', and she established a large circle of neighbours, relatives and friends. As a dear and helpful friend, she was allowed to walk into people's houses on a regular basis. No one associated her with the rather frequent regrettable deaths and illnesses that occurred among her circle of friends, since the 19th century was known for its high burden of disease and mortality. Therefore, no particular event stood out. It even remained unnoticed that Good Mie had advised all her acquaintances to buy funeral insurance from various burial funds (and if necessary, Good Mie solicited funeral insurance for others and paid the membership fee of 7.5 cents per week herself). The practice of purchasing funeral insurance for someone else without consent was not prohibited in the 19th century. Good Mie poisoned her insured loved ones with an anti-bed bug preparation, which contained one part of sulphur and four parts of arsenic, bought from the druggist and subsequently sprinkled in coffee, milk or pea soup. In total, Good Mie poisoned 102 people, of whom 27 died and 45 suffered from severe intestinal organ damage. After the victims' burial, she collected their insurance money, which was usually 50 guilders. She even poisoned her own parents, sister, brother-in-law and their children. In the end, the family killings raised the family doctor's suspicion and he sounded the alarm in 1883. Good Mie was imprisoned and brought to trial. The examining judge ordered the exhumation of the corpses at the graveyard and sent them for forensic laboratory examination. The presence of arsenic was indeed confirmed, and Good Mie's verdict in 1885 was life imprisonment.[17] The court trial attracted national and international attention in the news media. Good Mie's serial poisonings stirred imaginations that had been fed by arsenic's prominent role in 19th-century literary works from pulp fiction to classical literature. Most certainly, the best-known novel in which arsenic played a dark role was Gustav Flaubert's *Madame Bovary*. Iconography of the two magically potent snakes in a fatal stranglehold of the root of the tree of life used during the trial of murderous Mie and again in stage plays (see Figure 1.1) is most telling. Of course, the omnipotent presence of scientific evidence leaves no room for Good Mie's lucky escape.

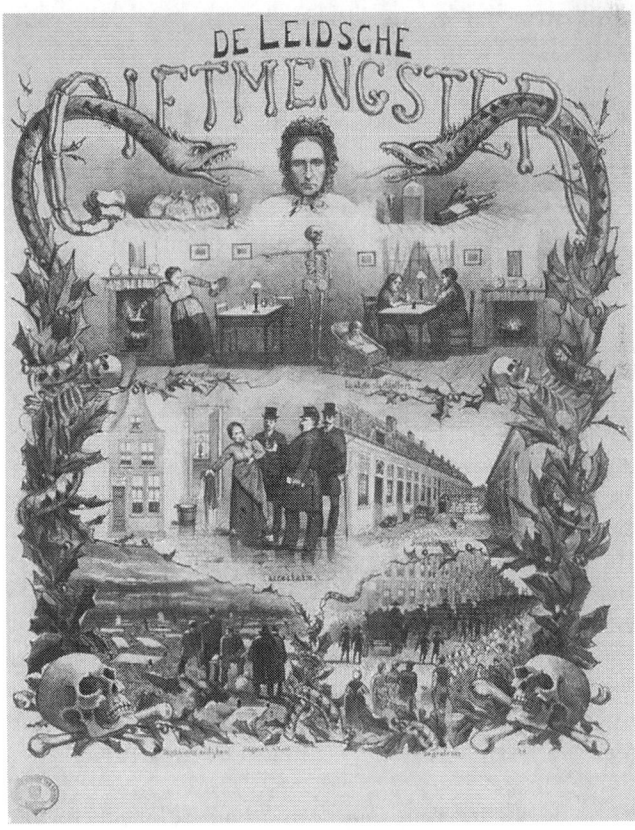

Figure 1.1 A 1883 lithograph of the life of 'murderous Mie' by R. Raar, Leiden University Library.

Handling God's own medicine

The heroic remedy and poisonous plant medicine with the longest history of use and abuse that is still used today is opium.[18] The word 'opium' is derived from the ancient Greek term *opos* (juice). Opium's use dates back as early as 4200 BC based on Carbon-14 dating records, and the earliest records of medicinal use are approximately 1500 BC in Egypt for the indication to 'stop a crying child'.[19] The Greeks and Romans added new indications for opium for treating female diseases, internal diseases and for anaesthesia. Knowledge about the medical use of opium was preserved in Islamic civilization and returned to Western medicine in the Renaissance with the Latin translations of the works of the Islamic physicians al-Rāzī (Rhazes (Latin), 854–925) and Ibn Sina (Avicenna (Latin), 980–1037). Once again, Paracelsus played a pioneering role in the circulation of knowledge about the medical use of opium and the development of a new preparation that was a potable concoction he called laudanum.[20] The basic innovation was to produce an extract of opium in brandy that empirically proved to be a more effective and easy-to-handle remedy, which could then be used both as an evacuant and as an anti-evacuant in a wide array of ailments: fevers, cough, diarrhoea, vomiting and preventing children from crying and causing disturbance. Laudanum was further popularized by Paracelsians and iatrochemists like the Flemish physician Jean-Baptiste Van Helmont (1580–1644) and subsequently standardized as a tincture of opium by the English physician Thomas Sydenham (1624–1689) who mixed opium with wine, saffron, cinnamon and cloves. According to Sydenham, of 'all the remedies it has pleased almighty God to give man to relieve his suffering, none is so universal and efficacious as opium'.[21] However, it was man-made, easy-to-handle concoctions that turned opium into a prominent home remedy. Just as the introduction of the hypodermic injection dramatically changed the medical landscape from the 1850s onwards, replacing opium with morphine and creating a new powerful and popular drug and poison, so the 17th- and 18th-century laudanum preparation innovations also had far-reaching implications.[22] Physicians were first in raising concerns about an excessive and indiscriminate use of laudanum. A growing number of cases of laudanum poisoning were reported, and the danger of iatrogenic opium poisoning was debated across Europe in the 18th century. According to the medical historian Andreas-Holger Maehle, from the early modern period onwards, a connection was made between experimental studies of opium – both animal studies and self-experimentation – and recommendations for its therapeutic use with warnings about the double-edged sword of benefits and harms.[23]

Although opium habituation did not go unmentioned, the modern concept of self-intoxication and addiction as a medical and social problem did not emerge until the second half of the 19th century.[24] Opium was generally a medicine for acute symptoms, in particular strong pains, diarrhoea, coughing and crying children; thus, it was used for rather short periods with a low risk of developing dependence. In Britain and on the continent, concerns were centred on the potential for acute dangerous intoxication by overdose, particularly in children.[25] In the 18th-century Netherlands, these concerns led to town-based legislation forbidding the open sale of *syrupus papaveris* (opium syrup) for use in children (mostly for the indication of *requies puerorum* [calming of children]) and restricting the sale to apothecaries on a prescription-only basis.[26] However, given the continuing child mortality in the Netherlands due to opium medicines far into the 19th century, the effectiveness of local legislation is doubtful. The same is true for the effectiveness of 19th-century national pharmacy acts across Europe and Great Britain.

Pure, simple and intoxicating

As far as the history of poisons is concerned, the 19th century can definitely be considered a watershed. The revolutionary changes in 18th-century chemistry and physics, e.g. Lavoisier's famous work on oxygen and James Watt's work on the steam engine, were at the core of the industrial and second scientific revolution that prepared the way for the creation and mass production of a new generation of chemical substances with medical or otherwise economic value, but with new toxic qualities as well. The new generation of man-made substances with new toxic effects and potencies did not undermine the premise that there is little to distinguish drugs from poisons except the dosage and the clinical need for antidotes or other treatments in cases of poisoning. The use of pure ingredients in precise dosages and known effects for all innovative formulations did not reduce the number of poison cases. As I will show, the new medications actually opened new avenues for mass poisoning in hospitals, households, nightlife, industry and the battlefield.

In 1804, the pharmacy apprentice Friederich Sertüner (1783–1841) isolated morphine. Subsequently, pharmacists Pierre Pelletier (1788–1842) and Joseph Caventou (1795–1877), in collaboration with the experimental physiologist and practitioner François Magendie (1783–1855), isolated and tested other alkaloids such as the convulsant strychnine ('given in all diseases of debility'), the febrifuge quinine and the vomiting-inducing substance emetine ('as a substitute for the common ipecacuanha preparations'). All these developments marked a new departure for the study of plant-based drugs and poisons and the maturation of the fields of pharmacology and toxicology.[27] Magendie played an important role in the dissemination of knowledge of these 'new substances, which chemistry and physiology hold out to us as valuable remedies'.[28] His multi-edition book *Formulary for the preparation and employment of several new remedies* was widely acknowledged in Europe and America. By the 1820s, apothecaries and druggists across the continent, Great Britain and the United States, produced and dispensed the new remedies on a commercial basis, thus laying the foundation for a burgeoning pharmaceutical industry.

As Magendie admitted, even enlightened practitioners initially regarded the new remedies with repugnance. Doctors had still to be convinced of the superiority of the pure alkaloids and clinical use increased only gradually on a trial-and-error basis to learn hands-on the do's and don'ts of dosing these 'heroic medicines' that were therapeutically effective, but also harmful in small doses. The poisonous quality of the new drugs was rather quickly appreciated by those people who wanted a non-arsenic choice to end their lives prematurely or as a tool for murder. It also spurred interest in the more direct, controlled application of the pure substances and resulted in the development of the hypodermic syringe in the 1850s.[29] The new medical injection technique gained quick acceptance as a more precise and seemingly safe alternative to oral forms of dosing. The availability and acceptance of the hypodermic syringe generated a significant increase in the demand for pure alkaloids and foremost popularized the use of morphine hydrochloride. Morphine injections were used to treat everything from post-operative pain, rheumatism and cholera to the pain of wounded soldiers on the battlefield. Misguided by the medical conviction that morphine was benign, morphinism as a modern form of iatrogenic self-intoxication made its way among the well-to-do of Europe and the United States, and war invalids. Until the end of the 19th century, little social stigma was attached to morphinism, as it was assumed that the addict had acquired morphine through medical treatment. By linking opiate intoxication with outcomes such as addiction, disease, incarceration and death, the boundary between a life-saving elixir and a poison became increasingly blurred. Gradually, therapeutically engendered opiate addiction became stigmatized. At the beginning of the 20th century, opiate use in general became internationally regarded as a social poison that threatened to undermine the health of nations.[30]

The genesis of the poisonous magic bullet paradigm

The modern investigation of poisons developed as part of experimental pharmacology and was closely connected to experimental physiology and the new field of forensics. Magendie's pupil and successor to the chair of physiology at the Collège de France, Claude Bernard (1813–1878), led the way in what materialized as the laboratory revolution in medicine.[31] In Bernard's laboratory, *in vitro* and animal experiments with the South American arrow poison curare showed that drugs and hence poisons act at specifically identifiable body sites.[32] Thus, Bernard and the later microbe hunters Louis Pasteur (1822–1895) and Robert Koch (1843–1910) (his illustrious contemporaries who separately identified the causative bacterial agents of at least 20 diseases) prepared the way for Paul Ehrlich's (1854–1915) dye experiments and the concepts of a 'magic bullet' (*wunder kugel*) and chemotherapy.

Ehrlich's idea that substances could be fixed in targeted organisms and visible when using dye, thus having diagnostic and subsequently therapeutic consequences, became the guiding principle for chemotherapy. In the case of an infectious disease, this meant specifically killing the microbes without harming the host.

The search for this magic bullet 'holy grail' as part of a target-oriented research programme became fundamental to later searches for synthetic drugs and poisons as well. Ironically, Ehrlich's pioneering efforts to find a miracle drug against a widespread and slowly destructive infectious disease like syphilis were hampered by the fact that most compounds that killed the microbe that caused syphilis, the spirochaete, *Treponema pallidum*, also appeared to be too poisonous for the host to tolerate. The substance that stood out for Ehrlich among the others in terms of effectiveness and that had a relatively 'low' toxicity was the organic arsenical compound 606, later known as Salvarsan and arsphenamine.[33] Salvarsan's trajectory of initial therapeutic expectations, rapid acceptance as a miracle cure and subsequent disrepute, since it turned out to be poisonous as a treatment for syphilis, illustrates the context-dependent and blurred status of most 20th-century drugs and poisons. At the moment of the introduction of Salvarsan, mercury was still regarded as the standard but rather poisonous treatment against syphilis. Salvarsan appeared to be benign compared to mercury, but unfounded praise resulted in the indiscriminate use of the drug by large numbers of patients who had not been treated initially with mercury and who experienced new alarming side effects when taking Salvarsan, such as deafness, and death.[34] The margin of safety and the line between a life-saving elixir and poison for the new generations of therapeutics – antibiotics, hormones, analgesics, antihypertensives, anti-inflammatories, antipsychotics, antineoplastics and biologicals – often appeared to be narrow. This was also true for a host of new molecules that were created and modified between the bench and the bedside and marketed by an increasingly successful and powerful pharmaceutical industry. The alluring promise of the magic bullet blinded researchers, doctors and patients alike, who for decades disregarded the necessity of exercising caution and promoting stricter rules for the testing and monitoring of medicines.[35]

The Seige-like cycle[36] of therapeutic optimism followed by disappointment that was manifest is exemplary for the repetitious nature of the therapeutic evaluation of most modern-day drugs. It starts with very optimistic reports about promising therapeutic results in specialized hospital environments for a specific target disease and patient population. Once the drug has been introduced, we see an expanding use of the drug outside of the original context of drug testing, accompanied by high expectations. Then comes rising criticism and disappointment due to unexpected and harmful side effects or to insufficient efficacy, which contracts use and limits application.

A drug can also reappear and start a new trajectory when it is used for a new diagnostic category, even in the case of a notoriously 'toxic' drug like thalidomide. The sedative thalidomide was banned from the global medical markets in the early 1960s as a result of a birth defects toxicity crisis. Following the thalidomide drug disaster, drug testing and safety standards and regulations were significantly strengthened. Yet, in the 1990s, the very same drug was reintroduced for the treatment of certain cancers and leprosy, under strictly controlled conditions that required women to use two forms of birth control and submit to regular pregnancy tests. Unfortunately, reported cases of thalidomide embryopathy still occur in poorly controlled healthcare contexts.[37] Drug therapies that work well in the capital of Brazil do not always work well in poor rural areas. To paraphrase, drugs that are effective and benign in specialized hospital environments can be ineffective and/or poisonous in general practice. The most telling historical example of a context-dependent modern-day drug and poison is the anticoagulant warfarin.

The thin line between rat poison and a life-saving therapy

Oral anticoagulation originated in the 1920s with the discovery of a hitherto unknown haemorrhagic factor which caused 'sweet clover disease' (a lethal condition with uncontrollable internal bleeding) in cattle on US and Canadian prairies. The investigating veterinary scientists, Francis Schofield (1889–1970) from Ontario and Lee Roderick from North Dakota, came to the conclusion that the cause was not a toxic substance, pathogenic organism nor a nutritional deficiency. Indeed, if the bleeding was not too serious, the disease was reversible by withdrawing spoiled sweet clover hay and transfusing fresh or defibrinated blood from healthy cattle. In 1931, Roderick showed that the physiology of the disease included a reduction of prothrombin activity (the precursor of thrombin); thus, the pathology and physiology of the condition were revealed, but the factor involved was still unknown.[38]

A long and arduous effort of trial and error followed in the search for the causative biochemical agent that might be turned into a 'magic bullet'. The protagonists in this story are the biochemists Karl Link (1901–1978) and Harold Campbell (1945–) at the Experimental Station run by the University of Wisconsin College of Agriculture. Part of the problem in isolating the factor was the lack of a reliable assay to quantitatively measure prothrombin activity in laboratory animals. In 1938, progress was made when the two biochemists succeeded in developing a reliable rabbit assay and managed to isolate the crystals of a potent anticoagulant. Additional support from the chemist Charles F. Huebner (1917–2012) resulted in the chemical identification and synthesis of 3,3-methylenebis (4-hydroxycoumarin). On the eve of the Second World War, Link and Huebner figured out that damp conditions can spoil sweet clover hay by bacterial action and the natural coumarin (which causes the smell of newly mown clover hay) becomes oxidized to 4-hydroxy-coumarin, followed by coupling to form a bis-coumarin or dicoumarol.[39] The Wisconsin Alumni Research Foundation (WARF), which was established upon the discovery of vitamin D, funded Link's laboratory research and helped to patent the chemical compound dicoumerol in 1941.

In 1945, while recovering in a sanatorium from 'wet pleurisy', Link had the idea to use coumarin derivatives as a rodenticide to cause rodents to die of internal haemorrhage. He reviewed all the chemical and bioassay data from his laboratory and selected analogues of dicoumarol that had been synthesized between 1940 and 1944 as candidates for potential 'better mousetraps (rat traps)'. He thought dicoumarol would be a poor rodenticide because it acted too slowly. Link and colleagues, still funded by WARF, began testing the most promising analogues. Number 42 of a list of 150 appeared to be a particularly active and effective rat poison – warfarin. However, it required significant salesmanship by Link and WARF to persuade companies to sell warfarin as a rat poison since it was a radical departure from previous practice. The novel concept used a slow-acting poison rather than the significantly more toxic conventional poisons that killed rats rapidly, such as the age-old arsenic and strychnine products. Nonetheless, eventually warfarin became a successful rat poison. Unfortunately, its reputation as a rat poison did not inspire clinicians to test the compound in humans, despite Link's urging that warfarin would also be a superior anticoagulant for humans.

European pharmaceutical companies were enthusiastic about coumarin and began developing more potent and safe dicoumarol analogues for clinical use. Roche and Geigy were each successful in launching competing drug compounds that would achieve blockbuster status in the 1960s: Marcoumar® (phenprocoumon) in 1954 and Sintrom® in 1955 (acenocoumarol), respectively. Faced with the European challenge, the resourceful Link started pushing American clinicians to test warfarin in humans. The first human trials with warfarin were started in 1953. Based on the preliminary results, Link, with the support of WARF officers, finally succeeded in convincing Endo Laboratories of New York to market the drug warfarin under the name 'Coumadin'. The pharmaceutical company was persuaded by warfarin's high water solubility and superior oral bioavailability. The drug was more potent and potentially more hazardous than dicoumarol, but it appeared that its anticoagulant effects could be reversed with the administration of high doses of vitamin K. However, a US president was needed to break the American rat poison spell. The fact that a publicly regarded 'rat poison' was successfully used to treat President Dwight D. Eisenhower after his coronary thrombosis (heart attack), in 1955, made a name for warfarin as a miracle drug. The press extolled warfarin as good for a war hero and the President of the United States as good for all, despite its use as a rat poison and potentially causing dangerous bleeding.[40] Over the years, accidental deaths and overdosing due to the improper use of anticoagulant drugs would receive increasing public attention. Worldwide anticoagulants have been identified as one of the top five drug types associated with patient safety incidents in the 1990s and 2000s.[41] Exemplary for the context-dependent nature of the blurry line between medicine and poison is the way in which the harmless ingredient garlic in the household kitchen can turn the taking of warfarin into a harmful event.

The harmful but addictive magic bullet fallacy of the cancer industry

It was Eisenhower's running mate, Richard Nixon, who as President added a new chapter to the mass consumption of powerful drug therapies that can cause life-threatening reactions, by signing the National Cancer Act of 1971 and officially declaring a 'War on Cancer'. Chemotherapy and oncologists are latecomers at the cancer scene. Cancer chemotherapy developed after the Second World War and had its origins in Ehrlich's testing of new specific antibacterial chemicals. According to medical historian John Pickstone, a scientifically innovative and promising third cancer modality was developed that relied on a new kind of clinical experimentalism developed from hospital-centred research laboratories and based on clinical trials and statistics.[42] Initially, government-funded institutions and war research programmes (e.g. programmes on mustard gas, on nutrition and on antibiotics), primarily in the United States, were central to the development of chemotherapy. The US National Cancer Institute and its clinical programme played a key role. The promise of a drug cure for cancer was highly appealing. Following Ehrlich's magic bullet paradigm, a major scientific screening programme would ideally generate drug compounds that could kill cancer cells without harming excessive quantities of normal tissues.[43] However, from the beginning, experimental drugs were hoped for but scientifically, with some exceptions, not considered curative for major killers like breast, prostate, lung and colon cancers with some exceptions. These drugs would be given until a relapse occurred, and then an alternative would be tried until no further therapy was available. Moreover, it appeared that the hope for a drug agent that would be specific and safe enough to restrict its action to cancer cells was elusive. After testing thousands of compounds – many coming from a list of highly toxic chemicals, including chemical weapons, pesticides, herbicides and dyes – it was accepted that chemotherapy would poison normal tissues as well as cancer cells. These normal tissues included rapidly dividing bone marrow cells, intestinal cells and hair follicles. Thus, the adverse effects of all of these cancer drugs were severe; the most significant and dose-limiting (i.e. life-threatening) problems were bone marrow suppression and renal and cardiac toxicity. Still, major advances in the treatment of a limited number of fast-growing tumours like childhood leukaemia, Hodgkin's disease, and testicular cancer kept the chemotherapy enterprise alive.[44]

The self-proclaimed War on Cancer even propelled the search for new 'cancer-killing' compounds with hundreds of millions of dollars being poured into cancer chemotherapy research. Over the years, tens of thousands of cancer patients have participated in clinical trials for experimental drugs in the hope that they would help fight a monstrous disease and that a lucky strike might occur. In the process, the high risk-benefit ratio of cancer chemotherapy became part and parcel of cancer therapy regimens. The pharmaceutical industry jumped on the bandwagon with all the major drug companies having a presence in the cancer treatment, which from the 1980s onwards became regarded as a promising medical market to exploit.[45] The global market for cancer drugs went from 200 million dollars at the end of the 1970s to 1 billion dollars in the late 1980s, then 10 billion dollars at the end of the 1990s and crossed the 100 billion dollar threshold in 2014.[46]

The cancer industry's exponential growth coincided with a growing commercial influence on medical research and publications, medical careers and the media. In the process, public criticism of the low success rate of the costly and harmful 'battle against cancer' in the late 1970s was essentially silenced. The benefits of the 'heroic' cancer therapies at monopoly prices became publicly accepted as outweighing serious side effects and even death. Under normal disease conditions, this kind of harmful drug profile would dissuade doctors, patients, regulators, pharmaceutical and health-insurance companies from encouraging the making, licencing and use of such drugs. But, in circumstances where there is little hope for a cure, the rules of the game appear to be unique and thus blur the medicine/poison line in dramatic ways.

Cancer care also puts a burden on the medical community's moral responsibility, which has barely coped with the ethical challenges of employing chemotherapy. 'First do no harm' is the oath that every physician supposedly swears to honour. Yet there is great difficulty in exercising therapeutic quality control on individual doctors who are trained and dedicated to healing while encouraged by desperate patients to defeat the cancer at any cost. Within this environment of high risk and unknown gain and an almost religious connection between doctor and patient, (semi-)criminal poisoning lurks, as a 2015 case report illustrates one of the most serious medical frights in history. One of Michigan's most respected cancer doctors, Dr. Farid Fata, intentionally prescribed over 9,000 unnecessary and potentially harmful chemotherapeutic injections and infusions to at least 553 patients, who had received bogus cancer diagnoses and prognoses over six years. These toxic treatments amounted to nearly 35 million dollars in insurance billings that he partly cashed, and a stunning mortality rate. This modern-day variation on the case of 'murderous Mie' should not be considered as a mere ludicrous exception according to a warning in *Newsweek* magazine. 'His actions appalling as they were, were not performed in isolation: they are emblematic of systematic issues' in cancer medicine and beyond.[47] These systematic issues concern the soft underbelly of evidence-based medicine with the pervasive power of the coalition between laboratory medicine and drug and insurance industries to monopolize information on the safety and efficacy of therapeutic drugs.[48] However, we should not only take into account the rather worrying immersion of medical practice in the activities of big industry, with doctors being compromised and subverted by commercial interests, but also the context-dependent nature of the benefits and risks of today's powerful drugs. Cancer drugs that are effective in terms of safety and efficacy within the high-tech environment of the Memorial Sloan Kettering Cancer Center can nevertheless have devastating effects as prescription drugs in general practice. The impressive rise of the use of the rather potent prescription drug methotrexate (originally developed and used for chemotherapy) in general practice for the treatment of rheumatoid arthritis and other autoimmune diseases, and the subsequent alarming rise in the number of reported serious, life-threatening side effects, should be a warning.[49] It is high time to rephrase Paracelsus' dose axiom about what constitutes the difference between a poisonous and a non-poisonous substance:

> What is there that is not a poison, all things are poison and nothing (is) without poison. The dose, the form of dosing and/or the context of use determines whether a thing is or isn't a poison.

Conclusion

By historically analysing the multidimensional and dynamic role of drugs as poisons and vice versa, from the 15th century to the current modern era of scientific medicine, I have been able to pinpoint a remarkable continuity in the blurred boundaries between medicine and poison. The hundreds of thousands of people dying each year in hospitals all over the globe from adverse reactions to medication bear witness to the rather frustrating way the trajectories of medical, social and criminal poisoning were and still are intricately intertwined.[50] What makes a poison is the sum of a context-dependent human-drug interaction that, however guarded by doctors, pharmacists and patients alike, was and is a rather high-risk endeavour with benefits that can be easily overshadowed by the negative medical and social effects. The most important lesson of history is that medical progress has done little to diminish the poison challenge; each newly developed medication multiplies the number of possible hazardous interactions. Patients, physicians, medical researchers, regulators and the pharmaceutical industry should all take heed of the poison past when looking towards the future.

Notes

1 Tomasetti C, Vogelstein B. Variation in cancer risk among tissues can be explained by the number of stem cell divisions. *Science.* 2015, 347(6217): 78–81.
2 Pieters T. *Interferon: The science and selling of a miracle drug.* (New York: Routledge, 2005), 162.

3 Conway A, McCarthy A, Lawrence P, Clarke RA. The prevention, detection and management of cancer treatment-induced cardiotoxicity: a meta-review. *BMC Cancer.* 2015, 15: 366–382.

4 Levy J. *Poison: A social history.* (Stroud, UK: The History Press, 2011).

5 Schelenz H. *Geschichte der Pharmazie.* (Hildesheim: Georg Olms, 1965).

6 Pagel W. *Paracelsus: An introduction to philosophical medicine in the era of the renaissance* (Basle: Karger, 1984).

7 Coley NG. Alfred Swaine Taylor, MD, (1805–1880): forensic toxicologist. *Medical History.* 1991, 35(4): 409–427.

8 Daughton CG, Jones-Lepp TL, eds., *Pharmaceuticals and personal care products in the environment: Scientific and regulatory issues,* Symposium series 791; American Chemical Society. (Oxford: Oxford University Press, 2001).

9 Parascandola J. *King of poisons: A history of arsenic.* (Washington, DC: Potomac Books, 2012).

10 In 1681 in the town of Utrecht, a citizen claimed to have successfully tested an arsenic antidote called 'orvietaen' based on a theriac mixture. This statement was evaluated by a committee of doctors and the town's apothecary; www. hetutrechtsarchief.nl/collectie/archiefbank/archieftoegangen/zoekresultaat? mivast=39&mizig=199&miadt=39&miaet=18&micode=34-4.U110a001&minr= 3347236&miview=ldt, accessed 1 July 2015.

11 Stoeder W. *Geschiedenis der Pharmacie in Nederland.* (Amsterdam: Schie-Pers, 1891), 121.

12 www.archieven.nl/nl/zoeken?mivast=0&mizig=210&miadt=236&miaet= 1&micode=2166&minr=1048692&miview=inv2, accessed 1 July 2015.

13 Ibid, 109.

14 Italie van L, Bijlsma UG. *Toxicologie en gerechtelijke scheikunde I.* (Amsterdam: Centen's Uitgevers, 1930), 7.

15 Ibid.

16 Moerman I. *Gif als goede gave. Maria Catherina van der Linden-Swanenburg/ Goeie Mie (1839–1915).* (Leiden: Leiden Promotie VVV, 2001); Nijgh L. Goeie Mie, de Leidse Gifmengster. *Het Vrije Volk,* 30 December 1989.

17 Ibid; in 1870, the death penalty in the Netherlands had been abolished.

18 Booth M. *Opium: A history.* (New York: St. Martin's Press, 1996).

19 Ibid, 16.

20 Ibid, 23–24.

21 Kramer JC. Opium rampant: medical use, misuse and abuse in Britain and the West in the 17th and 18th centuries. *British Journal of Addiction,* 1979, 74: 377–389.

22 Morson A. *Operative chemist.* (Amsterdam: Clio Medica, 1997), 83–121.

23 Maehle AH. *Drugs on trial: Experimental pharmacology and therapeutic innovation in the Eighteenth century.* (Amsterdam: Clio Medica, 1999), 127–222.

24 Padwa H. *Social poison: The culture and politics of opiate control in Britain and France, 1821–1926.* (Baltimore, MD: The Johns Hopkins University Press, 2012).

25 Berridge V. *Opium and the people – revised edition: Opiate use and policy in 19th and early 20th Century Britain.* (London: Free Association Books, 1999), 97–109.

26 Bosman-Jelgersma HA. *Vijf eeuwen Delftse Apothekers.* (Amsterdam: Meesters, 1979), 169–174.

27 Weatherall M. *In search of a cure.* (Oxford: Oxford University Press, 1990), 16–17.

28 Houlton J. *Formulary for the preparation and employment of several new remedies;* translated from the sixth edition (1827) of the *Formulaire* of M. Magendie. (London/New York: T. & G. Underwood, 1829), vii.

29 Morson A. *Operative chemist.* (Amsterdam: Clio Medica, 1997), 105.

30 Berridge V. *Opium and the people: Opiate use and policy in 19th and early 20th century Britain.* (– revised edition London: Free Association Books, 1999), 235–258; Courtwright DT. *Dark paradise: A history of opiate addiction in America.* (Cambridge, MA: Harvard University Press, 2001), 110–144; Booth M. *Opium: A history.* (1996); Padwa H. *Social poison: The culture and politics of opiate control in Britain and France, 1821–1926.* (Baltimore, MD: The John Hopkins University Press, 2012).

31 Cunningham A, Williams P, eds., *The laboratory revolution in medicine.* (Cambridge: Cambridge University Press, 1992).

32 Porter R. *The greatest benefit to mankind.* (London: HarperCollins, 1997), 337–341.

33 Weatherall M. *In search of a cure.* (Oxford: Oxford University Press, 1990), 55–67.

34 Greiling W. *Im Banne der Medizin; Paul Ehrlich.* (Düsseldorf: Econ-Verlag, 1954), 185–196.

35 Meyler L. *Schadelijke nevenwerkingen van geneesmiddelen.* (Assen: Elsevier, 1954).

36 Max Seige was one of the first to point out the cycle in 1912; see Snelders S, Kaplan C, Pieters T. On cannabis, chloral hydrate, and career cycles of psychotropic drugs in medicine. *Bulletin of the History of Medicine.* 2006, 80: 95–114.

37 Stephens T, Bryner R. *Dark remedy: The impact of thalidomide and its revival as a vital medicine.* (Cambridge, MA: Perseus Publishing, 2001).

38 Duxbury B, Poller L. The oral anticoagulant saga: past, present and future. *Clinical Applications Thrombosis Hemostasis.* 2001, 7: 269–275, 269.

39 Wardrop D, Keeling D. The story of the discovery of heparin and warfarin. *British Journal of Haematology.* 2008, 141: 757–763.

40 Lasby C. *Eisenhower's heart attack: How Ike beat heart disease and held on to the presidency.* (Lawrence: University press of Kansa, 1997), 75, 324–329.

41 www.nrls.npsa.nhs.uk/resources/?entryid45=59814, accessed 4 August 2015; www.jointcommission.org/assets/1/18/SEA_41.PDF, accessed 4 August 2015.

42 Pickstone J. Contested cumulations: configurations of cancer treatments through the twentieth century. In Cantor D. (ed.) *Cancer in the twentieth century.* (Baltimore, MD: The John Hopkins University Press, 2008), 164–196, 166.

43 Mann J. *The elusive magic bullet: The search for the perfect drug.* (Oxford: Oxford University Press, 1999), 143–152.

44 Moss RW. *The cancer industry.* (New York: Paragon House, 1991), 73–94.

45 Ibid.

46 www.imshealth.com/ims/Global/Content/Insights/IMS%20Institute%20 for%20Healthcare%20Informatics/Documents/The_Global_Use_of_ Medicines_Report.pdf, accessed 5 August 2015.

47 www.newsweek.com/farid-fata-farid-fata-sentenced-farid-fata-medical-fraud-oncology-cancer-352317, accessed 5 August 2015.

48 Kassirer JP. *On the take: How medicine's complicity with big business can endanger your health.* (Oxford: Oxford University Press, 2005); Pieters T. *Interferon: The science and selling of a miracle drug.* (New York: Routledge, 2005), 190.

49 Saeder EA, Brock B, Nielsen LP, Bonnerup DK, Lisby M. Identifying high-risk medication: a systematic literature review. *European Journal of Clinical Pharmacology.* 2014, 70(6): 637–645.

50 www.washingtonpost.com/wp-srv/national/health/daily/april98/drugs041598. htm, accessed 10 August 2015.

2 "First Behead Your Viper"

Acquiring knowledge in Galen's poison stories

Helen King

The work of Galen, the second-century AD physician, was highly influential in the history of understanding poisons. He combined and further developed the medical ideas of the writers of his favourite works of the Hippocratic corpus and of classical Greek philosophy. In the process, he developed the fullest form of humoral theory, which dominated Western medicine until the eighteenth century.[1] He both drew on and transformed existing knowledge of poisons and antidotes: his writings also informed many later discussions of these topics. He worked in large urban centres of the early Roman Empire – Rome and Pergamum – but also travelled slowly by land across the vast expanse of that empire and witnessed peasant practices *in situ* as well as when country people came into the big city.[2] He was well aware of both the traditional stories about how poisons and antidotes were discovered and the Roman 'poisoning culture' of the century or so before him. He made antidotes and developed theories about their operation; eventually, as a physician to the imperial family, he was responsible for overseeing the production of the emperor's theriac, the multi-ingredient drug that contained substances that could be poisonous and that acted as both panacea and antidote. This 'wild drug' was one answer to taming the wildness of poison, its name, from the ancient Greek for 'wild animal', evoking images of danger, pain and lack of control.[3] In addition, Galen used the imagery of poisoning to explain how diseases more generally affected the body.

He provides an important window on to the way that knowledge was transmitted in the Roman world, through technical treatises, stories and rumours and observation; he combined reading existing works on poison with going to watch antidotes being made and learned more from stories he had heard and patients he had treated. In this chapter, I shall present an overview of Galen on poison with a particular focus on how he knew what he knew. After situating him in an established Roman (and also Greek) tradition of stories of poison, poisoners, antidotes and immunity, I shall discuss how his theories about poison related to his wider views on the body. As I shall show here, Galen not only resisted any simple binary of drug and poison, but also expanded any binary into yet more categories.

Difficult dosage: poisons in Greece and Rome

Galen, of course, wrote in Greek, and if there is one thing that continues to be widely repeated about poison in the classical world, it is that the Greek word *pharmakon* means both healing drug and poison.[4] In Latin, the equivalent term *venenum* was similarly used in both senses, and in Roman law codes, it was specified that the recognised ambiguity of the word should be tied down by making it clear whether a 'good' or a 'bad' *venenum* is meant.[5] The *Digest* of Roman law issued in the sixth century AD explained that all drugs (Lat. *medicamenta*) can be considered *venena*, because a *medicamentum* is simply something that, by being applied, changes the nature of the thing to which it is applied.[6]

One way of tying down the ambiguity of *pharmaka* and *venena* is dosage, and it was well known in ancient medicine that one and the same substance will have different powers depending on how much of it is administered.[7] That this was common knowledge, rather than just physicians' lore, is illustrated particularly clearly by an Athenian legal speech dating to the period of 420–411 BC, in which we hear of the defence apparently used by a woman who thinks more must be better, when administering what she believes is a love potion.[8] Philoneos, a friend of the speaker's father, has decided to rent out his young mistress, a slave, as a prostitute in a brothel. The speaker's stepmother befriends this woman and tells her that she too is being wronged by a man (the speaker's father) and that both of them need to take action to restore the love of their partners. The stepmother announces that she has the means, but needs the slave to help her, and she hands over a *pharmakon* to the slave:

> Philoneos' mistress, who poured the wine for the libation … poured in the *pharmakon* with it. Thinking it a happy inspiration, she gave Philoneos the larger draught; she imagined perhaps that if she gave him more, Philoneos would love her the more: for only when the mischief was done did she see that my stepmother had tricked her.
>
> (Antiphon 1, *Prosecution of the stepmother for poisoning* 19)[9]

A poison given with the intention of inspiring love can have its own label in addition to the ambiguous *pharmakon*; it is a *philtron*, something which is in turn placed on a spectrum of possible ways of influencing another's desire, a spectrum that also includes spells and words.[10] Perhaps, in an even smaller dose, the unnamed substance added to the wine would indeed have been used as a *philtron*. In this law court speech, however, *pharmakon* is used. So, this is not presented as the story of a love potion that went wrong but as a poisoning inadvertently performed by a trusting and desperate woman. Receiving such a large dose, Philoneos died instantly, but the speaker's father was also taken ill and died 20 days later. If the slave had not given her lover so much to drink, it seems he would still have died from the drug. It looks like the stepmother's dosage recommendation was set at a level at which there would be a delayed effect, making it less obvious what the cause was and thus less likely that the culprits would be identified, but the younger woman's enthusiasm ruins the older woman's plan.[11] Here, as often in the classical world, women are associated with poison; not only does it require no physical force, but also it fits well with women's roles in food and drink preparation.

This story and others like it demonstrate why later Roman lawyers were always going to face problems in tying down the ambiguity of *venenum* into good/bad. It was never simple to know whether a death should be attributed to poisoning, or not; it depended on interpreting the event and its relationship to eating and drinking. The example I have discussed shows both that sudden deaths were most suspicious and that any death, whether rapid or gradual, could with hindsight be attributed to poison. Galen himself was adamant that there are no specific signs of poisoning a physician can detect; it is impossible to tell if something arises within the body or is due to material being added to that body (*Affected Parts* 6.5 and 6.6).

Even if a death was agreed to be the result of poison, the widely shared knowledge about the uncertainties of precise dosage made it hard to be certain about motive. Yet, in both Greek and Roman law, showing intent to kill was critical; at least for citizens, accidental poisoning merited a less severe penalty than deliberate poisoning.[12] Following the death of the two Athenian men, the stepmother is eventually brought to trial, but the young woman who poisoned the wine, being a slave, has long since been tortured and then executed.

It is in Roman rather than Greek history that poisoning features most heavily. From the Julio-Claudian dynasty, which as the first imperial dynasty demonstrated the risks of concentrating the rule of the state into a single person, the dangers posed to the incumbent emperor by anyone designated as his heir, and the perils of being so designated, come numerous poison stories, with which Galen was familiar.[13] The historian Suetonius (*Gaius* 49) includes the story of the emperor Claudius throwing his predecessor Caligula's poison collection into the sea, after which dead fish were thrown up on to the beach. There is a particularly fine set of poison stories around Claudius himself, and his fourth wife Agrippina is supposed to have hired a woman already convicted of poisoning – Locusta – to supply poisons. Paid by Nero, Agrippina's son by an earlier marriage, Locusta murdered Britannicus (a son of one of Claudius' earlier wives, and thus a rival heir for Nero), succeeding on the second attempt; the first only produced diarrhoea, but for the second one, the poison was in the water that was used to dilute an otherwise too fiery drink. This was a fast-acting poison which cleverly produced effects that could, at least initially, be attributed to Britannicus' existing epilepsy.[14] Locusta then provided Agrippina with a poison to accompany Claudius' favourite mushroom dish. According to one Roman historian, Tacitus, the physician C. Stertinius Xenophon helped the ailing Claudius to vomit but used a feather that was itself smeared with a rapid poison. Here, in the ultimate deception, poison is disguised as an antidote to poison.

In another example of poisoners taking advantage of the lack of any real line between 'drug' and 'poison', Suetonius states that Nero sent the Praetorian Prefect Burrus poison rather than the throat medicine he had promised him (*Nero* 35.5); this was then smeared on to his palate.[15] Horstmanshoff points out that it is possible that this was genuinely intended as a drug not a poison, and that only when it failed to work was Burrus' death then 'retrospectively attributed to the physician, or to Nero'.[16] This is a fair point, supported with the historian Dio Cassius's comment that Nero also 'killed his aunt Domitia with a *pharmakon*' (62.17.1).[17] Horstmanshoff notes that translating this as 'poison' may be wrong, because in Suetonius' Latin version of the same events, Nero 'bade the doctors give the sick woman an overdose of physic' (*Nero* 34.5), thus suggesting the issue here is once again dosage, which alone distinguishes a poison from a drug.[18]

Not only poison, but also fear of poison, was widespread under the Julio-Claudians. For example, Tacitus comments on Germanicus' sudden death in AD 19: 'the cruel virulence of the disease was intensified by the patient's belief that Piso had given him poison' (Tacitus, *Annals* 2.69).[19] The only solution to avoid being poisoned was to prepare your body in advance with an antidote. Agrippina, once she realised that her son Nero was intending to kill her, famously 'fortified her system by taking antidotes in advance' (Suetonius, *Nero* 34.2). As Horstmanshoff points out, what is key here is that these antidotes were firmly believed to be effective.[20]

Mithradatium

By the late twelfth century, *mithridatium* was called 'the mother of all antidotes'; the Greek word *antidota* has a broader meaning than our own, covering both prevention and cure.[21] For Galen, an antidote is something that cures disease by being taken into the body (as opposed to being applied externally) (*On Antidotes* 1, K 14.1–2).

Laurence Totelin has drawn attention to the very different accounts of the original *mithradatium* in ancient sources. The second-century BC king Mithradates VI Eupator was only one of the Hellenistic rulers of the kingdoms of Asia Minor who is described in Roman sources as highly interested in poisoning, using poisons on enemies and also testing antidotes on prisoners in the royal jails. The first-century AD writer Celsus gives a whole series of *antidota*, stating that the most famous of all is the antidote that Mithradates developed to be taken daily against the 'dangers of drugs' (*venenorum pericula*). When Celsus lists the ingredients, he gives a total of 36 including costly gums and spices such as myrrh; he includes precise quantities for all ingredients, such as 'hypericum, gum, sagapenum, acacia juice, Illyrian iris, cardamon, 8 grams each, anise 12 grams, Gallic nard, gentian root and dried rose-leaves, 16 grams each, poppy-tears and parsley,

17 grams each' and so on (*De medicina* 5.23.3). Another Roman medical writer of a similar date, Scribonius Largus, had at least 22 ingredients
in his recipe for theriac.[22] There was some concern about substitution of
cheaper ones, but the only solution was to taste or sniff for oneself. Pliny
the Elder has a slightly more complex process of preparing the royal body
for possible threats, crediting Mithradates with the idea of taking remedies,
then drinking a dose of poison every day, so that his body would gradually
become accustomed to it.[23] Mithradates' remedy was then adapted further
by Nero's physician Andromachos the Elder in the first century AD, with
viper flesh and opium being added to make what was known as 'theriac'.[24]

In terms of how knowledge of poison was developed and passed on, the
stories surrounding Mithradates make interesting reading. Pliny says that
the king collected books on medicine and also specimens, labelled with
their properties. Mithradatium is only one of the antidotes he discovered,
and he also mixed these antidotes with the blood of Pontic ducks, who
live on poison.[25] The king was, according to the ancient sources, in touch
with physicians (most notably Asclepiades, who practised at Rome) but also
with the famous root-cutter Crateuas.[26] This suggests access to two very
different traditions of knowledge on plant substances; the first left written
records, whereas the second did not.

When studying Mithradates, it is very hard to separate Roman imagination
from Greek reality, as constructing him as a particularly well-educated and
ingenious enemy made his eventual defeat even more impressive.[27] One of the
reasons why Romans told the story of Mithradates' experiments with poison
was precisely because the story goes that his immunity to poison proved to
be his downfall; when the Roman army defeated him, he tried to commit
suicide by taking poison but was unable to succeed. He therefore had to call
in a friend to cut his throat, meaning that his end was a violent one.[28] This is
really the key element of Mithradates' story: he overused the antidotes.

Totelin suggests that the story of his immunity – introduced by Galen with
the distancing device of 'They say…' – was created by Lenaeus, freedman of the
general Pompey the Great, who translated Mithradates' own pharmacological
library into Latin in the first century BC (Pliny, *Natural History* 25.3.5–7).
This collection of books seems to have been real, not a fantasy: it was later
kept in the Temple of Peace at Rome and was consulted by Aulus Gellius
(17.16.1–4). According to Pliny, the person who discovered Mithradates' own
personal recipes within this collection of books on drugs was Pompey himself;
he found a private notebook (Lat. *commentarius*) that included a remedy written in the king's own hand, mixing walnuts, figs, rue and salt, which conferred
immunity to poison for one day (*Natural History* 23.77.149).[29]

Epidemics and poison

Poisoning was not only the concern of prominent individuals cautious about
their chances of survival; it was also thought to be one explanation of epidemics. In humoral systems where individual balance is central, it is hard to

account for something that affects many, and very different, people at the same time. Other explanations were possible: for example, the air (shared by all) could be seen as the culprit, full of rot (Greek *sepsis*) and likely to cause disruption in bodies already full of viscous and thick humours, particularly in an atmosphere which is hot and wet. As the air is not something that can be changed – although the myth of Hippocrates trying to cure the plague of Athens by lighting bonfires shows one idea on how this could be attempted – physicians should instead try to change the bodies on which the air acts or break the link between the air and the body.[30]

But there is a long tradition of linking plagues to poison, and thus as something outside the remit of humoral medicine. The tradition goes back to the initial reaction of the fifth-century BC Athenians who, when the plague of Athens struck, initially assumed that their enemies the Spartans had poisoned the water supply (Thucydides, *Peloponnesian War* 2.48.2). The Romans had similar beliefs and, like the Greeks, also gendered poisoning as a female enterprise, a combination which explains why in Livy we find the story of a large number of deaths in 331 BC being attributed to poison (Livy 8.18). A female slave gave evidence that Roman women had been administering poison and around 20 were found in the process of making poisons; two who were questioned said these were actually 'good' *pharmaka* (Livy 8.18.8).[31] If the key distinction lies only in dosage, they may very well have been right. In time-honoured fashion, they were required to drink their own brew, and died. Another 170 were then found guilty. Romans were very quick to blame poison during plague; Livy has another account of around 3,000 people being put to death on charges of poisoning after a large number of influential Romans had died (Livy 30.37 and 43).

While accused poisoners in Rome were often women, this was not always the case; men also accused other men of poisoning their rivals, and motivations could be financial – to obtain an inheritance – as well as simply disposing of enemies.

Finding knowledge

So where was knowledge of poisons thought to come from, and how was it controlled? As with other substances used in medicine, for poisons and for their antidotes, Greeks and Romans drew on the tradition that drug knowledge originally comes from observation of animals. For example, Pliny describes how a scorpion touched by aconite – the fastest-acting of poisons[32] – uses white hellebore as an antidote (*Natural History* 27.2.6).

But in the case of poison, this imitation of the animal world is far from straightforward; Lucretius wrote that goats get fat on hemlock (*On the Nature of Things* 5.899). It may depend on what part of the plant is eaten; Pliny stated that the seeds, leaves and roots of hemlock are cold, which means they clot the blood, but the stems can be eaten either raw or cooked (*Natural History* 25.95.151–4). However, he added that in diluted form even the dangerous parts could be beneficial; for example, in eye salves (*Natural History* 25.95.153) or rubbed on the breasts to keep them firm (*Natural History* 25.95.154). Even the fast-acting poison of aconite could be used, for eye disease (Pliny, *Natural History* 27.2.9). If given in warm wine, aconite neutralises a scorpion sting: 'it is its nature to kill a human being unless in that being it finds something else to destroy' (Pliny, *Natural History* 27.2.5). This is an interesting understanding not only of how poisons can neutralise other poisons, but also of the mode of operation of poison, suggesting that the powerful aconite here heads for the sting rather than killing the person. As we shall see shortly when looking at Galen, this attraction of the aconite to the sting has analogies with Galen's comments on the action of food, drug or poison within the body.

Knowledge was also gained by working with others. Galen says it is easy to make theriac, so long as you learn by watching someone else doing it. He learned from the best: in particular, from Demetrios, his predecessor as doctor to Marcus Aurelius, who used a recipe that in turn went back to Andromachos the Elder (*On Antidotes* 1.2, K 14.4).[33] Essentially, you grind together all the dry ingredients, then mix the fluid ingredients with wine, and then add in the resins and honey and leave it to mature for two months (*On Antidotes* 1.2, K 14.6). Galen also experimented, finding that cockerels given theriac would survive snakebites (K 14.215).[34] He made it in huge quantities, and notes that he lost 'some eighty pounds of the famous theriac' in the fire that destroyed his books and his medical materials in AD 192 (*Avoiding Distress* 6).[35]

His views about theriac varied over time. In *On Theriac to Piso*, he is enthusiastic about it as a cure-all, but in other treatises, Stein has detected more caution.[36] Galen's concerns again hinge on dosage, which is a crucial element in ancient drug lore; if too much is given as a prophylactic, it will harm the body, but too low a dose means that it won't work (*On the Powers of Simple Remedies* 5.18, K 11.761–4).

To understand Galen's sources for his knowledge of poisons and of theriac, it is necessary to consider the authenticity and the relative dates of the key treatises already mentioned. There are several different authentic treatises of Galen which deal with poison. *On Antidotes*, for example, where in Book 1 he discusses the research into poison carried out by Mithradates, was written a little before AD 200; the other poison treatises are even later (Galen died, probably, in *c.* AD 216).[37] The date of *On Theriac to Piso* is disputed, but it was written after *On Antidotes*, with the plural reference to 'our present emperors' usually taken to mean that it was when Severus and Caracalla were co-rulers, with another reference apparently recalling an incident during the Secular Games of AD 204 (see K 14.212–4 and 217).[38] It was considered authentic in antiquity, but modern scholarship doubted this mainly because it was believed that Galen had died before this date; subsequently, with the dating of his death more recently modified to AD 216, this treatise has slipped back into the category of the genuine works.[39]

However, it may be about to slip out again, thus perhaps changing our views of the date of Galen's death once more; Robert Leigh dates it to after AD 203 and before 211 and argues that it was written by a Galenist, not by Galen himself.[40]

Returning to *On Antidotes*, Nutton argues that it reflects a revival of interest in theriac in the period of AD 200–210, when the drug – antidote and cure-all, remedy and prophylactic – came back into fashion. It is interesting that *On Affected Parts*, another late treatise by Galen, uses poison as an image of how a small amount of retained seed and menses can have such severe effects on the whole of a woman's body.[41]

When Galen uses this 'toxicological model' of disease causation, he often uses the stingray as an example, writing that 'Poison is characterised by an extremely violent destructive power' (*On Affected Parts* 6.5, K 8.422 lines 8–10).[42] I would therefore suggest that while references to poison occur throughout his works, Galen seems to have become particularly interested not only in toxicology and antidotes, but also in poisoning as a way of understanding disease, at the end of his life.

Galen and the snake catchers

For Galen, snakes seem to produce the paradigmatic type of poison, and one of the key components of his poison knowledge came from direct observation of both victims and antidote makers. Stein points out that even today there are around 40,000 deaths per annum from snakebites. Vipers remain the most significant snake risk in Europe today, and the bite is most commonly on the fingers, hand or arm; it causes cardiac arrest and stops the blood from clotting.[43] In *On Theriac to Piso*, Galen mentions the use of snakes in executions in Alexandria and the speed with which their poison took effect (*On Theriac to Piso* 8, K 14.237).

Galen's discussions of poison provide insight into his interactions with other groups in the ancient world associated with snakes and with healing. There are three named groups that feature in such discussions – the Ophiogenes, the Marsi and the Psylli – as well as various individuals with their own techniques, including the emperor's official snake catcher and performers at fairs. From such groups and individuals, Galen not only learned about poison but also obtained the viper flesh that had been an important ingredient of theriac since Andromachos the Elder added it to the recipe.[44] It is viper flesh that makes theriac both heating and drying, its action being understood as dissolving and excreting substances from the body.

We can trace something of the earlier stories Galen would have known. The Ophiogenes are mentioned by Pliny (*Natural History* 7.2.13), and his source is Crates of Pergamon – so, a writer from Galen's own home town. This group, no longer in existence a century before Galen, lived near Parium on the Hellespont, and their custom 'was to cure snake-bites by touch and draw the poison out of the body by placing their hand on it'. So, unlike

the Egyptians, who according to various ancient writers on natural history
had spells to bewitch snakes (Aelian, *Nature of Animals* 6.33), these groups
used their bodies rather than their words. Pliny also refers to Varro, who
wrote in the first century BC and who says there are still some individuals
in that area who use their saliva to neutralise snakebites.

Pliny then discusses the Psylli, for whom his source is the second-century
BC historian and geographer Agatharchides. They were a group, or race (Gk
ethnos), in Africa whose bodies produced a poison (Latin *virus*) deadly to
snakes, and their smell made snakes fall asleep (*Natural History* 7.2.14).
Touch, saliva, smell; in all these stories, there is a clear sensory dimension
to the action. Ancient writers said that while the Psylli were killed by an in-
vading tribe, or died out in a drought, some individuals survived.[45] Aelian,
a slightly later contemporary of Galen, also described the Psylli, again citing Agatharchides but giving rather more information. The Psylli cannot
be injured by any biting or stinging creature, but their smell sends the creatures to sleep, as though they have tasted a *pharmakon* (Aelian, *Nature of
Animals* 16.27). They apply their saliva to snakebites, and if the pain is
particularly severe, then the person will rinse his mouth with water and
give this to the sufferer to drink.[46] In his life of Cato the Younger, Plutarch
mentions two aspects of the Psylli; they can charm and deaden snakes with
incantations (so, here, they use words as well as touch), and they can take
in the poison through the mouth without it being absorbed into their bodies (*Cato Minor* 56.4). Galen, too, mentions doctors who draw out poison
with their mouths (*Method of Medicine* 14, K 10.896). But Pliny includes
one more method used by the Psylli: for even more serious cases, the healer
will lie naked beside the naked patient and press his skin to the patient's
skin (*Natural History* 16.28). So, here the bodies of the Psylli are effective
as a whole, skin to skin, not just through the mouth.

Finally, Pliny lists the Marsi, a group from central Italy claiming descent
from the Homeric sorceress Circe (*Natural History* 7.2.15, 25.5.11); they
can resist snakebites and are snake charmers (Lat. *dormitores serpentium*).
This group, he says, are still around.[47] He suggests it is not necessary to
be in one of these special groups to kill snakes; he notes that all people
'contain a poison available as a protection against snakes' in their saliva,
especially if they are fasting and if human saliva enters a snake's throat, it
kills the snake.

Galen knew all these stories. For example, in *De antidotis* 2.15 (K 14.193),
he quoted from material on the Psylli attributed to Damocratis. But he went
beyond the literary sources, stating that he personally consulted the Marsi
in Rome. He visited them to find out if there was a viper whose bite caused
intense thirst (*On Simple Medicines* 11.1, K 12.316) and to discuss how
many snakes were needed in an antidote (*On the Method of Healing, to
Glaucon* 2.12, K 11.143). In two treatises, he described how the Marsi
cut off the tails and heads of vipers (the most poisonous parts), and then
skin and wash them before eating (*On the Method of Healing, to Glaucon*

2.12, K 11.143–4; *On Antidotes* 1.8, K 14.45–9). Mattern suggests that the Marsi were used in the Roman army medical support 'probably to treat soldiers for snake and scorpion bites'.[48] In a recent study, Everett Wheeler notes that just three Marsi appear in inscriptions concerning the Roman army, probably in medical roles, and – supporting Galen's claim to have spoken to the Marsi – all of them date to the last 20 years of Galen's life, when he was most interested in poisons and antidotes.[49]

The Marsi, then, were for Galen not the stuff of legend, but fellow players in the medical marketplace. Aelian, as well as describing the Psylli, also writes about someone who rears snakes to show them off at fairs (*Nature of Animals* 9.62); he is a *pharmakotribês*, a medicine man. He lets an adder bite him, sucks out the poison, and then turns to his water pitcher to rinse his mouth, but someone through an act of treachery has spilled the water; he develops an ulcerating wound in the mouth and dies two days later. Horstmanshoff presents the Marsi as a subgroup of these market and fair 'exhibitors of wild beasts' (Gk *thêriodeiktai*), but I think Galen treats them more respectfully than this would suggest.[50]

Galen also learned from patients; for example, the peasant who is bitten on the finger but cuts off his finger and survives (*Affected Parts* 3.11, K 8.198); the emperor's snake catcher, who is bitten, tries the usual remedies but turns leaf green before Galen cures him with theriac (*Affected Parts* 5.8, K 8.355); the man who goes to the nearest city (Alexandria) and asks for the bitten finger to be removed (*Affected Parts* 3.11, K 8.197).

Therapeutic poison

Even snake venom, however, can have therapeutic effects in the right situation. Galen used it to cure patients with what the Greeks called elephantiasis. In his *Outline for Empiricism*, written in the 160s and surviving in the medieval Latin of Nicolaus of Reggio, he gives five different stories about this.

Two of these are stories he has heard in which this power of snake venom is a chance find. In the first, a village builds an isolated hut for a sufferer and takes his food to him there. A group of hunters passing through the area are brought wine in earthenware jars but find a dead snake in one; they donate this to the elephantiasis sufferer 'as if out of piety ... for they thought that it was better for him to die than to live. But he was cured by this potion in a miraculous fashion' as the affected skin sloughs off.[51] In the second, a girl gives her lover wine from a jar in which a snake has died, and he is cured.

The next two stories are accounts of Galen's own success 'based on my imitating these chance experiences'. Here, the effect of using such wine is to convert elephantiasis to leprosy, which in turn can be cured by 'the usual drugs'. In the second of Galen's own cases, the patient is himself a snake catcher and the treatment starts with purging and bloodletting and ends with the patient cooking some snakes, as one would eels, and eating them.

Finally, Galen describes a rich man who was told 'to take a daily portion of the snake drug' by Asclepius (*Outline of Empiricism* 10. 75–79); this suggests that temple healing, too, used snakes to heal, and not just in the symbolism of the sanctuary in which snakes could come to lick diseased bodies in the patients' dreams.[52]

In Galen's voluminous oeuvre, he twice tells the story of a drink intended to cause death but which, in fact, cures elephantiasis. In the version which opens this group of five stories in *Outline of Empiricism*, Galen says he has 'heard' the story, but then when he tells it for a second time in the 190s – during the period of his greatest interest in poison – he claims it as his own personal experience; it features in *On the Mixtures and Properties of Simple Drugs* in a list of his own experiences 'when I was still young, in Asia' (11.1.1, K12.312–13).[53] There is an earlier variant of the same story predating Galen's work; this appears in Aretaeus, *On Chronic Diseases* 4.13.20 (*c.* AD 50).[54] In what Nutton calls 'a charming story', a man's elephantiasis was cured when he was left to die in the wilderness and drank wine from a barrel of wine in which a viper had drowned.[55] Galen does not give Aretaeus as his source; indeed, he never refers to his writings.[56] Mattern therefore wonders if this is a local folk tale which Galen too had heard, or whether he simply took the story from Aretaeus.[57] Whatever the source of Galen's first telling of the story, 'with the passing of time a story that Galen had once read or heard became one in which he was a participant'.[58] This is not something unique to Galen, and it sounds a note of caution with regard to his stories, of poison and of other topics. The relationship between *historia* and *autopsia* – what you have discovered from your enquiries and what you have seen for yourself – was complex, and stories could pick up an 'I myself saw' during their transmission.

How does poison work?

In the last decades of his life, then, we have a clear picture of Galen experimenting with making theriac, observing and consulting snake experts who would otherwise be the stuff of folk tales, and even thinking about poisoning as a model for how disease happens, understanding the effect of small amounts of retained substances in the body as analogous to poison.

It was, however, earlier in his life that he began to think about poison as a model for disease and, indeed, for healing. The key treatise here is *Mixtures*, which dates to the period of Galen's second long stay in Rome, 169–75.[59] This was the same period in which he started his major pharmacological treatise, *The Mixture and Properties of Simple Medicines*.[60] In *Mixtures* book 3, Galen talks about 'potential' (*dynamis*), often translated as 'faculty'. This explains why a substance is medically considered 'hot', even though to the touch it is not hot. To be 'hot', it needs to be capable of being ignited, if given a little extra stimulus. Some things heat the body immediately, others take longer to burn; for example, a dry reed is easily lit, whereas green wood is not, although over time it can catch fire (*Mixtures* 3.1, K 1.653).

For Galen there are four faculties: attraction, retention, transformation and expulsion. A food is something which is assimilated, when all four qualities (hot, cold, wet and dry) act on the object to transform it; this means that the body is nourished by it, 'For nourishment consists merely in complete assimilation' (last line of 3.1, K 1.655, tr. Singer p. 270). Assimilation can take different lengths of time: wine is very quickly assimilated, while the flesh of birds is more quickly assimilated than that of animals (3.2, K 1.655). 'Now all those substances which are assimilated are called foods: all others are called drugs' (K 1.656). Galen says more about assimilation in a treatise written at a similar time, *On the Natural Faculties*. The faculties enable each part of the body to pull in the humour which is its own, and then the part completely assimilates this humour (*Nat. Fac.*, K 2.29.18–22). If what is taken in is not a food but a *pharmakon*, it will be drawn to any diseased part of the body – this is reminiscent of Pliny on aconite being 'attracted' to a scorpion sting.

In *Mixtures*, Galen then divides drugs into four types. In the first type, the body is overpowered by the drug. Galen notes, 'these drugs are of course deleterious and destructive to the animal's nature' (K 1.656, tr. Singer p. 271). The second type is also deleterious; it begins to respond to the body but then rots, and in the process also causes decay in the body. The third heats the body without harming it, and the fourth 'both acts [upon the body] and is acted upon [by the body]' (my brackets), so in both of these types, the drugs 'are gradually completely assimilated' to the extent that type 4 'falls into the category of both drugs and foods'.

How do we map our terms 'poison', 'drug' and indeed 'food' on to these four types? This is complex; not all drugs are food. *Mixtures* complicates the comments of those such as Mark Grant who, in his collection of translations of some other Galenic treatises on diet, comments that 'the same substance could act as a food or a drug', with drugs simply being more forceful and decisive than foods in their action on the body.[61] Grant also suggests that any drug can become a food 'through careful preparation, cooking and seasoning'[62]; according to *Mixtures*, however, this is not the case. And in *On the Powers of Food* book 1, Galen comments that some people say that when a substance is not 'active in the human body, but is only feeding it, this would not be included under the topic of medicine'.[63]

But perhaps what *Mixtures* is discussing is the line between poison and drug: the first two types of drug, the deleterious ones, act more like poisons and can never be transformed into food. Galen also discusses opium here. It is cooling, and the body does not manage to interact with it at all; its extreme cold simply overwhelms the body, even if the opium is heated up first. This is because the very nature of the juice of the poppy is 'cold' (K 1.666). But even this drug, taken in small amounts 'and in conjunction with other substances which are able to counteract the extreme nature of their cooling effect', can be of some value to the body (K 1.667). There is an example of this in Galen's later discussions of theriac: the ingredients of theriac, such as opium, may themselves be considered potentially as poisons, but the cooling effects of opium are then counteracted in the complex theriac recipe by castoreum.[64]

In *Mixtures*, Galen also states something else that later became important to his poison theories, particularly in his use of poison as an image for disease causation in *On Affected Parts*: the principle of a small amount of something causing a disproportionate effect. He uses as his examples in *Mixtures* stories of fire. In one story, a house burns down completely after a fire is started by sunlight igniting a window frame recently painted with resin and then setting alight pigeon droppings which were already putrefying and becoming warm. In another, Archimedes uses fire sticks to set the ships of the enemy fleet on fire. Galen also refers to rubbing stones together to make fire, and to Medea's poison which 'was of this nature; with the introduction of heat, this sets light to anything on to which it is rubbed' (tr. Singer p. 271; K 1.658). Here, the potential for heat exists, only needing a trigger.

This is a revealing example of Galen's interest in the character of Medea. He gives the recipe for Medea's poison as a mixture of brimstone and wet asphalt, adding, 'In fact this used to be performed as a magician's trick: one would extinguish a lamp and then light it again by bringing it into contact with a wall, or with a stone. The wall or stone had of course been covered in brimstone; and once this was realised the thing no longer appeared extraordinary' (tr. Singer p. 272). In *On the Doctrines of Hippocrates and Plato* book 3, he discusses theories of the psyche and, in book 4, their theories of the emotions.[65] Here, he refers to the Stoic Chrysippus' comments on Medea, picking up the charioteer image of the emotions from Plato's *Phaedrus*. At the point when Medea decides to kill her children, her psyche reveals the battle between reason and anger. She understands how terrible an act this is, but anger is like a horse dragging the chariot in a direction the charioteer does not wish to go in; reason pulls her back, anger pulls in the opposite direction, and then she makes her decision.[66] The philosopher Epictetus provides another example of using this Greek tragedy to show how people's judgements are mistaken, when he discusses the decision to kill the children as something that could have been changed if she had only been shown that she was making an error – and, in a further poison reference, he adds that her 'blind and crippled mind' meant that she 'changed herself into a viper' (*Dissertationes* 1.28.7–9).[67]

For Galen, while the language of Attic poetry was important to understand, poetry is a long way from science, and the poets tell us very little that is useful about the three parts of the soul.[68] He comments on Medea that when the chorus describes her in line 109 as *megalosplanchos*, this does not mean high-spirited but should be taken in the literal sense as 'having large internal organs' – so, her brain is large, making her intelligent, her liver is large, so her desires are strong and her heart is large, so her passions are powerful (*On Mixtures* 3.2, K 1.658 and K 5.317). This, for Galen, makes sense: her powerful desire for Jason meant that she betrayed her native land, her anger led her to murder her own children, and her plans were so well thought-out that she defied her enemies.[69] In *On Antidotes* 1

(K 14.33), he quotes a poem of Andromachos the Elder, which refers to the speed of action of Medea's lethal drugs.

Medea kills her husband Jason's new wife with a poisoned dress, and poisoned clothing, of course, is an example of non-internal action: the poison 'devours the flesh' of its victim (Euripides, *Medea* 1189). A poisoned tunic also features in Sophocles' *Trachiniai* where Heracles' wife Deianeira inadvertently sends him this gift, thinking that the ointment she puts on the clothing is a love charm. The poison is a *pharmakon* (*Trachiniai* 685) as well as a *philtron* (*Trachiniai* 584, 1142). Heracles' suffering is described as being like the bite of a viper (*Trachiniai* 770 f.). Medea the poisoner becomes a viper; one who is poisoned is like one bitten by a viper. Again, snake poison is the defining poison.

In *Mixtures* chapter 3, Galen goes on to consider substances which are food and do not damage the body when eaten, but when placed on the skin 'eat through it': mustard, pickles, onion and garlic (K 1.661). He lists many reasons why they do not have this corrosive effect when consumed; the process of digestion changes them, they are spread more widely across the body rather than being concentrated in one place, they are mixed with other fluids in the body, and they are quickly digested and the excess sharpness excreted. Other substances cause no harm externally but serious damage internally, while others sometimes cause harm internally and sometimes do not. Here again he refers to snake venom, which is less dangerous applied to the skin than when taken internally (K 1.665).

Conclusion

Galen, then, worked in a context. It was one in which everyone knew that poison and drug were the same substance; one in which everyone knew that individual deaths, sudden or gradual, and mass deaths, could be the result of poison. He knew what he knew from combining existing treatises on poisons and antidotes with a wider set of stories about extraordinary deaths and extraordinary powers of healing; from hands-on experience with the imperial snake catcher, the royal theriac maker, and various dodgier characters at the Roman markets; and from his knowledge of ancient Greek tragedy. From these different materials, he came to his own theories of the action of substances on the outside and the inside of the body, of the mode of operation of antidotes, and of disease causation as the result of an internal production of poison in the body.

Notes

1 For an assessment of the influence of humoral medicine, see Elisabeth Hsu and Peregrine Horden (eds), *The Body in Balance: Humoral Theory in Practice* (Oxford: Berghahn Books, 2013).
2 Susan P. Mattern, *Galen and the Rhetoric of Healing* (Baltimore, MD: Johns Hopkins University Press, 2008), p. 116 demonstrates that 'He is not isolated from peasant life'.

3 Véronique Boudon, 'La thériaque selon Galien: poison salutaire ou remède empoisonné', in *Le corps à l'épreuve. Poisons, remèdes et chirurgie: aspects des pratiques médicales dans l'Antiquité et au Moyen Âge*, eds. Franck Collard and Evelyne Samama (Langrès: 2002), 45–56: p. 45.

4 Perhaps most famously in Jacques Derrida's 1968 essay, 'Plato's pharmacy', in *Dissemination*, tr. Barbara Johnson (London and New York: Continuum, 1981), 98–110; Jasper P. Neel, *Plato, Derrida, and Writing* (Carbonsdale, IL: Southern Illinois University, 1986), 79–80.

5 *Digest* 50.16.236: *qui venenum dicit, adicere debet, utrum malum an bonum* (in the section *De Verborum Significatione*, http://droitromain.upmf-grenoble.fr/Corpus/d-50.htm#16, accessed 3 November 2015). See also H.F.J. Horstmanshoff, 'Ancient medicine between hope and fear: medicament, magic and poison in the Roman Empire,' *European Review* 7.1 (1999), 37–51: p. 44; Cheryl Golden, *The Role of Poison in Roman Society* (PhD dissertation, University of North Carolina at Chapel Hill, 2005), p. 6; Christopher A. Faraone, *Ancient Greek Love Magic* (Cambridge, MA and London: Harvard University Press, 1999), 25 n. 196 notes the 'almost identical' range of *venenum* and *pharmakon*.

6 *Digest* 50.16.236: *nam et medicamenta venena sunt: quia eo nomine omne continetur, quod adhibitum naturam eius, cui adhibitem esset, mutat.*

7 Faraone, *Ancient Greek Love Magic*, 129, Table 4, gives a useful list of substances which in small doses were used in love potions; in larger doses caused madness, sleep or intoxication; and in very large doses caused death.

8 Michael Gagarin, 'Athenian Homicide Law: Case Studies' (2003) notes that 'there can be a fine line between a love potion and a poison, and not only could no one prove which kind of drug this was, but it may, in fact, have had either effect depending on the dose given', www.stoa.org/projects/demos/article_homicide?page=all&greekEncoding=, accessed 20 August 2015. We should note here that the slave girl is dead at the time of the trial; we only read her intentions ('she imagined perhaps...') through the words of the male speaker.

9 In the translation given in the Loeb Classical Library, which I am using here, *pharmakon* is translated as 'poison' on this occasion; earlier in the story, it is translated 'draught' (1.17). For similar cases from Athens, see Faraone, *Ancient Greek Love Magic*, 116.

10 Derek Collins, *Magic in the Ancient Greek World* (Oxford: Blackwell, 2008), p. 136; on Plato, *Laws* 933a–d, see Michael A. Rinella, *Pharmakon: Plato, Drug Culture, and Identity in Ancient Athens* (Lanham, MD: Lexington Books, 2010).

11 Faraone, *Ancient Greek Love Magic*, 115 (on Antiphon 1.9.2) points out that the stepmother had previously tried to use *pharmaka* to kill her husband, and when caught in the act had then used the 'it was only a love potion' defence. He cites [Aristotle] *Magna Moralia* 16, 1188b30–38, a later anecdote of a woman acquitted on a charge of murder with a *philtron* because 'she gave it to him for affection, but missed her mark'.

12 *Digest* 48.8.3.2, from Aelius Marcianus in the early third century AD; what matters is 'that which is possessed for the sake of killing a person'. This explicitly extends 'bad *venena*' to include 'what are called love potions'.

13 See, for example, Louise Cilliers and F.P. Retief, 'Poisons, poisoning and the drug trade in ancient Rome', *Akroterion* 45 (2000), 88–100. One unanswered question concerns whether the fears of poisoning were justified; while we do not have the bodies of Roman emperors to examine, a possibly comparable case is discussed by Gino Fornaciari et al., 'A medieval case of digitalis poisoning: the sudden death of Cangrande della Scala, lord of Verona (1291–1329)', *Journal of Archeological Science* 54 (2014), 162–7; here, modern toxicological analysis of the hair, bowel contents and liver showed 'digoxin and digitoxin concentrations measured in the tissues of the Prince at death time were well above the lethal

concentrations' which would fit with Cangrande della Scala's symptoms, so the authors conclude that deliberate poisoning is the most likely hypothesis.

14 Horstmanshoff, 'Ancient medicine between hope and fear', pp. 40–1.

15 *Burro praefecto remedium ad fauces pollicitus toxicum misit.*

16 Horstmanshoff, 'Ancient medicine between hope and fear', p. 43.

17 The Loeb translates this as 'poison', but the Greek is simply *pharmakon.*

18 Horstmanshoff, 'Ancient medicine between hope and fear', p. 43. In the Loeb, this is 'bade the doctors purge the sick woman too aggressively' which is a better translation of the Latin *praecipitque medicis ut largius purgarent aegram.*

19 Horstmanshoff, 'Ancient medicine between hope and fear', p. 370.

20 Horstmanshoff, 'Ancient medicine between hope and fear', p. 42.

21 Laurence Totelin, 'Mithradates' antidote: a pharmacological ghost', *Early Science and Medicine* 9.1 (2004), 1–19: p. 1, quoting the *Antidotarium Nicolae*; Françoise Skoda, 'Désignations de l'antidote en grec ancien', in *Docente Natura. Mélanges de médecine ancienne et médievale offerts à Guy Sabbah*, eds. Armelle Debru and Nicoletta Palmieri (Université de St-Etienne, 2001), 273–91.

22 The first part of the recipe is lost: Ann Ellis Hanson, 'Roman medicine', in *A Companion to the Roman Empire*, ed. David S. Potter (Oxford: Blackwell, 2006), 492–523: p. 510. On theriac, see Dusanka Parojcic, Dragan Stupar and Milica Mirica, 'La thériaque: Médicament et Antidote', *Vesalius* 9 (2003), 28–32.

23 Michael Stein, 'La thériaque chez Galien: sa préparation et son usage thérapeutique', in *Galen on Pharmacology. Philosophy, History and Medicine. Proceedings of the Vth International Galen Colloquium. Lille, 16–18 March 1995*, ed. Armelle Debru (Leiden, New York and Cologne: Brill, 1997), 199–209: p. 201.

24 Galen, *De antidotis* I, 6 (XIV. 32–34 K); Totelin, 'Mithradates' antidote', p. 2.

25 Totelin, 'Mithradates' antidote', p. 3; Pliny, *Natural History* 25.3.5–7.

26 Totelin, 'Mithradates' antidote', p. 4.

27 Totelin, 'Mithradates' antidote', p. 3. Like another eventually defeated enemy of Rome, Cleopatra (Plutarch, *Life of Antony*, 27.4–5), Mithradates was credited with knowledge of many different languages.

28 Galen, *On theriac to Piso* 16 (K 14.283–4). As Totelin, 'Mithradates' antidote', p. 6 notes, the earliest version of this was in Livy, *Periocha* 102.

29 Alain Touwaide, 'Galien et la toxicologie', in *Aufstieg und Niedergang der Römischen Welt* II. 37.2, ed. Wolfgang Haase (Berlin: de Gruyter, 1994), 1887–1986: p. 1942. On the Temple of Peace library, see Richard Neudecker, 'Archives, books and sacred space in Rome', in *Ancient Libraries*, eds. Jason König, Katerina Oikonomopoulou and Greg Woolf (Cambridge: Cambridge University Press, 2013), 312–31: pp. 328–9.

30 Armelle Debru, *Le Corps respirant: La pensée physiologique chez Galien*, Studies in Ancient Medicine, 13 (Leiden and New York: E.J. Brill, 1996), pp. 238–9; on the use of bonfires, see J. Rubin Pinault, *Hippocratic Lives and Legends*, Studies in Ancient Medicine, 4 (Leiden and New York: E.J. Brill, 1992), pp. 37 and 45.

31 David B. Kaufman, 'Poisons and poisoning among the Romans,' *Classical Philology* 27 (1932), 156–67: pp. 156–7.

32 Pliny writes that 'death occurs on the same day if the genitals of a female creature are but touched with it', *Natural History* 27.2.4. He notes that M. Caelius accused Calpurnius Bestia of using aconite to murder his wives while they slept, and alludes to a reference in Caelius' speech against Calpurnius to the somewhat unsavoury role of Calpurnius' finger here.

33 Stein, 'La thériaque chez Galien', p. 208.

34 Touwaide, 'Galien et la toxicologie', p. 1903.

35 Tr. Vivian Nutton, in P.N. Singer (ed.), *Galen: Psychological Writings* (Cambridge: Cambridge University Press, 2013), p. 79.

36 Stein, 'La thériaque chez Galien', p. 204.

37 Alba Aguilera Felipe, Los venenos en la Antigüedad: Corpus Toxicologicum, www.academia.edu/5283381/Los_venenos_en_la_Antiguedad_Corpus_Toxico-logicum, accessed 22 August 2014; Touwaide, 'Galien et la toxicologie', p. 1901.

38 Touwaide, 'Galien et la toxicologie', pp. 1902–3, summarises the position in 1994, but this has since changed; see below.

39 *On Theriac to Piso* was seen as authentic in antiquity; see Pinault, *Hippocratic Lives and Legends*, p. 51. *On Theriac, to Pamphilus* is not authentic; Vivian Nutton, 'Galen on theriac: problems of authenticity', in *Galen on Pharmacology. Philosophy, History and Medicine. Proceedings of the Vth International Galen Colloquium. Lille, 16–18 March 1995*, ed. Armelle Debru (Leiden, New York and Cologne: E.J. Brill, 1997), 133–51: pp. 137–8 and 140–1. See further Vivian Nutton, 'Galen *ad multos annos*', *Dynamis*, 15 (1995), 25–39: pp. 33–34, concluding 'There are, I suggest, not good grounds for supposing that *Ad Pisonem* is spurious, and an overwhelming case in favour of authenticity' (p. 37). Nutton dates it between 204 and 211.

40 See Caroline Petit on www.medicineancientandmodern.com/?p=210, accessed 1 July 2015. For fuller discussion, see Robert Leigh's 2013 Exeter PhD thesis, https://ore.exeter.ac.uk/repository/handle/10871/13641, shortly to be published as *On Theriac to Piso, Attributed to Galen: A Critical Edition with Translation and Commentary*, Studies in Ancient Medicine, 47 (Leiden and New York: E.J. Brill, 2016), p. 18 and 53.

41 On the date of this treatise, see Touwaide, 'Galien et la toxicologie', p. 1898. On retained seed and menses, see Helen King, 'Galen and the widow. Towards a history of therapeutic masturbation in ancient gynaecology', *EuGeStA: Journal on Gender Studies in Antiquity*, 1 (2011).

42 Debru, *Le Corps respirant*, p. 228; Touwaide, 'Galien et la toxicologie', p. 1973.

43 Stein, 'La thériaque chez Galien', p. 199; see also C. H. Campbell, 'The effects of snake venoms and their neurotoxins on the nervous system of man and animals', *Contemporary Neurology Series* 12 (1975), 259–93 on how snake venom acts at the neuromuscular junction, disrupting the function of the brain and the nervous system, usually causing paralysis.

44 *On Antidotes* 1.1 (K 14.2); *On Theriac to Piso* 5 (K 14.232); Leigh, *On Theriac to Piso*, p. 25 on how in *On Antidotes* 'The importance of viper's flesh [to theriac] is apparent ... from the fact that it is the only change to the recipe which Galen specifically identifies', a statement with which whoever wrote *On Theriac to Piso* agrees.

45 For the drought version, see Herodotus 4.173.

46 Daniel Ogden, *Drakon. Dragon Myth and Serpent Cult in the Greek and Roman Worlds* (New York and Oxford: Oxford University Press, 2013), p. 210.

47 Ogden, *Drakon*, pp. 213–4.

48 Susan P. Mattern, *Prince of Medicine: Galen in the Roman World* (Oxford and New York: Oxford University Press, 2013), p. 217.

49 Everett L. Wheeler, 'Pullarii, Marsi, Haruspices, and Sacerdotes in the Roman Imperial Army', in *A Roman Miscellany: Essays in Honour of Anthony R. Birley on his Seventieth Birthday*, eds. H.M. Schellenburg, V.E. Hirschmann and A. Krieckhous (Gdansk: Foundation for the Development of Gdansk University, 2008), 185–201: pp. 188–9.

50 Horstmanshoff, 'Ancient medicine between hope and fear', p. 46.

51 *Outline for Empiricism* 10.75–7; Richard Walzer and Michael Frede, *Galen. Three Treatises: On the Nature of Science, on the Sects for Beginners, an Outline for Empiricism* (Indianapolis, IN: Hackett Publishing, 1985), pp. 39–40.

52 *Outline for Empiricism* 10.77–8; Walzer and Frede, *Galen*, pp. 40–1. On snakes at the temple, see Ogden, *Drakon*, pp. 368–70.

53 ἔτι νέος γενόμενος.

54 *Corpus Medicorum Graecorum*, p. 90.

55 Vivian Nutton, *Ancient Medicine*, 2nd edition (London and New York: Routledge, 2013), p. 210; Stein, 'La thériaque chez Galien', p. 204.

56 Hence, the alternative dating that would see them as contemporaries, perhaps writing without knowledge of each other, Nutton, *Ancient Medicine*, p. 210.

57 Mattern, *Galen and the Rhetoric of Healing*, p. 38.

58 Nutton, *Ancient Medicine*, p. 210. Something similar happens when the sixth-century Aetius of Amida repeats as his own experience a story taken from Galen; Armelle Debru, 'La Suffocation hystérique chez Galien et Aetius: réécriture et emprunt de "je"', in *Tradizione e ecdotica dei testi medici tardoantichi e bizantini*, ed. Antonio Garzya (Naples: M. D'Auria, 1992), 79–89: pp. 85–9. See further King, 'Galen and the widow', p. 222 and Peter Pormann, 'New Fragments from Rufus of Ephesus' *On Melancholy*', *Classical Quarterly* 64.2 (2014), 649–56.

59 His time in Rome, which began in 162, was interrupted by an outbreak of plague, during which he went back home to Pergamon, and by a summons from the emperor to come with him to Germany.

60 Philip van der Eijk, 'Galen and the scientific treatise: a case study of *Mixtures*', in *Writing Science: Medical and Mathematical Authorship in Ancient Greece*, ed. Markus Asper (Berlin and Boston, MA: de Gruyter, 2013), 145–76: p. 150 describes it as 'one of the most rigorous and tightly argued works in the Galenic corpus'.

61 Mark Grant, *Galen on Food and Diet* (London: Routledge, 2000), p. 7.

62 Grant, *Galen on Food and Diet*, p. 7.

63 Grant, *Galen on Food and Diet*, p. 73.

64 Stein, 'La thériaque chez Galien', p. 207.

65 *On the Doctrines of Hippocrates and Plato* 3.3.13–18 (CMG p. 188); 4.2.7 (CMG p. 244); 4.6.19–23 (CMG p. 274).

66 CMG V 4, 1, 2, tr. de Lacy; III 2.17 = K 307; quoting *Medea* 1078–79; Christopher Gill, 'Did Chrysippus understand Medea?', *Phronesis*, 28.2 (1983), 136–49.

67 Philip DeLacy, 'Galen and the Greek poets', *Greek, Roman and Byzantine Studies*, 7 (1966), 259–66.

68 DeLacy, 'Galen and the Greek poets', p. 263.

69 DeLacy, 'Galen and the Greek poets', p. 266.

3 Mining for poison in a devout heart

Dissective practices and poisoning in late medieval Europe

Montserrat Cabré and Fernando Salmón

In recent years, historiography has drawn our attention to the need to consider poisons fully as part of medieval culture. Medical, social and legal historians have approached medieval concerns about poisons from a variety of perspectives: from the analysis of treatises dealing with the workings of poisons or the therapeutic strategies for dealing with them, to the relatively frequent charges of intentional poisoning and how the construction of the crime manifested tensions within the community, which in turn shone a light on power relations.[1]

In this chapter, we would like to address medieval understandings of poisoning from a rather particular stance. We will attempt to explore the significance for the history of poisons of an important source that has hitherto passed unnoticed by medical historians and that may well contain the earliest-known Western illustration of the opening of a body in a case of poisoning—a domestic dissection of a young woman's corpse. The rich narrative of our story is contained in a Spanish 13th-century collection of miracles, the *Cantigas de Santa María* (Songs of the Holy Mary). Its intriguing and dense report articulates in a single account elements that invite us to bring into dialogue various histories that more often than not do not cross paths: the history of poisons and the domestic pursuit of knowledge of the body. In light of the work by Katharine Park on the history of dissection, we believe that our story may be read not just as a mere anecdote but interpreted as carrying significant meanings about 13th-century understandings of poisoning.[2]

A poison story in 13th-century Castile

The *Cantigas de Santa María* is a compilation of 420 miracles written in the scriptorium of Alfonso X the Wise, King of Castile and León between 1252 and 1284. Its production was a complex process of collection and composition of miracles, involving the selection and importation of narratives as well as the creation of versified texts and visual accounts. The compilation was not only produced by a team of poets, scholars, scribes and illuminators under the king's auspices but also with his direct involvement, which is acknowledged in a handful of songs. Alfonso X is well known as a lyricist and musical poet in Galaico-Portuguese, the language of the Cantigas in which learned poetry was written in 13th-century Castile. Despite the fact that the *Cantigas* is one of the most well-known sources from the second half of 13th-century Iberia, as far as we know the historical significance of the story told in song number 188, *The Image that was Found in a Young Girl's Heart*, has as yet gone unnoticed.[3] The narrative of the song, both the lyrics and the accompanying musical notation, is preserved in two of the four extant manuscripts containing Alfonso's *Cantigas*. Fortunately for us, one is the richly illuminated *Códice rico* today held in the Library of San Lorenzo del Escorial and known as manuscript T[4]; it is this codex that we will be using as a source in this essay (Figure 3.1).[5]

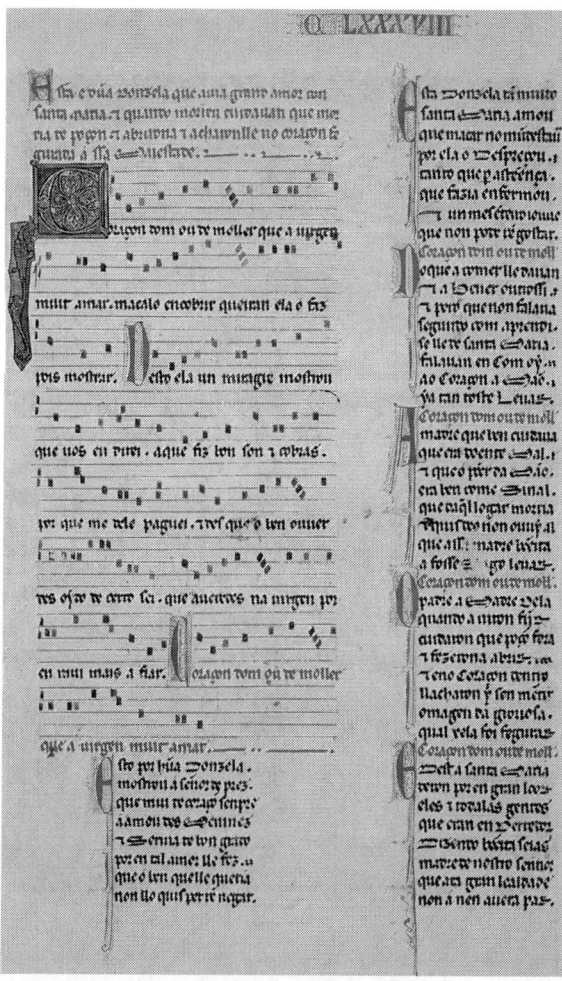

Figure 3.1 Full image of Cantiga 188. Library of San Lorenzo del Escorial, manuscript T. © Patrimonio Nacional.

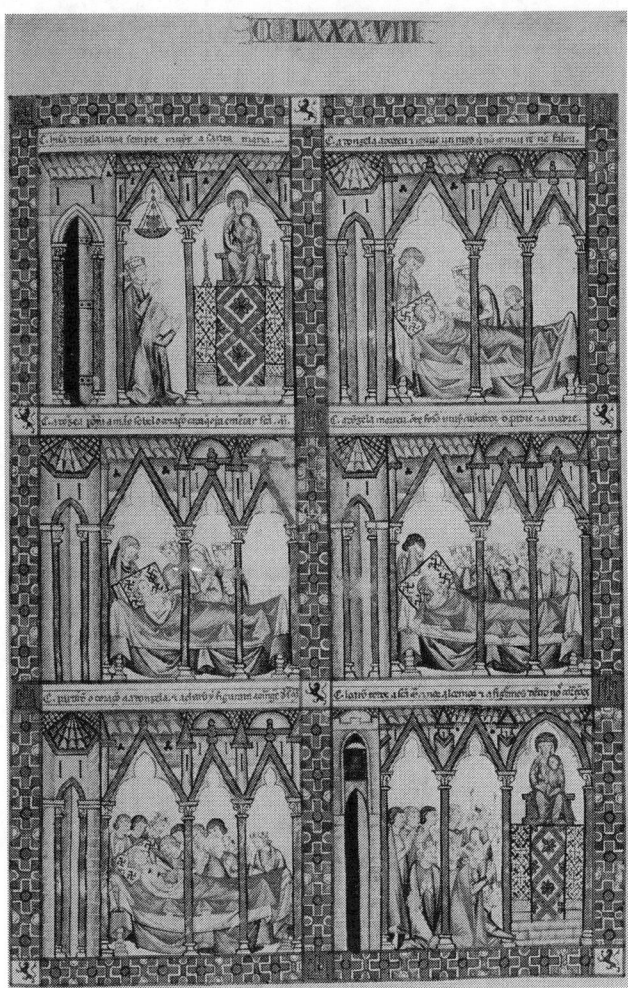

Figure 3.1 (Continued).

Cantiga 188 is a virelai in sol whose layout follows the structural pattern in which the songs are organized in the *Códice rico*. The verso of folio 246 contains the title, the musical notation with the lyrics of the chorus and the first stanza, and six more stanzas to be chanted in the same way as the given example. Next, the recto of folio 247 offers a series of six miniatures illustrating the story, organized in two columns, each image identified with its own caption.

The narrative recounts the story of a young woman, a maiden who was a devotee of the Virgin Mary. The text states that since she was a child, she had loved Holy Mary and served her with all her heart. The first image represents the young woman kneeling before an image of the Virgin, with her mother standing at her back. The girl lived in the world, but she despised it so much, for the Virgin's sake, that she endured intense abstinence; because of such fasting, she fell ill and lay for a whole month without being able to taste what they gave her to eat or to drink. Indeed, the second illustration depicts her in bed, surrounded by a young boy and an adult bearded man—perhaps her brother and father. Her mother stands by her side holding a bowl with her left hand, while she tries to feed her daughter with a spoon with her right hand. The maiden was unable to speak, but if her relatives spoke to her about Holy Mary, she raised her hand immediately pointing to her heart. Her mother, who took good care of her—as the song highlights—was convinced that it was a serious illness and that her putting her hand there was a sign that she was about to die from a disorder in that place. Actually, the third miniature in the series represents the young woman naked in bed signaling her heart with her right hand, while a group of five people surround her—her mother, the young boy, two women and a non-bearded man. Nothing could be done to avoid death, for it was God's will to take her with Him to His Blessed Mother. And when the father and the mother of the girl saw her expire, the text states that they thought that it had been caused by a poison (*cuidaron que poçón fora*).

In the death scene, the crying father and mother are accompanied at the bedside by the young boy and five other women. And as the text clearly states, immediately following her demise, her parents had her cut open: *e fezérona abrir* (Figure 3.2).

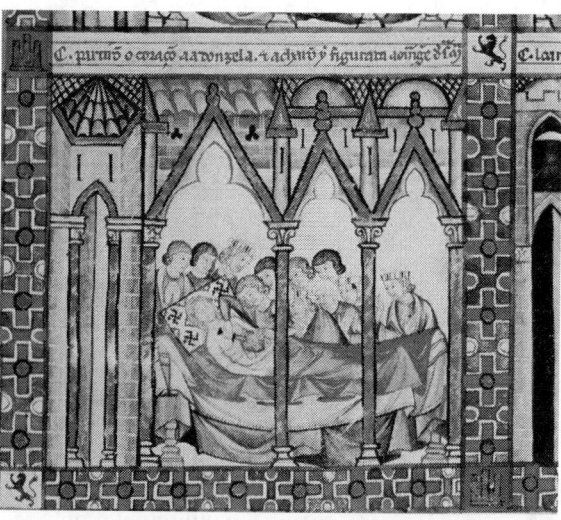

Figure 3.2 Post-mortem vignette from Cantiga 188. Library of San Lorenzo del Escorial, manuscript T. © Patrimonio Nacional.

According to the illustration, her heart was dissected in the same bed where she died, before the interested eyes of a group of four men and five women. A male figure performs the post-mortem procedure. In the attending crowd, we can see in the foreground next to the dissector the women who had tended her. The young boy who had witnessed all the illness is not present in this scene, whereas three adult men accompanying the father appear at the bedside for the first time. The dissector, with no other iconographical attribution but a knife in his right hand, occupies the central place of the scene. The gestures of all the characters appearing in this vignette are remarkable: their heads and bodies are ostensibly leaning toward the corpse, showing their curiosity about the procedure. And when the young woman's heart was dissected, they swear they found inside "a likeness of the Glorious one, which She [Holy Mary] had graven there".[6] The story ends with the girl's relatives and all the crowd gathered there giving great praise to Holy Mary for the graven image, happily saying, "Blessed be You, mother of our Lord, for your great constancy has not, nor ever will have, equal".[7] And finally, the last miniature depicts this praise by showing the group who attended the dissection—five women and four men—praying devoutly in church before an image of the Virgin with her Son.

The compilation of the *Cantigas* was a long process that extended for years, and it was the product of some complex teamwork done at Alfonso's court, probably while in Seville.[8] The courtly dimension is an important feature as it gave the effort a collective nature, not only in the actual composition of the songs by diverse troubadours and in the execution of the scribal and iconographical programs, but also in the very identification and selection of the miracle stories that went into the compilation. Although the precise dating of the production of the collection is still debated, *cantiga* 188 clearly belongs to a second stage of the process of the compilation, when the initial cluster was extended to 200 songs. The only chronological frame we have for our story is then the production of manuscript T, the earlier of the extant two that contain the miracle; the latest studies conclude that the *Códice rico* was initiated around 1280 and was finished before Alfonso's death in 1284.[9]

There are certain traits that distinguish *cantiga* 188 as peculiar in the framework of the collection. Most of the Marian stories that are included contain geographical identifications of the places where they took place. Alfonso was particularly interested in showing that his kingdom had been profusely distinguished by the Virgin and the *Cantigas* are a rich source with which to document local miracles. However, our story is devoid of any context, and there is no internal clue as to where it happened. Neither does the text provide any idiosyncratic feature to identify the circumstances of the maiden's family. In addition, many of the miracles compiled are found in earlier or contemporary collections, from the *Liber miraculorum* of Gregory of Tours to the *Liber Mariae* of the Franciscan Juan Gil de Zamora (*c.* 1241–1318), who collaborated closely with the Wise king. Nevertheless, scholars of the *Cantigas* have found no textual parallel for *cantiga* 188 in any Iberian or European miracle collection. Furthermore, they agree on attributing an oral source to this particular song.

The story of the devout maiden was not copied from another text, but it was rather transformed into a song by Alfonso's direct intervention, and it has been signaled as the one out of four songs that most clearly shows the authorship of the king.[10] His voice emerges distinctively, addressing the listener and stating his particular inclination for the story:

> Concerning this, She performed a miracle, which I shall tell you. I set it into melody and verse, because it delighted me so, and when you have heard it, I know for certain that you will have even greater trust in the Virgin.[11]

> [*Desto ela un miragre mostrou que vos eu direi,*
> *a que fiz bon son e cobras porque me dele paguei.*
> *E des que o ben ouverdes oiso, de certo sei*
> *que averedes na Virgen por én mui máis a fiar.*][12]

Alfonso's interest in legitimizing it personally is evident, and he insists on quoting an oral source:

> Although she did not speak, *according to what I learned*, if they spoke to her of Holy Mary, she raised her hand immediately to her heart, *as I heard*.[13]

> [*e pero que non falava, segundo com' aprendi*
> *se lle de Santa Maria falavan én, com' oi,*
> *ao coraçon a mão ia tan toste levar.*][14]

Although there is no trace in the text about how the story came to his ears, it is certain that he trusted the means through which he knew the story, at least as much as any other of the written or contextually framed miracles included in the collection. The narrative recounts the course of the events as if they were following a common, logical order of causation. In particular, the decision to open the body because poison was suspected is stated in the same verse: "*cuidaron que poçon fora e fezerona abrir*" [they thought that it had been caused by a poison and had her cut open].[15]

There is no other similar story compiled in the miracles contained in the *Cantigas*. There are three other songs where poisons have a part in the stories, as they imply a suspicion of animal or human intentional poisoning.[16] However, Mary's intervention in these cases is to heal the poisoned individual rather than to show her greatness through bodily presence. For the broader European context, we have been unable to identify any other similar poison story, either contemporary or from an earlier period.[17] However, the account contains many elements which give cultural plausibility to the story it tells, even beyond the credibility that the king himself gave to the story he had heard.

The story embodies important themes solidly grounded in the religious culture of the time. Manifestations of the divine through material or physical impressions abounded in 13th-century Europe, and there are other miracles in the *Cantigas* involving the impression of sacred images in stone.[18] In addition, the emergence of Franciscan spirituality gave currency to the motif of the inscribed heart, a phenomenon shared by many contemporary saints, both male and female.[19] Nevertheless, although most famously attributed to saint Ignatius of Antioch—in whose heart was found the name of Jesus Christ—the phenomenon particularly concerned women and became part of the rich female imaginary of embodied piety.[20]

Cantiga 188 depicts a post-mortem procedure, a domestic autopsy commissioned privately, not by a judicial court. There is no clue as to who performed it, but no medical practitioner is mentioned either as attending the illness, and the miniaturist did not attribute to the dissector any particular trait beyond those identifying an adult male. We have no traces either of domestic autopsies being carried out in Castile at that time, or, for that matter, in any other Iberian territory.[21] The scattered documents we have regarding the dissection of corpses are from a later period and come from judicial sources, not from domestic private practices that sought *to know* or *to know more* about the cause of a death as a way to make sense of an individual's demise, as our miracle tells.

Most of the *Cantigas* tell us exactly where the events of the miracles took place. This is the case not only with local events, but also with imported accounts from all over Europe. Since the context of our story is totally blurred, it is plausible to think that the king's oral source was reporting a story that came from afar, either far in time or in space, or both, as it is likely that a story that had taken place in his own kingdom would have reached Alfonso's ears with more geographical precision. The story that so delighted the king had not necessarily had to have happened in Castile; an account from a foreign land could have easily reached him. A very learned king, he could have heard the story from many people at his court, including European travelers—diplomats or scholars. His relationships with Italy were close and many. Frederick II Hohenstaufen, King of Sicily, was a cousin and legal tutor of his mother, Elisabeth (renamed Beatrice) of Swabia, who spent her childhood at his court until she left to marry Alfonso's father, and the relationship with the Castilian monarchy lasted until Frederick's death in 1250. Between 1256 and 1275, Alfonso was committed to becoming elected as Holy Roman Emperor, and embassies and diplomatic contacts between Castile, Rome and the Italian cities were frequent and might have had a direct impact on the compilation of the *Cantigas*.[22] Ten of the collected miracles actually happened in Italian cities or bear Italian themes,[23] and scribes of Italian provenance—and probably illuminators—are documented as working at Alfonso's scriptorium.[24]

As with the case of domestic autopsies, we have no record of post-mortem procedures taking place in 13th-century Castile. Indeed, there are very few documented instances of post-mortem dissections in continental Europe before the 14th century. However, practices of embalming and evisceration developed earlier in the context of funerary practices, although local and dynastic traditions seem to greatly vary.[25] Recent work on techniques of the conservation of the corpse in medieval Castile shows that these practices were not generalized in the Iberian Peninsula and that the embalming of both, Alfonso X and his mother Elisabeth of Swabia, was an exception rather than a rule. Alfonso was also atypical in programming a double burial for his body and heart, as this practice was growing elsewhere but it was not current in the Hispanic Kingdoms.[26]

In contrast with these trends, Katharine Park's work has shown that in late 13th-century Italy, however infrequent, dissection practices were rich and diverse. Domestic autopsies have been documented among the well-to-do Florentines only in the 15th century,[27] but there is no reason to think that they could not have been performed earlier, as our story suggests. Italian sources indicate that early dissection practices emerge often in connection with the flourishing women's religious movements that gave rise to forms of embodied sanctity in the form of relics, most prominently in the well-documented case of Clare of Montefalco, whose heart was dissected in 1308 by her fellow nuns who found inside a cross and other instruments of Christ's passion.[28] On the other hand, Caroline Bynum has shown that fasting was a crucial trait of 13th-century women's spirituality.[29] The behavior toward intake shown by the anonymous girl of *cantiga* 188 was certainly in fashion at the time, and the domestic, non-institutional character of her distinguished religiosity may have prevented her story from offering a precise context to her deed. We have no evidence of the existence of a significant movement of women's fasting in 13th-century Castile, but the Franciscan ideals spread giving new impetus to already-significant forms of women's dedication to the religious life, such as that of *mulieres religiosae*, and independent and extreme modes of female piety were not unknown.[30]

By definition, miracles express the workings of divine power in a narrative frame that needs to embody recognizable traits of daily life where the extraordinary outcome of an ordinary situation may be clearly distinguished. If the origin of our story suggests an Italian provenance, it is interesting to note that neither a comment of surprise nor an explanation of the facts was added in the king's reworking of the story. Since the collection was addressed to an Iberian audience, we can assume that neither the extreme fasting of the girl nor the petition of the domestic autopsy in connection with the suspicion of poisoning seemed to be alien to Castilian sensitivities. And independently from where it originated and how it traveled to Alfonso's court, once it was written and illuminated in the *Cantigas* the story was surely heard, seen and heard by many in the Castilian kingdom, chanted as a song.

Searching for poison in the heart

No less intriguing than its origin is the content of the story itself that we would like to explore in what follows. The song explains that the actual motive behind the decision to open up the young woman's body was the mother's suspicion that, after evaluating the course of her daughter's illness, led to her thinking that the cause of death had been poisoning. But why? And even if the suspicion of poisoning can be seen as a rather plausible inference for the relatives of the fasting girl to make, we need to ask about another important inference they make in relation to that. Namely, what they do to investigate their suspicion: ask for her to be cut open, with the belief that in her insides they would be able to see the material traces of poisoning.

The source tells that the young girl fell ill due to intense fasting, and once she was ill, for a month she could not eat or drink what they gave to her. The narrative goes further and explains that she was also unable to speak, and when she heard talking about the Virgin, she pointed to her heart. This made her mother think that the cause of her dying lay in there: "the mother thought ... that she was dying from that place" (que daquel logar morria).[31]

Just by following the narrative of the symptoms reported, various culprits could be pointed out as responsible for the death such as the extreme fasting itself or the excess of spiritual love. The sources recounting the lives and experiences of holy fasting women describe the harmful effects on their bodies of their behavior and explain the fact that they may live on by direct divine intervention.[32] There was also a growing cultural interest in lovesickness and manifestations of both earthly and spiritual love flourished in 13th-century Europe. Affective piety and excessive human love were profoundly distinct in nature; however, their sufferers shared certain effects on the body caused by their afflictions. Mary Wack has shown the physical analogies of these two forms of love and how they could be confused in practice.[33] Although learned medicine highlighted the erotic nature of lovesickness, its definitions of the affliction and its consequences were broad and could encompass both physical and spiritual love. The obsessive fixation with the love object prevented the sick person from sleeping or eating; as a result, she might undergo general debilitation and could even die.[34] It might also be the case that the effect of lovesickness could be taken for another illness, as happened to the sisters of the 13th-century mystic Juliana of Mont Cornillon, who mistook her sickness of divine love for a physical illness.[35]

But the logical narrative of the closing of the song in a celebratory praise of a miraculous Holy Mother needs to call upon an ailment that both affects the heart and whose effect left a material trait that can be seen in the heart by dissection. Poison here seems the obvious candidate, and it would be historiographically rewarding to explore why.

Historiography has pointed out the growing cultural and intellectual interest in poisons from the late 13th century onward.[36] The court of Castile was not an exception in this interest, and a treatise on poisons was produced by the Franciscan scholar Juan Gil de Zamora, who had strong links with the king Alfonso X and who, as we have seen, was involved directly and indirectly in the compilation of the *Cantigas*.[37] At the end of the 13th century, he produced a *Liber contra venena et animalia venenosa* that he dedicated to Raymond Geoffroy, minister general of the order of St. Francis, a text that reflects, as most of the contemporary and later works on the topic do, the influence of Avicenna's theoretical knowledge about poisons both within and outside strictly medical circles[38]—a knowledge that can help us to evaluate the narrative plausibility of the suspected poisoning as told in *cantiga* 188.

Avicenna discusses the issue of poisons in two places in his *Liber Canonis*: in Lib. I, fen 2, doct. 2, cap. 15 "De iis que proveniunt ex his que comeduntur et bibuntur"[39] and in lib. IV which devoted fen 6 specifically to "De venenis".[40] In Liber I, he offers what would become a very handy concept in medieval disquisitions about the action of drugs—medicines and poisons alike—that of the specific form or entire substance. Avicenna explains that anything we take in works inside the body in three different ways: through its quality, through its matter and through its entire substance (*tota substantia*).[41] Medicines can act through quality; for instance, a hot medicine alters the body qualitatively, by heating it, while the medicine itself remains unaltered. Food can act in the body through matter by transforming itself into bodily matter and also qualitatively through the quality that dominates that particular food stuff. But some drugs or ingested food can also act through its entire substance or specific form, through a property that does not depend on the qualities of the simples that compose them but that is specific to the entire compound. These substances may have therapeutic effects on the body, such as theriac, or on the contrary, like poisons, may have harmful effects.[42] The property that results from the specific form of a compound is a quality peculiar to that individual compound, and can be determined only through experience. It is not predictable, as are the properties of a compound derived from its simples.[43]

This general frame supports Avicenna's classification of poisons, developed later in book IV of the *Canon*, based on the rationale of their functioning. He divides poisons according to three broad criteria: the principle of their action, the extension of their action and the speed and timespan of the action. Focusing on the principle that explains their actions, poisons were divided into two types: poisons that act through their quality (*inflammans* through their hot quality, *infrigidans* through their cold quality, etc.) and poisons that act through the specific form or *tota substantia*. According to the extension of their action on the body, they can be divided into those that act upon one particular member, like the cantharides upon the bladder, or into those that affect all the body, like opium. And also, poisons could be divided into fast or slow according to the speed of the appearances of their effects, and into those that act immediately or, on the contrary, in a deferred manner.[44]

But in addition to the explanatory basis for understanding the effects of the poison on the body, Avicenna's section *De venenis*, like other chapters or monographs devoted to the topic by the many medical and non-medical authors who contributed to the long tradition of medieval interest in poisoning, was concerned in giving practical advice such as how to avoid it, when to suspect it, how to recognize the particular poison involved in the intoxication and how to handle it once the poisoning has taken place.[45]

Some historians have connected the growing emergence of a medieval literature on poisons to the real fear of poisoning felt in the medieval courts.[46] Despite Umberto Eco's suggestion, the space of the monastic life seemed somehow safer.[47] However, the protection of the life of the minister general of the order of St. Francis to whom Juan Gil de Zamora's treatise was dedicated was the reason given in its prohemium to justify its composition[48] maybe not just rhetorically.[49]

Intentional poisoning has attracted the attention of historians and the public with juicy stories of crime and power and of colorful preventive measures at the rich courtier dining tables such as the presence of ornate serpent horns, but less attention has been paid to cases of accidental poisoning.[50] However, as happens in Avicenna's book IV, the treatises on poisons take this possibility seriously into account by giving some advice on how to store food and drinks to avoid accidental poisoning due to an unnoticed contamination by venomous animals. Advice that in some cases extends to recommending caution in the accusation of intentional poisoning in order to avoid the wronging of innocents.[51]

So, we can assume that when in our *cantiga* the mother expressed her suspicion of poisoning as the cause of death of her daughter, there was no need for the hearers of the song to believe that a crime was feared.

At first sight, more intriguing for us could be the possibility of poisoning in someone who has not eaten or drunk for a month. Medieval theories of poisoning, though, again make the story plausible. As mentioned before, our maiden's case could be one of the actions of a poison of deferred effect. Medical sources reflect on this possibility, and judicial cases of this type have been reported for a later period.[52] Poisoning obviously could happen through it being taken in with food or drink or by itself when swallowing internally, and also externally by the bite or by the touch of a venomous animal. But in the medieval understanding of poisoning, the body was thought widely porous and the poisoning could also happen through a glance, a sound or a smell. The venomous glances of the basilisk, the hiss with which certain serpents kill the birds or the poisonous odor of certain fungi, furnished not just the treatises on poisons but a long literary tradition as well.[53] And even without any external factor, the ability of the humoral body to poison itself through the corruption of its humors was an accepted commonplace.[54]

The *cantiga* does not say much about the symptoms of the girl's illness: she lay in bed and was not able to speak, to eat or to drink. Other contemporary descriptions of signs and symptoms of poisoning were much more florid: sudden paleness or redness of the face, excessive salivation, bad taste in the mouth and changes of color in the tongue, bad breath and bad bodily odor, vomiting and contortion of the bowls and acute pains in the stomach, palpitation, lower pulse, cold sweating, redness of the eyes or white eyes with disappearance of the pupils, etc. appeared recorded both in treatises on poisons and in chronicles and legal records.[55] It is true that in some cases, namely in those due to poisons that act through their entire substance, the symptoms could be just a general body weakness, cold sweat and syncope,[56] symptoms that could be more in tune with the general state described in the song. However, the mark of the poisoning was clearly revealed to the hearers of the song not so much through the symptoms but when the mother interpreted the raising of her daughter's hand toward her heart as the locus of the ailment that would cause her death.

The relationship between the heart, the movements of the blood and poisoning is a common theme in the ancient and medieval traditions on poisons. In fact, the fantastic approach to the origin of the Latin word for poison popularized through the *Etymologies* of Isidor of Seville (*c.* 560–636) reflected this connection, affirming that "venenum" owes its name to the fact that it runs in the veins and that it is only when mixed with the blood that it kills.[57] Various popular maneuverings in the case of poisonous bites, such as the sucking of the wound and the spitting out of the blood, or the application of a tourniquet, were advised in order to prevent the poison reaching the heart.[58] The same rationale lies behind the explanation of the effect of the antidotes that work by deterring the poison from reaching the heart.[59] And some medieval physicians concluded that what all the poisons have in common is the fact that all of them harm the heart and that death does not occur unless this damage is produced.[60]

There are indirect signs that support this connection, such as the alteration of the pulse, the *tremor cordis* and syncope just mentioned, that are common in cases of poisoning, or even the deadly sign of changes in the nails' color, since these were thought to be produced by the vapours emanating from the heart.[61] But more important for our story is the possibility of opening the cadaver to explore direct signs of the heart's damage.

Treatises on poisons do not recommend opening a cadaver to confirm the effect of the poison visually. However, some of the authors explained the effect of poisons in the heart with powerful images that suggested direct observation in humans or animals. Juan Gil de Zamora, in his treatise on poisons, following *verbatim* Gilbertus Anglicus' medicinal compendium (1250s),[62] refers to the coagulation of blood in the heart as an effect provoked by a cold poison. It is true that the image of coagulation or freezing could just be a logical inference made by someone trained in the Aristotelian mode of thought, since it is simply logical that something of a cold quality, like a cold poison, can thicken something of a hot nature like the blood and the heart. But Zamora's reflection pointed out openly that the proof (*signa eius*) that cold poisons act in this way is the fact that in those dead due to poisoning, coagulated blood can be found near the heart and inside it.[63] That the blood coagulates in the heart seems a commonplace, and authors refer to it without explaining the mechanism in full, but the analogies that they offer to describe this phenomenon are suggestive of a visual examination. The blood coagulates around the heart by the action of a poison as "the milk coagulates", says the 10th-century physician Ibn al Jazzar, in his influential *Viaticum* when advising the use of theriac to avoid or dissolve that coagulation.[64] A powerful image—that of curdled milk— one that stresses the likeness of an eye-witnessed phenomenon.

Franck Collard, using French chronicles and legal documentation, seems to contradict this interpretation by calling our attention to the ambiguity of the sources in order to properly understand the kind of examination carried out in the evaluation of someone dead from poisoning. In most cases, it seems that the exam was done by medical practitioners. However, these latter were called to do an external evaluation of the corpse or to help as experts in embalming processes but not to do an autopsy to confirm the poisoning.[65]

Some historians have pointed out geographical differences on this issue. While autopsies with a medical-legal aim would be relatively common in some parts of Italy and southern France, they would be rarer on the rest of the continent.[66] In fact, some of the first documented autopsies in cases of poisoning are of Italian provenance.[67]

But, irrespective of local traditions, Collard asks a puzzling question that is relevant to our story and needs to be addressed: why do an autopsy when the external signs and symptoms of poisoning were evident or, on the contrary, when there were none? It seems that the practice of the autopsy could be justified to confirm further poisoning as the cause of death due to the consequences that a wrong evaluation of the cause of the decease would entail for a third party.[68] But, if we think about poisoning not necessarily as the result of a crime, the question might be less puzzling. What if the autopsy was carried out purely due to the desire to know differently what was already known? In his influential *De venenis* from the first decade of the 14th century, Pietro d'Abano recalled a story that would support this hypothesis. While explaining the action of mercury, he recounts one example in which an autopsy was performed in the case of an apothecary who in the middle of the night and being very thirsty took by mistake a flask of mercury, drank from it and died. The death scene was clear for those who found the corpse, since the flask was nearby the corpse and mercury was coming out from his anus. Irrespective of this evidence, however, "anatomizatus fuit", and it was found that the blood near the heart was coagulated and so was the heart, and in the stomach, almost a pound of mercury was found.[69] It is difficult to explain this autopsy as a way to ascertain a cause of death. Rather, it seems more likely that what led to the anatomical dissection was the desire to know not through inference of signs and symptoms but directly from the material traces of poisoning inside the body.

Working primarily with legal records, historians have shown that in the 14th and 15th centuries, autopsies were gradually performed in southern Europe as a method of identifying or discarding poisoning as the cause of death, particularly in cases where intentional poisoning was suspected, involving medical practitioners and legal prosecutors alike. However, our source documents practices of dissection being performed earlier and outside the judicial and medical realms, in a domestic setting and with no other obvious goal but the wish to know more, and differently, about a relative's death. Certainly, the story that so pleased king Alfonso was not ordinary: a miracle took place. It is not our intent to suggest that similar stories of domestic post-mortem dissection were frequently happening in Italy, Castile or elsewhere. But the rich narrative of *cantiga* 188, with the exuberant iconography and musical notation accompanying the poetry, encoded culturally plausible traits that, however infrequent, were perceived as sound and conceivable. Learned theories of the workings of poisoning inside the body explained its dramatic effects in the heart, a knowledge that in light of our story seems to be widely shared. *Cantiga* 188 suggests that a wish to experience visually the inner material marks of poison could have been motivated by different aims than those of claiming a crime, and that this commitment was handled independently from an institutional setting. In the world that Alfonso's illuminator depicted, such an experience was attractive to a good number of people, both women and men. Looking at the heart could fulfill the very human aim to make sense of death.

Acknowledgments

Our work has been enriched by suggestions received from Jean Dangler, Jack Hartnell, Josemi Lorenzo, Therese Martin, Ángela Muñoz, Katharine Park, Sara Ritchey and Miriam Shadis. Research leading to this chapter has been funded by project HAR 2015-63995-P (MINECO/FEDER).

Notes

1 An updated reflection in Franck Collard, "Des poisons au Moyen Âge", *Cahiers de recherches médiévales et humanistes*, 17 (2009): pp. 1–5.
2 Katharine Park, *Secrets of Women. Gender, Generation and the Origins of Human Dissection* (New York: Zone Books, 2006).
3 We use the English short title given in *The Oxford Cantigas de Santa María Database*: http://csm.mml.ox.ac.uk/index.php?p=poemdata_view&rec=188 (consulted 24 September 2015).
4 The other is manuscript E, known as *Códice de los músicos* and also kept in San Lorenzo de El Escorial where *cantiga* 188 is found in fols. 175r–176r. Antonio G. Solalinde, "El códice florentino de las 'Cantigas' y su relación con los demás manuscritos", *Revista de filología española*, 5 (1918): pp. 143–179 (p. 167).
5 There are many editions and modern versions of the *Cantigas*, but the first critical edition is Alfonso X el Sabio, *Las Cantigas de Santa María: Ms. T-1-1, Real biblioteca del Monasterio de San Lorenzo de El Escorial*. Dirección científica y coordinación del proyecto, Laura Fernández Fernández y Juan Carlos Ruiz Souza. Vol. I. Edición crítica de Elvira Fidalgo (Madrid: Patrimonio Nacional—Testimonio Compañía Editorial, 2011); *Cantiga* 188 is found on pp. 441–443.
6 *Songs of Holy Mary of Alfonso X, The Wise. A translation of the Cantigas de Santa María*. Translated by Kathleen Kulp-Hill, with an introduction by Connie L. Scarborough (Tempe: Arizona Center for Medieval and Renaissance Studies, 2000), p. 225.
7 Ibid., p. 225.

8 Laura Fernández Fernández, "'Este livro, com'achei, fez á onr' e á loor da vir-gen Santa Maria'. El proyecto de las Cantigas de Santa María en el marco del escritorio regio. Estado de la cuestión y nuevas reflexiones" in Alfonso X el Sabio (ed.), *Las Cantigas de Santa María: Ms. T-1-1, Real biblioteca del Mon-asterio de San Lorenzo de El Escorial.* Dirección científica y coordinación del proyecto, Laura Fernández Fernández and Juan Carlos Ruiz Souza. vol. II. Es-tudio (Madrid: Patrimonio Nacional—Testimonio Compañía Editorial, 2011), pp. 45–78 (pp. 66–67).

9 Ibid., pp. 76–77.

10 Manuel Pedro Ferreira, "Alfonso X, compositor", *Alcanate*, 5 (2006–2007): pp. 117–137 (pp. 128–130).

11 *Songs of Holy Mary*, p. 225.

12 Alfonso X el Sabio, *Las Cantigas de Santa María*, p. 442.

13 *Songs of Holy Mary*, p. 225, our emphasis.

14 Alfonso X el Sabio, *Las Cantigas de Santa María*, p. 442.

15 Ibid., p. 442; *Songs of Holy Mary*, p. 225.

16 These are *cantigas* 189, 314 and 334; the search engine of *The Oxford Cantigas de Santa María Database* allows cross-scrutiny of the themes in the miracles: http://csm.mml.ox.ac.uk/?p=database188 (consulted 24 September 2015).

17 Albert Poncelet's index of Marian miracles from the 6th to 15th centuries is fully searchable through *The Oxford Cantigas de Santa María Database*: http://csm.mml.ox.ac.uk/index.php?p=pon_list (consulted 24th September 2015).

18 Rocío Sánchez Amejeiras, "'Imagines sanctae': Fray Gil de Zamora y la te-oría de la imagen sagrada en las Cantigas de Santa María", in Miguel Romaní Martínez and María Ángeles Novoa Gomez (eds.), *Homenaje a José García Oro* (Universidade de Santiago de Compostela, 2002), pp. 515–526; Rocío Sánchez Amejeiras, "Imaxes e teoría da imaxe nas *Cantigas de Santa María*", in Elvira Fidalgo (ed.), *As cantigas de Santa María* (Vigo: Edicións Xerais, 2002), pp. 247–330.

19 Marie-Anne Polo de Beaulieu, "La legende du coeur inscrit dans la litterature religieuse et didactique", in *Le "Cuer" au Moyen Âge: Realité et Senefiance* (Aix-en-Provence: Centre Universitaire d'Études et de Recherches Médiévales d'Aix, 1991), pp. 219–312; Eric Jager, *The Book of the Heart* (Chicago, IL: Chicago University Press, 2000), pp. 87–102.

20 Jager, *The Book of the Heart*, pp. 93–97; Caroline W. Bynum, *Holy Feast and Holy Fast: The Religious Significance of Food to Medieval Women* (Berkeley: University of California Press, 1987), pp. 210–212.

21 The few documented examples of post-mortem dissections in Iberia involve cases of poisoning prosecuted by judicial courts. The first we know of oc-curred in 1385, when six practitioners including distinguished university professors examined a corpse in "all members and places which must be searched and seen according to the art of medicine". Manuel Camps Sur-roca; Manuel Camps Clemente, "La violencia en el medio familiar en Lérida. Siglo XIV", *Gimbernat*, 12 (1989): pp. 29–52 (pp. 46–47); Manuel Camps Surroca; Manuel Camps Clemente, "L'activitat forense dels antics mestres de la Facultat de Medicina de Lleida", *Gimbernat*, 30 (1998): pp. 91–101 (p. 100, note 23). For 15th century Valencia, see Carmel Ferragud, "Los peritajes médicos en la Valencia bajomedieval: los casos de envenenami-ento", *Dynamis*, 36.1 (2016): pp. 119–141 (pp. 132–139).

22 Julio Valdeón, "Alfonso X y el Imperio", *Alcanate*, 4 (2004–2005): pp. 243–255.

23 Laura Molina López, "Viaje a Italia a través de las Cantigas Historiadas de Al-fonso X el Sabio", *Anales de Historia del Arte*, volumen extraordinario (2011): pp. 319–330.

24 Fernández Fernández, "Este livro, com'achei, fez á onr' e á loor da virgen Santa Maria", pp. 70–72.

25 Immo Warntjes, "Programmatic Double Burial (Body and Heart) of the European High Nobility, c. 1200–1400. Its Origin, Geography, and Functions", in Karl-Heinz Spies and Immo Warntjes (eds.), *Death at Court* (Wiesbaden: Harrassowitz Verlag, 2012), pp. 197–259.

26 Margarita Cabrera, "Técnicas de conservación *post mortem* aplicadas a los miembros de la realeza hispánica medieval", *Edad Media. Revista de Historia*, 16 (2015): pp. 175–198 (p. 181).

27 Park, *Secrets of Women*, pp. 122–129.

28 Katharine Park, "Relics of a Fertile Heart: The 'Autopsy' of Clare of Montefalco", in Anne L. McClanan and Karen Rosoff Encarnacion (eds.), *The Material Culture of Sex, Procreation and Marriage in Premodern Europe* (New York: Palgrave, 2002), pp. 115–133.

29 Bynum, *Holy Feast and Holy Fast*.

30 Ángela Muñoz Fernández, "Oria de Villavelayo, la reclusión femenina y el movimiento religioso femenino castellano (siglos XII–XVI)", *Arenal. Revista de Historia de las Mujeres*, 5.1 (1998): pp. 47–67.

31 Alfonso X el Sabio, *Las Cantigas de Santa María*, p. 442; *Songs of Holy Mary*, p. 225.

32 One extreme case is that of Alpaïs of Cudot, who supposedly lived 40 years on the Eucharist alone, see Bynum, *Holy Feast, Holy Fast*, p. 134. Fasting and illness were frequently indistinguishable.

33 Mary Wack, *Lovesickness in the middle ages. The Viaticum and its commentaries* (Philadelphia: University of Pennsylvania Press, 1990), pp. 24–26, esp. p. 25, note 71.

34 See Introduction to Arnau de Vilanova, *De amore heroico. De doi tyriacalium medicinarum*, introduction and edition by Michael McVaugh in *Arnaldi de Villanova Opera Medica Omnia* (Barcelona: Universitat de Barcelona, 1985), pp. 11–39. See also, Arnau de Vilanova *Tractat sobre l'amor heroic*, Introduction, edition and Catalan translation of the Latin text by Michael McVaugh and Sebastià Giralt (Barcelona: Barcino, 2011), pp. 5–45.

35 *Fête-Dieu (1246–1996). 2. Vie de Sainte Julienne de Cornillon*. Edition critique par Jean-Pierre Delville (Louvain-la-neuve: Université Catholique de Louvain, 1999), I.26, p. 74.

36 Frederick W. Gibbs, *Medical understandings of poison circa 1250–1600* (PhD dissertation). (Madison: University of Wisconsin, 2009), esp. pp. 57–115.

37 Juan Gil de Zamora, *Liber contra venena et animalia venenosa de Juan Gil de Zamora. Estudio preliminar, edición crítica y traducción*. Cándida Ferrero Hernández (introduction, edition and Spanish translation of the Latin text) (Barcelona: Reial Acadèmia de Bones Lletres, 2009), pp. 22–33.

38 Joël Chandelier, "Théorie et définition des poisons à la fin du Moyen Âge", *Cahiers des recherches médiévales et humanistes*, 17 (2009): pp. 23–38. In the case of Juan Gil de Zamora's treatise, it has been argued that Avicenna's teaching on poisons can come directly and also indirectly through Vincent de Beauvois' *Speculum Maius*, cf. Juan Gil de Zamora, *Liber contra venena et animalia venenosa*, pp. 52–55. Our comparison of the most theoretical parts of Juan Gil de Zamora's work with the popular Gilbertus Anglicus' *Compendium Medicine* shows an almost verbatim similarity that suggests that the *Compendium* could have been for Juan Gil another route of incorporation of Avicennian thought on the topic. Gilbertus Anglicus, *Compendium medicine Gilberti anglici tam morborum universalium quam particularium nondum medicis sed et cyrurgicis utilissimum* (Lyons, 1510), fols. 348va–351ra.

39 Avicenna, *Liber canonis tocius medicinae* (Venice, 1527. Repr., Brussels: Medicinae Historia, 1971), fols. 28va–29rb.

40 Ibid., fols. 367rb–377ra.

41 "Quod comeditur et bibitur in corpore humano tribus operatur modis. Aut enim in ipso sola sui qualitate operationem efficit aut sui materia aut operationem facit tota sui substancia" Ibid., fol. 28va.

42 Ibid., fols. 28va–29rb.

43 See Introductions to Arnau de Vilanova, *Aphorismi de gradibus*, introd. and ed. by Michael McVaugh in *Arnaldi de Villanova Opera Medica Omnia* (Granada and Barcelona: Universitat de Granada, 1975), esp. pp. 17–18; to Arnau de Vilanova, *De dosi tyriacalium medicinarum*, introd. and ed. by Michael McVaugh in *Arnaldi de Villanova Opera Medica Omnia* (Barcelona: Universitat de Barcelona, 1985), esp. pp. 60–65; and to Arnau de Vilanova, *Epistola de reprobacione nigromantice ficcionis (De improbatione maleficorum)*, introd. and ed. by Sebastià Giralt in *Arnaldi de Villanova Opera Medica Omnia* (Barcelona: Universitat de Barcelona/Fundació Noguera, 2005), esp. pp. 83–91 and 158–172. See also, Sebastià Giralt, *"Proprietas*. Las propiedades ocultas según Arnau de Vilanova", *Traditio*, 63 (2008): pp. 327–360.

44 Avicenna, *Liber canonis*, fol. 367va.

45 Prevention is a constant feature in the literature on poisoning and most of the treatises open with some recommendations to avoid intentional and accidental poisoning that run from detecting mischievous servants and suspicious foods to avoiding the storage of food and drink in places where poisonous animals could have easy access. On the practical uses of preventive measures at some rich medieval dining tables, see Franck Collard, *Le crime de poison au Moyen Âge* (Paris: PUF, 2003), pp. 83–91.

46 Lynn Thorndike, *An history of magic and experimental science* (New York: Macmillan, 1923–1958), vol. III, pp. 525–545.

47 Franck Collard, *"In claustro venenum*. Quelques réflexions sur l'usage du poison dans les communautés religieuses de l'Occident medieval", *Revue d'histoire de l'Église de France*, 88 (2002): pp. 5–19.

48 "Quoniam uita uestra quam a longis temporibus totis amplector uisceribus sicut nouit almifluus ac dulcifluus Dei Filius Ihesus Christus toti mundo est necessaria et salutifera, idcirco ad eius custodiam, cum diuino adiutorio, mitto uobis libellum contra uenenosa communia et uenena mortifera, cuius haustu et contactu occubuerunt multi uiri probissimi, quos mundus abiecit, Deus recepit" Juan Gil de Zamora, *Liber contra venena et animalia venenosa*, p. 71, ln. 9–15.

49 Cándida Ferrero Hernández, "Regimen sanitatis zelantibus?", *Cahiers de recherches médiévales*, 17 (2009): pp. 7–21.

50 Collard, *Le crime de poison au Moyen Âge*; Idem, *Pouvoir et poison. Histoire d'un crime politique de l'Antiquité à nos jours* (Paris: Seuil, 2007).

51 See, for example, Bernard de Gordon's reflection:

> Et tamen cavendum est quod aliquis incusetur sine culpa quia aliquando accidit quod aranee et scorpiones et similia animalia venenosa ceciderunt in ollam aut scutellam aut in pastam aut in dolium aut in vas ubi est vinum, hoc enim potest fieri propter immunditiam locorum aut quia cibus fuit absconsus in nemore aut inter paleas aut inter loca subterranea et multa consimilia que oblivioni tradere non debemus et ut caveamus et ut alios iniuste non accusemus.
>
> Bernard de Gordon, *Lilium medicinae* (Paris, 1542), f. 27v

52 "Venenosa quedam interficiunt statim infra tres horas. Quedam non statim, sed post tres dies; quedam post annum; quedam medio modo" Juan Gil de Zamora, *Liber contra venena et animalia venenosa*, p. 183, ln. 81–83; Collard, *Le crime de poison au Moyen Âge*, pp. 75–76.

53 Pietro d'Abano reflects this tradition in his classification of poisons according to how they can interact with humans.

> Secundo modo consideratur venenum relatum ad nos et secundum hoc dixerunt: Venenum aliud est assumptum intra corpus et aliud extra. Quod vero est assumptum intus est de genere potiorum perniciosarum, datum sub specie cibi vel potus vel medicinae [...] Quod vero extra est, dicitur reptilium morsus sicut cum visu, aut auditu aut gustu aut tactu aut odoratur sentitur venenum.
>
> Pietro d'Abano, *Libellus de venenis*
> (Venice, 1565. Rpr. Padua: Antenore, 1985), fol. 263va

54 See Fernando Salmón and Montserrat Cabré, "Fascinating women: the evil eye in medical scholasticism", in Roger K. French, Jon Arrizabalaga, Andrew Cunningham and Luis García Ballester (eds.), *Medicine from the Black Death to the French Disease* (Aldershot: Ashgate, 1998), pp. 52–84.

55 Usually, there is a distinction of signs and symptoms according to the hot or cold quality of the poison. See, Juan Gil de Zamora, *Liber contra venena et animalia venenosa*, pp. 184–185. Collard, *Le crime de poison au Moyen Âge*, pp. 76–80.

56 "Et si non apparent nisi casu virtutum et sudor frigidus et sincopis, tunc est de venenis que contraria sunt rebus cum tota substantia et est deterius eorum" Avicenna, *Liber canonis*, f. 367vb. This description appeared repeated almost in the same way in numerous treatises contemporary of our *cantiga*, see in the *Compendium medicine*: "Si autem contingat casus virtutis et sudor frigidus et sincopis, signum est quod venenum est a tota substancia ut est napellus" Gilbertus Anglicus, *Compendium medicine*, f. 350ra. Following *verbatim* this last one, see, Juan Gil de Zamora: "Si autem contingat casus uirtutis et sudor frigidus et sincopis, signum est quod uenenum est a tota substancia ut est napellus" Juan Gil de Zamora, *Liber contra venena et animalia venenosa*, p. 184, ln. 129–131.

57 "Venenum autem dictum, eo quod per venas vadit [...] Vnde non posse venenum nocere, nisi hominis tetigerit sanguinem" *Etymologiarum* XII, 4, n. 41 and 42 in *San Isidoro de Sevilla, Etimologías* (Edición bilingüe. Libros XI–XX). José Oroz Reta and Manuel A. Marcos Casquero, ed., trans. and intro. (Madrid: B.A.C., 1994, 2ªed), vol. II, p. 88. For a detailed analysis of the ancient physiological frame that supports Isidoro's approach to *venenum*, see Alain Touwaide, "De la matière à la nature: Les transformations d'un concept pathologique, de l'Antiquité aux débuts du Moyen-Âge: *venenum* chez Isidore de Séville, *Etymologiae*, XII, 4", in Armelle Debrú and Guy Sabbah (eds.), *Nommer la maladie. Recherches sur le lexique gréco-latin de la pathologie* (Saint-Étienne: Publications de l'Université de Saint-Étienne, 1998), pp. 143–159.

58 "Quem tyrus momorderit [...] et nisi succurratur veneno cor incenditur et periclitatur. Incipiendum est a medicina ut loca morsure stricte ligentur statim ne venenum vias perforet ad membra principalia; post, ore sugatur et cum sugens sit fatur os eius cum oleo et vino lavetur, locus tactus cum spongia calida fumigetur nimisque scarificetur ut venenum egrediatur, utilis autem est incisio illius loci si in loco sit qui incidi possit sicut in digitis et in similibus locis" Ibn al-Jazzar, *Viaticum* in *Gerardus de Solo Commentum super Viatico* (Venice, 1505), f. 182vb.

59 "Sunt medicine que contrarie sunt veneno quare non permittunt ipsum pervenire ad cor" Avicenna, *Liber canonis*, f. 368ra.

60 "[Avicenna] Docet venena operativa a proprietate et iterum ponit diversas species venenorum, secundum diversitatem eius in quo agunt. Nota quod omnia communicant in lesione cordis. Ratio est quia omnia venena occidunt et hoc

non fit nisi leso corde" Gentile da Foligno, *Primus Canon Avic. cum argutissima Gentilis expositione* (Pavia, 1510–1512), f. 149ra.

61 "Notandum quod arterie directe extenduntur a corde ad digitos unde ungues fiunt. Ungues enim fiunt vapore cordis unde cum venenum cor petit statim digiti mutantur et ungues inficiuntur et hoc est signum mortale, presumitur enim cum pervenit infectio ad exteriora quod iam infecta sunt interiora" Gerardo de Solo, *Gerardus de Solo Commentum super Viatico*, f. 182vb.

62 Michael McVaugh, "Who was Gilbert the Englishman?", in George H. Brown and Linda E. Voigts (eds.), *The Study of Medieval Manuscripts of England: Festschrift in Honor of Richard W. Pfaff* (Tempe: ACMRS, 2010), pp. 295–324 (pp. 309–314).

63 "Et in genere ueneni calidi, secundum Isaac, est uenenum tiri. Et ex genere ueneni frigidi est uenenum aranee et scorpionis. Et quemadmodum uenenum calidum resolvit humiditatem cordis et dispergit calorem et spiritus in aduentu ipsius, sic uenenum frigidi coagulat humiditatem et congelat in ipso spiritus. Et signum eius est quod mortuis ex ueneno inuenitur sanguis coagulatus circa cor et in ipso corde" Juan Gil de Zamora, *Liber contra venena et animalia venenosa*, p. 183, ln. 74–81.

> Et in genere veneni calidi, secundum Isaac, est venenum tiri. Et ex genere veneni frigidi est venenum aranee et scorpionis. Et quemadmodum venenum calidum resolvit humiditatem cordis et dispergit calorem et spiritus in adventu ipsius, sic venenum frigidi coagulat humiditatem et congelat in ipso spiritus. Et signum eius est quod mortuis ex veneno invenitur sanguis coagulatus circa cor et in ipso corde.
>
> Gilbertus Anglicus, *Compendium medicine*, f. 349ra

64 "Detur eciam tyriaca maior ut sanguinem dissolvat et coagulari prohibeat quia venenum sanguinem cordi coagulat sicut lac coagulatur. Sed calore tyriace dissolvitur /183ra et cor inde expellendo confortatur sicut flamma ignis in expulsione fummi" Ibn al-Jazzar *Viaticum*, f. 182vb–183ra.

65 Franck Collard, "Ouvrir pour découvrir. Réflexions sur les expertises de cadavres empoisonnés à l'époque médiévale", in Franck Collard and Évelyne Samama (eds.), *Le corps à l'épreuve: Poisons, remèdes et chirurgie: Aspects des pratiques médicales dans l'Antiquité et au Moyen-Âge* (Langres: Guéniot, 2002), pp. 177–190.

66 Katherine Watson, *Forensic Medicine in Western Society: A History* (London: Routledge, 2011), p. 34.

67 Katharine Park, "The criminal and saintly body: autopsy and dissection in Renaissance Europe", *Renaissance Quarterly*, 47 (1994): pp. 1–33 (pp. 4–5).

68 Collard, "Ouvrir pour découvrir. Réflexions sur les expertises de cadavres empoisonnés à l'époque médiévale", pp. 183–190 (p. 183)

69 "Mineralia igitur venena quedam sunt a natura, quedam ab arte procurata. A natura quidem que in ventre terre generantur et horum unum est argentum vivum, quod intus assumptum quandoque interficit sua humiditate putrefacere faciente humiditatem cordis naturalem, quandoque autem interficit sua frigidate actuali congelante cor. Cuis signum est quod quidam apothecarius cum de nocte tempore magni estus sitiret, tentans invenit ampullam plenam argento vivo quod bibit et mane inventus est mortuus et invenientes argentum vivum exire de ano. Anatomizatus fuit et inventus fuit sanguis circa cor coagulatus et ipsum cor similiter. Inveneruntque in stomacho fere libram unam argenti vivi." Pietro d'Abano, *Libellus de venenis*, f. 263vb.

4 *Pestis Manufacta*

Plague, poisons and fear in mid-fourteenth-century Europe

Jon Arrizabalaga

Fear in time of plague is one of the greatest chapters in the cultural history of this emotion in Old Regime Europe, as Jean Delumeau stressed in his classical study on this topic.[1] Anticipation of an almost certain death was the main cause underlying this intense and ambiguous fear, which prevailed under multiple masks and which explained social behaviour when people were faced with words like plague (*pestis*), pestilence (*pestilentia*) and other similar terms. Needless to say, in the past, all these words evoked not only the fearsome infectious disease caused by the *Yersinia pestis* bacterium B, but also any human ailment, not necessarily contagious, involving a great mortality. Indeed, the condition nowadays known as 'plague' emerged in the late nineteenth and early twentieth centuries in the context of the reformulation of infectious diseases successfully promoted by the followers of the germ theory.[2] In contrast, the terms 'plague' and 'pestilence' referred in pre-modern Europe to 'any malignant disease with which men and beasts are stricken', particularly an 'infectious disease or epidemic attended with great mortality', and to any 'affliction', calamity, evil, 'scourge', often with reference to 'the ten plagues of Egypt', as the authoritative *Oxford English Dictionary* reminds us.[3]

Artificial reproduction of epidemic infections, together with biological warfare, only became frightening realities in the course of the twentieth century, thanks to progress in biotechnology and genetic engineering.[4] Yet, the feasibility of such a risk fed the human imagination long before. The belief in human agency in this and other social evils (like mass poisoning, cannibalism and infanticide) was already widespread by the outbreak of the Black Death in 1348,[5] and it enjoyed a long cultural life in pre-modern Europe both before and after this epidemic disaster. This supposed human agency in bringing about plague was projected onto rather disparate social groups – lepers, mad individuals, beggars, pilgrims, foreigners, members of religious orders (Templars, Franciscan spirituals), members of religious minorities (Jews and Muslims, heretics), prostitutes and even public health officers – by virtue of exacerbated anxieties in specific social groups and of their emotional use in peculiar circumstances. Thus, different groups of 'others' were used as scapegoats by blaming them – either on their own or in different mutual associations (e.g., lepers and Jews under the instigation of

Muslim kings in South France in 1321, the anti-Jewish pogroms in 1348) –
for conspiring to cause diseases, poisonings and other social scourges to
eradicate Christendom, so that they were subjected to social exclusion and
violence in different places and times.[6]

This chapter explores the fortune of the idea of human agency in causing
plague in Old Regime Europe, that is, during what is traditionally known
as the 'second plague pandemic' that repeatedly struck Europe over almost
four centuries – from the mid-fourteenth-century Black Death (1346–1353)
to the Plague of Provence (1720–1721). More specifically, a number of
mid-fourteenth-century pieces of evidence traditionally employed in order to illustrate the belief in 'artificial' plague – *pestis manufacta* – will
be reviewed in order to better characterise this idea in its own historical
context.[7] For this purpose, I will assess the role played by the notion of
poison – whether closely bound to pestilence or not – and examine the ways
in which different social actors allegedly operated.

Bacteriological war avant-la-lettre?: *Gabriele de' Mussi on the siege of Caffa*

The well-known account of the siege of Caffa – an allegedly crucial early episode in the spread of the Black Death across Europe – is part of the *Ystoria
de morbo sive mortalitate que fuit anno Domini MCCCXLVIII*, an account
by the Italian lawyer Gabriele de' Mussi (d. 1356), who witnessed the epidemic from Piacenza, the northern Italian city where he lived.[8] According to
De' Mussi, in 1346, the Tartar army besieged Caffa (now Feodosiya, Crimea),
a Christian city fortified by the Genovese, where Italian traders took refuge
after having escaped by sea from Tana (now Azov) after it had been conquered
by the Tartars. Surrounded by a countless enemy army, the crowded Christians
at Caffa could hardly breathe, but they managed to resist the siege for almost
three years, thanks to the slight hope a ship with provisions gave them.

Allegedly, the Tartar army was destroyed during the siege by a 'pestiferous disease' that greatly weakened them by daily killing countless thousands
of people. The scourge looked like arrows falling down from the heavens to
crush the arrogance of the Tartars who 'were suddenly dead, their bodies'
joints being marked with a humour that coagulated in their groins, and a
putrid fever following on', this all without hope of recovery. Made desperate
by such a great calamity and seeing that they were hopelessly dying, the
Tartars ordered the corpses of the dead to be thrown into the interior of
Caffa by means of their catapults, so that 'its inhabitants lose their strength
due to their unbearable stench'. Despite the besieged Christians striving to
throw into the sea as many corpses as possible of those fallen upon them,
they could neither cope with doing this nor hide themselves or escape.

> And since the whole air was soon infected and the waters poisoned with
> the putrid rottenness, the stench became so strong that hardly one soldier

out of thousands attempted to run away from the remnants of the Tartar army. Moreover, the few fugitives, because they were infected, spread the poison out everywhere and passed on the disease to any person in any place, and none knew nor could find any remedy for it.[9]

The slaughter resulting from this 'pestiferous disease' was so sudden and massive in the Orient – De' Mussi emphasised that 'wounded by a very violent arrow making their bodies swell, almost all its victims got weak and perished from a sudden death' – that 'between 1346 and 1348 most Eastern peoples –Chinese, Indians, Persians, Medes, Cilicians, Armenians, Tarsians, Georgians, Mesopotamians, Nubians, Ethiopians, Turcomans, Egyptians, Arabs, Saracens, Greeks – suspected that the Day of Judgement had arrived at their nations'.[10]

After this dramatic account, the Piacenza lawyer described in a more detailed way the scourge's accidents (cold rigor, hard and painful swellings in armpits and groins, very acute putrid fever, and unbearable stench), its signs of good and bad prognoses and its eventual treatment. He attributed it to 'God's warnings' that put under risk of death all healthy people of both sexes. His interpretations were fully in agreement with those of university medicine at the time. But it is remarkable that a 'poison' (*venenum*) fallen from the heavens allegedly played a central role as a transmitter of the 'pestiferous disease' on a large scale (through air and water), as well as on a small, interpersonal one, even through the sight. To explain how the poison infected each individual, De' Mussi claimed that the scourge's victims felt the 'shooting pricks of arrows as if a lance had gone through them'. On the other hand, he pointed out that an unbearable stench was the clearest sign that poison had taken possession of their bodies.[11]

De' Mussi claimed that the scourge's poison could be neutralised and expelled from the infected bodies by means of the series of remedies university physicians then used to resort to in case of plague, namely (1) theriac because of its antidote effect, (2) bloodletting proximal to the swellings as soon as they showed signs of external softening, (3) emollient remedies like mallow or marshmallow poultices applied locally to ease their ripening and (4) direct incision of the swellings in order to evacuate the remaining venomous humour.[12]

In summary, human agency was instrumental in spreading 'natural' plague into Caffa by infecting the city's atmosphere with the stench from the catapulted corpses of victims of this plague. In all other respects, De' Mussi's account of this condition entirely fits contemporary medical practitioners' views about plague.

Water and food poisoning

Accusations of poisoning waters in wells, springs, fountains and rivers, as well as foods, get us more properly inside the territory of 'artificial' plague.

These accusations that had circulated, mostly against lepers, in the Kingdom of France on the occasion of the Shepherds' Crusade (1320–1321),[13] spread widely throughout all Europe on the occasion of the Black Death. Here, I will mostly focus on mid-fourteenth-century sources from Germany, Switzerland, France and Spain.[14] They raise two major questions. On the one hand, it was debated whether this poisoning was a part of the pestilential infection or not and, in case its effects were independent of the plague, whether they contributed to spreading that infection or not. On the other, the poisoning was attributed to a deliberate action by different actors who were seeking to harm the population in a country or town (e.g., by the enemies of France, by underprivileged people such as beggars, and so on), or more generally, the Christians (e.g., by their religious rivals, namely Jews and Muslims).

On 10 April 1348, Arnau Derill, the governor of Rousillon and Cerdagne, writing from Perpignan to the King of Aragon, Pere III el Ceremoniós (1336–1387), reported that the delegates of the French royal court in Carcassonne and Narbonne had certified a 'great infinity' of deaths in the regions of both cities. These deaths were attributed to the poisoning of all the waters – even the holy water – vegetables and other foods by 'wicked persons' who had already confessed their crimes. These individuals had even smeared with their poisonous preparations (*metzines*) the benches 'where people sit or put their feet' so that they became impregnated with them. The governor reported to his monarch that in various cities of Roussillon (Salses), great numbers of deaths had happened as a result of these poisonings, so that he had ordered a search for every stranger in order to rule out that they were carrying any poison. He pointed out that the poisoners spread everywhere and were usually dressed as penitents and unfortunate people.[15] Eleven days after, the King echoed all this news in a letter in which he ordered the butler of his daughters to transfer them from Tarragona to Montblanc in order to protect them from the 'disease better known as epidemic' (*malaltia appellada epidèmia*) that, according to his information, was spreading 'over the coastal areas'.[16]

Moreover, between these two dates, on 17 April 1348, André Benezeit (*Andreas Benedicti*), the representative of the Viscount of Narbonne, answered an information request by Girona's town councillors about the great mortality (*de mortalitate gentium*). According to what they had heard, it was beginning to strike the regions of Avignon, Narbonne and Carcassonne. It seems that these councillors wanted to know whether this mortality was caused by potions or poisons put in different places by some individuals or could rather be attributed to some other cause; they also wanted to have details of any arrest, confession and punishment of poisoners. Benezeit confirmed that during the previous Lent, the regions of Narbonne, Carcassonne and Grasse might have lost a quarter of their population as a result of that great mortality. He also informed them about the arrest of 'many poor persons and beggars of diverse nations bringing with them powdered potions that they were putting in waters, houses, churches, and foods with the intention of killing people' in Narbonne and other places, by means of the 'aromatic scent of the said potions or poisons'. The arrested people had confessed, either spontaneously or after having been tortured, that these 'lethal potions' had been given to them in different places by people whose identity they did not know – without daring to say for certain, Benezeit revealed his suspicion that they were enemies of the Kingdom of France – and that they had been induced to disseminate the poison in return for money. For this reason, eleven individuals had been executed, namely four in Narbonne, five in Carcassonne and two in Grasse.[17]

Interestingly enough, despite the fact that some people persisted in associating those mortalities with natural causes of astral origin, Benezeit tended to attribute them to the concurrence of effects between planets and potions, and he held the contagious condition of diseases to derive from these causes. Furthermore, he argued that when someone had died as a result of any of these diseases in a house, his/her servants, friends and family ended up suffering from the same ailment and usually died in three or four days.[18]

To summarise, while Arnau Derill (our first source) had exclusively attributed the great mortality to a poisoning resulting from deliberate human action, André Benezeit (our third source) tended to consider it as a combined effect of a poisoning and a harmful planetary influence, and to defend the high contagiousness of the diseases as having caused this mortality. Finally, to King Pere el Ceremoniós (our second source), the mortality was attributable to both causes, albeit in different ways.

Incidentally, the Aragonese monarch's views were not very different from those held by the university physician and lecturer in the *Studium Generale* at Lleida, Jacme d'Agramont (d. 1348) in the *Regiment de preservació a epidímia o pestilencia e mortaldats*, which he finished writing in the Catalan vernacular on 24 April 1348 – just three days after the above-mentioned royal letter – at the request of Lleida city council. There, Agramont clearly distinguished the great mortality caused by the 'epidemic' (*epidímia*) that was then striking southern France and dangerously approaching Lleida, from other 'many deaths' which had happened in the French Midi – he referred to Colliure, the regions of Carcassonne and Narbonne, the barony of Montpellier, Avignon and the whole of Provence – as well as 'in some nearer regions'. While Agramont characterised the former as a 'universal pestilence' caused by a substantial corruption of the air, he attributed the latter to the action of 'wicked men, sons of the devil, who, by means of very false ingenuity and wicked skill, are corrupting foods with various poisons and medicines'.[19]

Of all the above-mentioned accounts, only those by Derill and Benezeit gave details about the identity of the poisoners by pointing at individuals dressed like 'penitent and unfortunate people', and 'poor and beggars', respectively. An account of the difficulties two dignitaries of the Spanish province of the Order of Hermits of St Augustine had to cope with while crossing Catalonia in May 1348 on the way to Pavia to attend the general chapter of their order also confirms the spread of suspicion about poisoners swarming through Catalan lands. In Barcelona, these priests were warned that no clergyman could then safely travel through that area since in many places all religious travellers were searched and even arrested, and their personal belongings were confiscated because of the rumour going around that 'men disguised as priests were infecting the waters and putting down potions'.[20] Despite the warnings, these hermit friars continued their travel to three leagues beyond Girona, where they eventually decided to turn round after having repeatedly received news that a great mortality was raging in Perpignan and Avignon; that hostels were not lodging travellers, particularly foreigners; and that if any of them fell ill there, he would be expelled with no medical help and would die alone.[21]

Accusations of poisoning waters and foods were widespread throughout Europe at the time. In many places, the supposed perpetrators of these crimes were identified with Jews, as seems clear in a number of sources from Savoy, Alsace, Switzerland, Germany and even the papal city of Avignon. Yet, as Ernest Wickersheimer pointed out in the 1920s, these accusations had preceded the arrival of the Black Death, while the pogroms subsequently unleashed were very often coincidental with the epidemic. And the panic provoked by the epidemic would have facilitated the association of ideas between both circumstances and caused the breakout of persecution of this religious minority.[22]

Specifically, between August 1348 and September 1349, the magistrate of Strasburg gathered in a dossier the answers given by various neighbouring cities to his letter requesting any evidence that Jews were poisoning the wells, as well as about the measures taken against the guilty persons. The replies he received confirmed that many Jews, as well as some Christians influenced by them, had confessed to the crime, mostly by torture but sometimes even spontaneously. Various Jews living in Savoy (five at Villeneuve and another five at Châtel), who had been jailed in the castle of Chillon, were charged with 'poisoning wells, springs and other places as well as with putting poison in foods in order to destroy and eradicate the whole Christian religion'. Their confessions, collected through September and October 1348, appear to have been presented altogether as evidence of an authentic plot involving members of a wide network of Jewish communities in the region. Moreover, two rabbis of Chambéry – Jacob of Toledo and Peyret – were repeatedly blamed for being leading members of that plot through asserting their religious authority and using bribes to recruit disseminators of the poison among their faithful. A reference was even given to a meeting of plotters before Pentecost (8 June 1348) in order to organise the poisonings. All the Jews who had confessed, as well as their accomplices who they had denounced in their statements, were allegedly executed.

Because of its peculiar interest, I will focus for a while on some details of the statement by a Jewish surgeon called Balavigny, who lived in Thonon. He confessed that rabbi Jacob of Toledo had sent him, by means of a Jewish boy, a leather bag about the size of an egg that was full of a venomous powder. The delivery was accompanied by a letter commanding him, in obedience to the Jewish law and under pain of excommunication, to put the bag in the largest and most commonly used wells in order to poison the people using them, and to keep everything secret. The surgeon ended up confessing that the boy had showed him many similar letters he was carrying for numerous Jews living in different towns on the banks of Lake Leman (Villeneuve, Montreux, La Tour de Vevey and Évian les Bains) and its surroundings (Monthey and San Mauricio), and that rabbis had warned him and other Jews not to drink water from the poisoned springs until nine days after the poison had been put in them.[23]

Balavigny declared that he had secretly placed the venomous powders – the colour of which was red and black – in various springs of these towns. First, one afternoon he had put them under a stone in a spring of Thonon and forbade his wife and children to use it – though without telling them why. Then he left, inside a spring close to Montreux, an amount of poison about the size of a nut, wrapped in a linen rag that Aquetus, a Jew of Montreux, had given to him. According to Balavigny, Mussus, a Jew of Villeneuve, had told him he had also placed the poison in two public fountains close to the custom houses of Villeneuve and Chillon. According to the informer, a legal investigation into the latter fountain led to finding there part of that poison, and this was proved because of the death of a Jew who had been given some of it.[24] The surgeon also gave evidence of his conviction – endorsed by 'expert physicians' – that any person infected with the poison could pass on it to other people by contact, above all through sweat and breath. Balavigny allegedly claimed to believe that the poison was a product derived from the basilisk – a mythological beast that captured human imaginations in Antiquity and the Middle Ages because of its supposed lethal power – and only effective, to the best of his knowledge, when the proper procedure had been followed.[25]

Balavigny's subsequent statements reported accusations against a great number of Jewish plotters who had allegedly devoted themselves to poisoning numerous wells in different towns of the region.[26] The details given by other Jews' confessions fit a similar pattern, with small variants like the colour of the poison (red and black, green and black, white), the material (linen, leather or cloth rags, paper cornets, pieces of net with little holes) of the container being used to wrap it, or the place where it was put in (springs, wells, fountains, 'other things used by Christians', and so on). The accusations were extended to other supposed accomplices such as the wives and children of those involved in the poisonings,[27] as well as to several Christians whom the plotters had bribed. Moreover, two denounced Jews testified that they had carried the poison to other parts of Europe. One of them, Agimeto of Geneva, confessed that he had been commissioned by rabbi Peyret of Chambéry to put poison in wells, springs and cisterns of freshwater in Toulouse and Italy (Venice, Calabria, Apulia), while the other, Iconetus of Châtel, conceded that he had placed it in springs of various Belgian cities (Brussels, Hainault, Tinimont, Mons), disguised as a beggar and commissioned by a very rich and powerful Jew.

These accusations against Jews and the subsequent repressive measures taken against the perpetrators of the supposed plot were echoed throughout all Europe, although different surviving accounts give an uneven credit to their plausibility.[28] One of the most interesting ones is included in a universal chronicle up to 1349 written by the Franciscan friar Hermann Gigas from Franconia. Everything he wrote on the occasion of the year 1347 was about the Black Death (*pestilentia et mortalitas fere in toto mundo*), its causes and its consequences. Then, after having described the devastation provoked by the scourge all over Europe, Gigas related that some attributed the 'pestilence' to air corruption, while others attributed it to the poisoning of all the wells and water sources by Jews with intent to eradicate the whole of Christendom through poison. Gigas added that, according to the testimony of many tortured Jews, in order to prepare that poison they had bred spiders and toads in pots and pans and bought poison in overseas regions. He claimed that many evidences of this supposed plot had been found all over Germany so that in 1349 the wickedness of the Jews was being punished by fire in most places.[29]

Finally, two additional testimonies provide evidence about how mentally unstable individuals might fuel fear of plague infection by human agency. The first was given by Heinrich Seuse (*c.* 1295–1366), a mystic Dominican, disciple of Master Eckhart and preacher in Konstanz. In his autobiographical *Leben*, he reported that on the occasion of a journey along with a lay brother who was 'mentally unbalanced', he had at the last minute escaped being lynched by the mob. This was a result of being blamed by the mob – after some soldiers made a similar accusation against him – of having been entrusted by the Order with 'a bag of poison to sink in the wells, here and there in the country as far as Alsace, whither he is now bound', as well as of having a 'large sack which is full of these bags of poison and with the gold pieces, that he and his Order have got from the Jews to pay him for committing these crimes'.[30]

While Seuse's account might suggest that deliberate water poisoning was also attributed in Germany at the time of the Black Death to conspiratorial associations between Jews and Dominican friars, an account from Mallorca refers to a Turkish slave of a 'G. Brassa' whose behaviour kept people terrified in 1348 in the Alcudia Bay area. His master might have been a relative of Guillem Brassa, the earliest documented victim of plague in the island, who had just died in late March that year at Alcudia. After his corpse was buried on the small island of Porros, belonging to the neighbouring town of Santa Margarida, fear of plague infection in the region fuelled a major controversy between the mayors of both towns that forced Mallorca's royal lieutenant and bishop to intervene. At all events, fear of plague had made the slave become a scapegoat for it, and people in Alcudia wanted him to be expelled from the town. He was said to have threatened 'to kill all the people in Alcudia' if he was not freed, and to have intimidated everybody there by going bathing in the sea, taking sea water in his mouth, and spewing it out in the hallways of hostels. Although the slave was arrested for a while, at the end of April, the royal lieutenant still protected his safety as G. Brassa's property, against other citizens' demands to expel him from the island without first buying him.[31] It might make sense to think that the social overreactions against this slave were led by a combination of circumstances like his Turkish origin, his presumably being a property of the family of the earliest victim of plague in Mallorca, and the fear that the sea water he spewed out from his mouth might be contaminated by Guillem Brassa's burial in Porros' little island.

Air poisoning

The feasibility of artificially reproducing an epidemic infection transmissible through the air was imagined by at least one university physician during the mid-fourteenth-century Black Death. The testimony comes from Montpellier, and it was included in the *Epistola et regimen de pestilentia*, a brief work written about 1349 by Alfonso de Córdoba, a 'master in liberal arts and medicine' who might have also been lecturing at the local *Studium generale*.

Alfonso de Córdoba distinguished three different pestilences in 1348, namely two attributable to natural causes and another to artificial ones.[32] The first pestilence consisted of a 'natural infection of the elements' as a result of an astral constellation –a lunar eclipse in Leo associated with an unfortunate planetary conjunction – and which spread throughout 'every Christian region'. The second pestilence was caused by a major earthquake in Italy and 'the overseas regions on the opposite angle to the triangle of the house of Europe', although it lasted for just one year and its effects were not so disastrous.

The third pestilence, however, was due to an artificial and deliberate infection of the waters, especially non-flowing ones, by which foods and drinks had been contaminated. This artificial pestilence was properly the subject of Alfonso de Córdoba's *Epistola*, allegedly written in 'compassion towards the faithful Christians' – its main victims – with the aim that those 'pious and good' people could protect themselves from 'so many imminent dangers and evils'. He claimed that this terrible scourge was preventable and curable despite the fact that no 'advice of wise physicians' had benefitted or helped those suffering from it. To prevent it, Alfonso de Córdoba first recommended going away from the places affected by this pestilence and keeping oneself safe from infection by every living thing (*rerum vitalium*).[33] Then, he prescribed taking before every meal, because of its antidote effect, one dose of theriac of *terra sigillata* – or an alternative electuary, the recipe of which he gave – since it provoked vomiting in case of ingestion of any infected food or drink. Finally, for curing the artificial pestilence, he recommended taking, in addition to the already-mentioned remedy, a drug made of *tiriaca maior* and a concoction of various plants on an empty stomach and inside a warm bath to promote the removal of poison through sweating.

Moreover, Alfonso de Córdoba even considered the feasibility of an artificial pestilence by a deliberate infection of the air. To him, this was the worst pestilence ever imaginable, and he appears to have given credit to the idea that it was then actually operating and raging. Its prevention, according to him, was only possible for experts and was based on two alternative kinds of pills – the 'pestilential' kind, and others using aromatic plants, the preparation of which he described in detail. It also required fumigations of chambers using 'clean coals' (*mundi carbones*) upon which one pill of the second kind had to be placed. For its cure, he recommended taking the *tiriaca maior* inside a warm bath, without omitting the treatment of the eventual 'apostemes' by means of bloodletting, cupping glasses, drugs and surgery.

For our purposes, the greatest interest of this part lies in Alfonso de Córdoba's description of the procedure to provoke a pestilential infection of the air through human artifice:

> air can be infected by means of artifice, as when a preparation is made in a glass amphora. When this preparation is well fermented, whoever wishes to produce this evil [*illum malum*] will wait for a strong and steady wind coming from any world region. Then he will walk against the wind, and will put his amphora near a stony place opposite the city or town which he wishes to infect. Going back against the wind, so as not to be infected by the vapour, with the amphora neck covered up, he will throw the amphora with violence against the stones. As soon as the amphora is broken, the vapour will spread out and disperse in the air. Whoever is touched by this vapour will die very soon as if he were touched by the pestilential air.[34]

Certainly, the quoted passage recalls another one from the account by Dio Cassius (AD 155–235) on the Antonine Plague or the Plague of Galen (AD 165–180) which originated, according to a very popular contemporary account, in the temple of Apollo at Babylon. There, a Roman soldier unintentionally broke a chest from which a pestilential spirit (*spiritus pestilens*) emanated that invaded the Parthian Empire and the whole world.[35] Yet, Alfonso de Córdoba went further in asserting that a 'pestilence' could be artificially unleashed in any place and moment by means of a controlled spreading of pestilential vapours issued from an *ad hoc* preparation.

Unfortunately, he neither gave any ingredient of the preparation – though spiders, toads and basilisks may be presumed from the above-mentioned testimonies – nor any authoritative source to support his view. Yet an early fifteenth-century documentary source – the *Collectum de peste* (1411) by the Lübeck physician Heinrich Lamme – provides us with a likely answer. Among the diverse sources of the insidious air infection behind the plague that led Lamme to write that work, were not only the familiar celestial and terrestrial causes, but also corpses in wars, some toxic herbs and even – he claimed – 'the poison found by the Polish wise man as shown at the passage of his work where he teaches how to make this preparation with which a city or even a whole region could be infected'.[36] Most probably, Lamme was referring to Niklas von Mumpelier or Nicholas of Poland (1235–1316), a Dominican friar who might be connected to educational centres of his order at Montpellier between 1250 and 1270, although this quotation has not been found. Niklas wrote *Experimenta magistri Nicolai* – a compilation of his medicaments based on alleged extraordinary virtues of toads, scorpions, lizards, snakes and so on – and the *Antipocras* or *The book of empirical things* – a fierce invective against scholastic medicine and in favour of an unorthodox medical empiricism, which caused a scandal near Cracow in 1278.[37] Lamme continued his report by collecting three other authoritative accounts – by an 'English soldier' (*miles Anglicanus*), Guy of Chauliac and Galen himself – about the feasibility of lethal air infection by different means, in order to emphasise the analogy between the great mortality caused by the 1348 plague and the one arising from infection by snakes, dragons and basilisks.[38]

Whatever the ingredients of Alfonso de Córdoba's preparation were, his recipe included a process of fermentation. The notion of this process came from the ancient world and spread in medieval Europe through at least two ways. On the one hand, the concept of a metallurgical 'ferment' passed from ancient literature into the alchemy of the Arabs and in the early fourteenth century into the Latin alchemical *corpus*. On the other, Aristotle doubtless had in mind a fermentative process when, in explaining the formation of the foetus, he compared analogically the performative role of semen upon the material basis of menstrual blood with the effect that rennet produces when acting upon milk. Albert the Great was expressing something very similar when he wrote that 'eggs grow into embryos because their wetness is like the wetness of yeast'.[39] Again, Avicenna applied the idea of 'fermentation' to medicinal drugs. He emphasised that each compound drug contained not only the sum of the properties (*virtutes*) of the simples constituting it but also other unique and specific properties that derived from its 'specific form' and which appeared as a result of a 'fermentation'. The 'specific form' of any compound could be learned only through experience. Avicenna also thought that the *virtus* of any fermented product became doubled, which implied that the intensity of its expected effect doubled too.[40]

Alfonso de Córdoba probably took this important idea from Avicenna, for in his dual role as university physician and probable lecturer at a medical school, he would have been well acquainted with Avicenna's pharmacological doctrine. Certainly, the traces of Avicennan thought in Alfonso's discussion are unmistakable. Nevertheless, this does not affect the high significance of this discussion in mid-fourteenth-century Europe. And this for at least two reasons. On the one hand, Alfonso de Córdoba was to my knowledge the only physician dealing at this time with such a question in a plague treatise. On the other hand, his remarks do not refer just to poisoning of food and drink – perfectly possible, and in fact usual at the time – but to air poisoning on a large scale, and with the purpose of provoking nothing less than a 'pestilence'.

At the time, Alfonso de Córdoba's view that natural conditions that caused a 'pestilence' could be reproduced through human artifice meant first a significant reaffirmation of human power over nature; second, the legitimation of natural philosophy as a useful instrument by which to attain this power over nature – a clear reason why kings and other rulers were interested in alchemy, natural philosophy, and whatever other knowledge could be employed to get or to increase their political power; and third, the possibility of using medical and natural philosophical knowledge in a double direction (good-evil), namely in order to achieve health and the public good or to cause destruction and death.

Furthermore, Alfonso de Córdoba's work is a valuable direct testimony about the acquiescence, if not complicity, of some sections of the Montpellier academic community in the accusation that the origin of this second 'pestilence' lay in a human artifice. He qualified this artifice as deriving from the 'depths of an evil discovered through the most subtle practice of profound iniquity' and noted that it mostly victimised Christians. In other words, he was providing a rational interpretative basis – leaning on scholastic medicine and natural philosophy – for the charge that the pestilence had been deliberately caused by the enemies of the Christians. Potentially, they could be identified with Jews as much as with Muslims. Yet, the aggressive tone of phrases like 'deep wickedness' and 'a very sharp and cruel art' coincides with culturally significant ways among fourteenth-century Christians of referring to Jews, and the context of production of the work – Montpellier – points in the same direction of blaming the Jewish minority for having deliberately caused that mortality.

By way of conclusion

The enormity of the mortality provoked by the Black Death in mid-fourteenth-century Europe plunged its population into panic and desolation and fuelled and exacerbated collective anxiety which was projected onto various socially excluded groups who became scapegoats and were subjected to stigmatisation and violence.

University physicians began to perceive the Black Death as a particularly serious 'pestilential fever' whose terrible effects evoked the *topoi* of ancient epidemics like the plague of Cranon or that of Athens (as described by Thucydides), and they came eventually to consider it as a new epidemic phenomenon, not a return of any previous catastrophic disease. From the very beginning, they coped with this phenomenon as a medical problem and constructed it by means of intellectual and technical resources taken from their university education, their professional experience when confronted by other lethal epidemics, and the views of the ancient and medieval medical authorities. Yet, gradual changes in their perceptions led them to pay a growing attention to the specificities of the causes and signs of epidemics in different places and times.[41]

While the infectious condition of the pestilence was almost universally recognised, there is a dialectical tension in the early medical testimonies à propos the nature, either putrid or specifically venomous, of the matter transmitting the infection.[42] In both circumstances, the infected bodies would be faced with death by collapse of their vital forces whenever the exposure time to the cause was long enough. However, these two kinds of morbid matter operated in different ways: while the putrid matter acted by altering the properties deriving from the humoral mixture, the poisonous one did it through an 'occult property' – its 'venenosity'.

Irrespective of university doctors' discussions about the condition, either exogenous or merely endogenous, of the place where the poison had been generated, the increasing influence through time of the notion that pestilential matter or vapours had a poisonous condition was not only in tune with their need to explain the fierce and massive effects of the new pestilence. It also fuelled in the collective imagination the scope for human action in the artificial production of plague. This circumstance would help to explain the omnipresence of poisons in medical culture from the fifteenth century as well as to assist the development in early modern Europe of an ontological theory of infectious disease.

Seen in a retrospective way, it may be said that the mid-fourteenth-century Black Death paved the way for a profusion of conspiratorial views of plague in early modern Europe as deliberately caused by a broad spectrum of actors ranging from witches and religious dissenters to public health officers and/or those destitute people (usually poor foreigners) who were contracted as plague workers during the outbreaks.[43]

Acknowledgements

I am indebted to José Luis Gil-Aristu for his help in accurately translating the quotations from Gabriele de' Mussi, to Lluís Cifuentes for valuable bibliographical references he provided me with, and to Andrew Cunningham for his revision of the English style of this work.

Notes

1 Jean Delumeau, *La peur en Occident (XIVe–XVIIIe siècles. Une cité assiegée* (Paris, 1978), pp. 98–142.
2 Andrew Cunningham, 'Transforming plague: The laboratory and the identity of infectious disease', in Andrew Cunningham and Perry Williams (eds.), *The laboratory revolution in medicine* (Cambridge, 1992), pp. 209–244.

3 *The compact edition of the Oxford English Dictionary. Complete text repro-duced micrographically* (Oxford, 1987), 3 vols.: vol. II, p. 2193.

4 Stefan Riedel, 'Biological warfare and bioterrorism: A historical review', *Bay-lor University Medical Center Proceedings*, 17 (2004): 401–406.

5 Guy de Chauliac's well-known *Digressio de mortalitate* inserted in his *Chirur-gia magna* (1361) provides a detailed account about the popularity of the *pestis manufacta* idea during the 1348 Black Death by a privileged witness:

> De causa istius ingentis mortalitatis multi haesitaverunt. In aliquibus locis crediderunt quod Iudaei venenassent mundum, et ita interfecerunt eos; in aliquibus, pauperes truncati et effugabant eos; in aliis, nobiles, et ideo dubi-tabant ire per mundum. Finaliter ad tantum devenit quod tenebant custodes in civitatibus et villis, et nullum permittebant intrare nisi bene notum; et si alicui invenissent pulveres, aut unguenta, timentes quod essent pociones, faciebant eos transglutire.

See Michael R. McVaugh (ed.), *Guigonis de Caulhiaco (Guy de Chauliac) In-ventarium sive chirurgia magna. Volume one: Text* (Leiden, 1997), p. 118, lines 22–28.

6 Philip Ziegler, *The Black Death* (Harmondsworth, 1969), pp. 98–111; Carlo Ginzburg, *Ecstasies: Deciphering the Witches' Sabbath* (London, 1990), pp. 33–86. R. I. Moore has framed these features in the context of a gradual transformation of Western Europe since the eleventh and twelfth centuries in a repressive society where 'deliberate and socially sanctioned violence' was directed 'through estab-lished governmental, judicial and social institutions' against not only individuals but also 'groups of people defined by general characteristics as race, religion or way of life'. See R. I. Moore, *The formation of a persecuting society. Power and deviance in Western Europe, 950–1250* (Oxford, 1987), pp. 5, 135, 152–153.

7 Séraſine Guerchberg's continues to be the classic work on this question: 'La controverse sur les prétendus semeurs de la «Peste Noire» d'après les traités de peste de l'époque', *Revue des Études Juives*, 108 (1948): 3–40. English trans-lation: 'The controversy over the alleged sowers of the Black Death in the con-temporary treatises on plague', in Sylvia L. Thrupp (ed.), *Change in Medieval Society. Europe North of the Alps, 1050–1500* (London, 1965), pp. 208–224.

8 A. W. Henschel (ed.), 'Document zur Geschichte der schwarzen Todes', *Archiv für die gesammte Medicin*, 2 (1842): 26–59; A. G. Tononi (ed.), 'La peste dell'anno 1348', *Giornale Ligustico de Archeologia, Storia e Letteratura*, 11(1884): 139–152. For an English version, see Rosemary Horrox (ed.), *The Black Death* (Manchester, 1994), pp. 14–26.

9 'Et ecce morbo Tartaros invadente totus exercitus perturbatus longuebat et cottidie infinita millia sunt extincta. Videbatur eis, sagittas evolare de celo, tangere et opprimere superbiam Tartarorum, qui statim signati corporibus in iuncturis, humore coagulato in inguinibus, febre putrida subsequente, expira-bant. Ex tanta clade et morbo pertifero fatigati, sic deficientes, attoniti et un-dique stupefacti, sine spe salutis mori conspicientes, cadavera, machinis eorum superposita, intra Caffensem urbem precipitari jubebant, ut ipsorum fectore intollerabili, omnino deficerent. Sic proiecta videbantur cacumina mortuorum, nec Christiani latere, nec fugere, nec a tali precipicio liberari valebant, licet def-functos, quos poterant marinis traderent fluctibus inmergendos. Moxque toto aere infecto, et aqua venenata, corrupta putredine, tantusque fetor invasit ut vix ex millibus unus, relicto exercitu fugere conaretur qui eciam venenatus aliis ubique venena preparans, solo aspectu, loca et homines, morbo infficeret uni-versos. Nec aliquis sciebat, vel poterat viam invenire salutis' (Henschel, 'Docu-ment', pp. 48–49).

10 "Sic undique Orientalibus, et meridiana plaga, et qui in Aquilone degebant, sagita percussis asperima, que corporibus crepidinem inducebat, morbo pressis pestifero, fere omnes, deficiebant, et morte subita corruebant. Quanta, qualisque fuerit mortalitas generalis, Cathaijnj, Indi, Perses, Medi, Cardenses, Armeni, Tarsenses, Georgianj, Mesopotami, Nubiani, Ethijopes, Turchumani, Egiptij, Arabici, Saraceni, Greci et fere toto oriente corrupto, clamoribus, flectibus et singultibus occupati, a supra dicto millesimo, usque ad millesimum cccxlviiii in amaritudine commorantes, extremum deij Judicium suspicantur' (Henschel, 'Document', p. 49).

11 'Existentes sani, utriusque sexus, nec mortis pericula formidantes, iiii^{or} ictibus asperimis carnibus vexabantur. Et primo eos quidem rigor algens, humana subito corpora commovebat que quasi lancea perforati sagittarum pungentes aculeos senciebant. Ex quibus quosdam, in iunctura brachii subter lagenam, quosdam in inguinibus, inter corpus et cossiam, ad modum cuticelle durissime grosse et quandoque grosioris, dirus impetus affligebat, cuius ardore mox in febrem acutissimam et putridam, cum dolore capitis incidebant. Qua nimium prevalente, aliis fetorem intollerabilem relinquebat; aliis sputum ex ore sanguineum; aliis inflaturas iuxta locum precedentis humoris, post tergum, et circha pectus, et iuxta fêmur, et alia acerbitate precipua ingerebat. Quidam vero inebriati sopore, non poterant excitari. Ecce bulle Domini comminantis' (Henschel, 'Document', p. 55).

12 Henschel, 'Document', pp. 55–56.

13 David Nirenberg, *Communities of violence: Persecution of minorities in the Middle Ages* (Princeton, 1996), pp. 43–68.

14 Guilleré, 'La peste noire à Gérone (1348)', *Annals de l'Institut d'Estudis Gironins*, 27 (1984): 103–105, 141–143 [the first of the two documents edited by Christian Guilleré was first published by Jaime Villanueva, *Viage literario a las iglesias de España* (Madrid, 1803–1852), 22 vols.: vol. XIV, pp. 270–271]; Ginzburg, *Ecstasies*, pp. 63–86; Horrox, *The Black Death*, pp. 207–226; Jon Arrizabalaga, 'Facing the Black Death: Perceptions and reactions of university practitioners', in Luis García Ballester, Roger K. French, Jon Arrizabalaga and Andrew Cunningham (eds.), *Practical medicine from Salerno to the Black Death* (Cambridge, 1994), pp. 237–288; Nirenberg, *Communities of violence*, pp. 231–249.

15 Josep Coroleu, *Documents històrics catalans del segle XIV* (Barcelona, 1899), p. 69:

> algunes malycens persones se son levades e matzinen totes les aygues e la salpassa e la ortalissa e totes les viandes que poden, e encara posen les dites metzines en los banchs on hom seu o ten los peus, per ço que aquells qui aquí seuran recuyleguen les dites metzines. (...) E sobre açó, mon senyor, jo he fetes provissions que faç escorcoyar tot hom estrany qyich venga, per saber si portarien metzines ... com jo haya entès que les dites persones malvades s'escampen per tota la terra. Aquestes persones, mon senyor, van meses a manera de gent de penitencia e d'estrugament.

The document comes from the Archivo de la Corona de Aragón (ACA), Canc. Reg., 1128, fols. 178–179.

16 Coroleu, *Documents històrics catalans*, p. 70.

17 'Et fragante dictarum potionum seu menzinarum crimine plures reperti et capti extiterunt in Narbona et alibi diversarum nationum pauperes et mendicantes portantes, ut dicebant et videbatur, potiones pulverizatas quas in aquis, domibus, ecclesiis et rebus victualibus ponebant ad finem gentes interficiendi' (Guilleré, 'La peste noire à Gérone', p. 141).

18 'Et licet aliqui naturales adhuc asserant hoc provenire ex duabus planetis nunc regnantibus, credimus esse certi quod planete et potiones concurrant et dictas

mortalitates inducant. Scientes quod infirmitates que ex predictis evenerunt sunt contagiose, quoniam defuncta una persona in aliquo hospicio, servitores, familiares et parentes illius modo et morbo consimili afliguntur et infra tres vel quatuor dies comuniter moriuntur' (Guilleré 'La peste noire à Gérone', p. 142).

19 'Per altra rahó pot venir mortaldat e pestilència en les gents, ço és a saber, per malvats hòmens fiylls del diable qui ab metzines e verins diverses corrompen les viandes ab molt fals engiynn e malvada maestria, ja sie ço que pròpriament parlan, aytal mortalitat de gents no és pestilència de la qual ací parlam, mas he·n volguda fer menció per ço car ara tenim temps en lo qual s'a[n] seguides moltes morts en alcunes regions prop d'ací axí como en Cobliure, en Carcassès, en Narbonès e en la baronia de Montpesler e a Avinyó e en tota Proença'. See Jon Arrizabalaga, Luis García Ballester and Joan Veny (eds.), *Jacme d'Agramont. Regiment de preservació de pestilència* (Barcelona, 1998), p. 56.

20 'Affectantes complere obedientiam sui ordinis, ad locum de Papia predictum ut interessent dicto capitulo, prout decet, iter acceperunt et, quamvis Barchinone illis fuisset, ut asseruerunt, intimatum quod sine magno periculo dictum iter facere non poterant, quia in locis pluribus licenter apparebantur homines ex toto expoliebantur et prescrutabantur et pro modica occasione capti tenebantur precipue religiosi, cum sacerdotalia facientes esset suspicio quod homines sub habitu religionis aquas inficiebant et potiones imponebant, ideo non erat securum alicui religioso iter illud accipere' (Guilleré, 'La peste noire à Gérone', pp. 142–143).

21 'Et cum audivissent tantam mortalitatem quod nullus poterat exprimere, et revertentes homines una cum eis audissent asserentes quod hospicia non inveniebantur nec erat qui ad hospicium aliquem extraneum vellet recipere et si alicui extraneo aliquid infirmitatis contingebat, statim extra loca sine medicina ponebantur et ibidem moriebatur absque solietate cuiscumque, prout eis dictum et narratum, ut asseruerunt, fuit' (Guilleré, 'La peste noire à Gérone', p. 143).

22 Stephanus Baluzius, *Vita Paparum Avenionensium*, ed. G. Mollat (París, 1914), 2 vols.: vol. I, pp. 251–252; Ernest Wickersheimer, 'Les accusations d'empoisonnement portées pendant la première moitié du XIVᵉ siècle contre les lepreux et les juifs; leurs relations avec les épidémies de peste. Communication au Quatrième Congrès International d'Histoire de la Médecine (Bruxelles, avril 1923)' (Antwerp, 1927); Hans Witte and Georg Wolfram (eds.), *Urkundenbuch der Stadt Strassburg. Fünfter Band: politische Urkuden von 1332 bis 1380* (Strasbourg, 1896), pp. 164–165, 167–174, 178–179; Horrox, *The Black Death*, pp. 210–220.

23 Witte and Wolfram, *Urkundenbuch der Stadt Strassburg*, pp. 168–170; Horrox, *The Black Death*, pp. 212–214.

24 In the chronicle by Heinricus Dapifer de Diessenhoven (1316–1361), John XXII's papal chaplain, echoing these accusations against Jews as well as the subsequent repression of their communities in the German countries, it is pointed that in 1348, a poison whose toxic condition was experimentally tested had been found in a Jew's house in the Swiss-German city of Zofingen (repertum fuit venenum in domo Iudei dicti Tröstli quod consules civitatis ibidem inquirentes reperierunt, et per experienciam probant esse fore toxicum). See J. F. Boehmer (ed.), *Fontes Rerum Germanicarum* (Stuttgart, 1843–1868), vol. IV, p. 69.

25 Witte and Wolfram, *Urkundenbuch der Stadt Strassburg*, p. 169; Horrox, *The Black Death*, p. 214. To Isidore of Seville, the basilisk was the 'king of serpents so that they all scape from it because it kills them with its breath, and does it to men with its sight' in the same way as it does to any bird flying in its presence, even being far away. See Isidore, *Etymologies*, lib. 12, Chap. 4, ver. 6:

> Basiliscus Graece, Latine interpretatur regulus, eo quod rex serpentium sit, adeo ut eum videntes fugiant, quia olfactu suo eos necat; nam et hominem vel si aspiciat interimit. Siquidem et eius aspectu nulla avis volans inlaesa transit, sed quam procul sit, eius ore conbusta devoratur.

The poisonous gaze of the basilisk and that of the so-called 'Venomous Virgin' were analogously related to that of a patient dying from pestilence in the *Tractatus de epidemia* (Montpellier, *c.* 1348–1349) signed by 'a certain practitioner of Montpellier'. See Arrizabalaga, 'Facing the Black Death', pp. 263–264.

26 Witte and Wolfram, *Urkundenbuch der Stadt Strassburg*, pp. 168–169; Horrox, *The Black Death*, p. 213.

27 Witte and Wolfram, *Urkundenbuch der Stadt Strassburg*, pp. 168–171; Horrox, *The Black Death*, pp. 213, 215–216.

28 Compare the contents of the universal chronicle by the Franciscan Hermann Gigas (for its reference, see below) with other sources having exonerated Jews from such accusations and having defended their protection and called for an end to their prosecution. These are, among others, the cases of the letter sent – in reply to the enquiry of Strasburg city – by the consistory of Cologne in January 1349 to defend Jews' innocence, and of Clement VI's papal mandate protecting Jews. See Witte and Wolfram, *Urkundenbuch der Stadt Strassburg*, pp. 178–179 (doc. no. 190) (English translation in Horrox, *The Black Death*, pp. 219–220); Shlomo Simonsohn, *The Apostolic See and the Jews. Documents: 492–1404* (Toronto, 1988), pp. 397–398 (doc no. 373) (English translation in Horrox, *The Black Death*, 221–222).

29 'Istam pestilentiam quidam dicunt ex corruptione aeris evenisse, alii vero Judaeos totam Christianitatem voluisse veneno extinguere, ubique terrarum puteos et fontes intoxicasse. Et hoc Judaei multi tormentati confessi sunt, quod araneas et bubones nutrierint in ollis et cacabis, et quod venenum de ultramarinis partibus sibi comparaverint, istudque scelus non omni Judaeorum plebi constare, sed tantum potentioribus, ne videlicet divulgaretur'. See Herman Gigas, *Flores temporum seu Chronicon universal* (Leiden, 1750), pp. 138–139. English translation in Horrox, *The Black Death*, p. 207.

30 Horrox, *The Black Death*, pp. 223–226 (quotations from pp. 224–225); Henry Suso, *The life of the servant* (London, 1952). For the original German text, see 'Das Leben Heinrich Suso's von ihm selbst erzählt', Chapter xxvi, in Heinrich Suso (known as Amandus), *Leben und Schriften*, ed. Milchior Wiepenbrock (Regensburg, 1837), pp. 58–61 [https://archive.org/details/heinrichsusos-ge00grgoog (14 April 2015)].

31 'N Arnau de Lupià, donzell ..., al amat lo battle d Alcudia o a son lochtinent. Salut e dilecció.

> De part del senyor rey, e per auctoritat del offiçi que usam, vos dehim e expresament manam que en continent, vistes les presents, quens informets deligentment si lo catiu turch den G. Brassa ses banyat en la mar e si aportava de la aygua de la mar en la bocha, e si aquella escupia ne gitava per los portals dels alberchs del dit lloch d Alcudia, e si es stat en la villa de Polensa. E si lo dit catiu ha dit que si nol giten de catiu que farà morir tots quants son en Alcudia, e encare de totes alters coses que lo dit catiu haia fetes ne dites e a vos sien denunciades....

Datum Mairicarum III idus aprilis MCCCXLVIII'. See Álvaro Santamaría Arández, 'La peste negra en Mallorca', in *VII Congreso de Historia de la Corona de Aragón* (Valencia, 1969), vol. I, pp. 103–130 (at p. 130).

32 Karl Sudhoff, 'Epistola et regimen Alphontii Cordubensis de pestilentia', *Archiv für Geschichte der Medizin*, 3 (1909–1910): 223–226.

33 'Et est alia causa quam naturalis et propter hoc et propter compassionem fidelium, quae praecipue patiuntur, descripsi istam epistolam et regimen cum medicinis ne pii et boni tot periculis subiciiantur et sciant sibi praecavere de tantis periculis et malis imminentibus praecipue christianis in ista pestilentia. Ante omnia praecavendum est ab omni cibo et potu quae infici possunt et

intoxicari ab aquis praecipue non fluentibus, quia ista potissime possunt infici. Experientia docuit quod ista pestilentia non vadit ex constellatione aliqua
et per consequens nullam naturalem infectionem elementorum, sed vadit ex
profundo malitiae per artificium subtilissimum profundae iniquitatis inventae,
quare consilium sapientium medicorum non proficit nec iuvat illos detentos
isto pessimo crudeli et pernicioso morbo, unde hoc summum remedium est,
fugere pestem, quia pestis non sequitur fugientem, aut praecavere ab omni<-
bus> rerum vitalium infectione in quantum possibile est' (Alfonso de Córdoba,
'Epistola', p. 224).

34 '... aer potest et infici per artificium, ut quando praeparetur quaedam confectio in amphora de vitriaco et quando fuerit illa confectio bene fermentata, ille
qui illud malum velit facere, exspectat quando fuerit ventus fortis et lentus ab
aliqua mundi plaga, tunc vadat contra ventum et locat amphoram suam iuxta
lapides contra civitatem vel villam quam velit inficere et zona longa alligata re-
cedendo contra ventum ne eum inficeret vapor, trahat fortiter amphoram super
lapides et amphora fracta se vapor effunditur et dispargitur in aere et quem-
cunque tetigerit ille vapor, ille morietur tanquam de aere pestilentico et citius'
(Alfonso de Córdoba, 'Epistola', pp. 224–225).

35 '... et nata fertur pestilentia in Babylonia, ubi de templo Apollinis ex arcula
aurea, quam miles forte inciderat, spiritus pestilens evasit, atque inde Parthos
orbemque complesse'. See Dio Cassius, *Historia Augusta* (Loeb Classical
Library 139: Cambridge, MA–London, 1921), vol. I, book 5, p. 222.

36 'Sic igitur versus orientem serpens [novus aer] venit nunc in Saxoniam, quod
similiter est interdum ac si de cadaveribus bellorum fuisset progenita vel aliqua-
rum herbarum intoxicatarum vel veneno a sapiente pol. invento, ut patet in suo
libro ubi talem confeccionem docet facere, ex qua una civitas vel una tota regio
possit intoxicari' (Karl Sudhoff, 'Pestschriften aus den ersten 150 Jahren nach
der Epidemie des 'schwarzen Todes' 1348', *Archiv für Geschichte der Medizin*,
11 (1918–1919): 149).

37 On Nicholas of Poland, see William Eamon, 'Antipocras. A medieval treatise
on magical medicine by brother Nicholas of the Preaching Friars (c. 1270)'
(s.l., 2014) and the bibliography referred to there. [https://nmsu.academia.edu/
WilliamEamon/Texts-and-Translations (15 April 2015)]

38 Sudhoff, 'Pestschriften', pp. 149–150:

>Scribit enim miles anglicanus, in yndia fore arbores, que portant farinam,
>qui gustantur de ea, citius morientur, de quibus diffamati erant Judei, quon-
>dam christianos intoxicasse, cum fuerit illa prima magna pestilentia, de qua
>scribit Gwido, quod fuerat anno Domini 1348, et dicit eam fuisse quasi per
>totum mundum, sicut etiam mortalitas ex inficientibus serpentibus, draconi-
>bus et basiliscis, ut exemplificabat Galienus de iuvamento anhelitus, quamvis
>proprie not sit stilus eius, de tribus militibus volentibus interficere basiliscum,
>quorum cuiuslibet hasta tangebat equum alterius, ac si unus eum non inter-
>ficeret, ut alius faceret, quia omnes tres mortui sunt sola aeris infeccione.

39 Joseph Needham, et al., *Science and civilisation in China. Vol. V: Chemistry
and chemical technology. Part V: Spagyrical discovery and invention: Apparatus, theories and gifts* (Cambridge, 1980), pp. 366–367. For more information,
see Amanda Jane Leep, *The rooster's egg: Maternal metaphors and medieval
men* (Ph.D. Dissertation, University of Toronto, 2010).

40 Avicenna, *Canon medicinae*, lib. V, Tractatus scientialis, De qualitate composi-
tionis (Venice, 1527), fols. 391r-v; Avicenna, *De viribus cordis*, tract. II, cap. IV
(De differentibus laetificandi et confortandi repertis in medicinis) (in *Canon*,
fol. 427v). Also see Michael R. McVaugh, *Arnaldi de Villanova Opera Medica
Omnia. Vol. II: Aphorismi de gradibus* (Granada-Barcelona, 1975), pp. 18–19;

John M. Riddle and James A. Mulholland, 'Albert on stones and minerals', in James A. Weisheipl (ed.), *Albertus Magnus and the Sciences. Commemorative Essays 1980* (Toronto, 1980), pp. 203–234: 206, 208; Sebastià Giralt, '*Proprietas*: las propiedades ocultas según Arnau de Vilanova', *Traditio*, 36 (2008): 327–360, particularly pp. 343–347.

41 Melissa P. Chase, 'Fevers, poisons, and apostemes: Authority and experience in Montpellier plague treatises', in Pamela O. Long (ed.), *Science and Technology in Medieval Society* (New York, 1985), pp. 153–169.

42 Chase, 'Fevers, poisons, and apostemes'; Arrizabalaga, 'Facing the Black Death', pp. 259–264.

43 On early modern conspiratorial views of plague, see, among others, A. Lynn Martin, *Plague? Jesuit accounts of epidemic disease in the 16th century* (Kirksville, 1996), pp. 104–111; William G. Naphy, *Plagues, poisons and potions. Plague-spreading conspiracies in the Western Alps, c. 1530–1640* (Manchester-New York, 2002); Alessandro Pastore, *Veleno. Credenze, crimini, saperi nell'Italia moderna* (Bologna, 2010), pp. 52–57.

5 Alchemy, potency, imagination

Paracelsus's theories of poison

Georgiana D. Hedesan

'All things are poison, and nothing is without poison', declared the maverick Swiss physician Theophrastus Bombastus von Hohenheim, called Paracelsus (1493–1541) in a late defence of his works.[1] This affirmation sounds harshly dualistic and, like much of Paracelsus's rhetoric, is intended to shock its reader. Nevertheless, it also contains in a nutshell the core theory of poison that he expressed at least ten years before and remained essential to his philosophy.

Paracelsus has long been recognised as one of the chief exponents of the medical Renaissance of the sixteenth century. He was much more radical than other reforming physicians: while most contemporary efforts were directed at humanist reappraisals of ancient medicine, he rejected authority in favour of personal experience and practice.[2] He was scathing of the Galenic medical system of his era, and particularly of the theory of four humours on which it was based. Instead, he proposed a new medical framework based on four pillars of knowledge (philosophy, astronomy, alchemy and virtue); amongst other things, his approach led to the gradual acceptance of chemical medicine in the medical pharmacopoeia. His emphasis on treating the causes of disease rather than its symptoms also led to major change in medicine. Certainly, many of his ideas were not new, but the emphasis he put on them and the influence he had on the next generations of medical practitioners made him a central figure of medical reform.

Despite the recognition of Paracelsus's medical innovations, classical historians of science have hesitated to approach his ideas in detail. There are three main types of difficulties in reading Paracelsus: the first is his style that alternates clear pronouncements with obscure references, the second is the apparent inconsistency of ideas across treatises and the third is the framework, which is often radically different from that of modern medicine. Thankfully, due to the extraordinary research of dedicated scholars like Karl Sudhoff, Kurt Goldammer and the late Joachim Telle, we now understand that many of Paracelsus's inconsistencies can be explained by intellectual development or misattribution. At the same time, and with all the effort made by scholars like Walter Pagel or Charles Webster, we are still a long way from grasping Paracelsus's system of thought.

A case in point is Paracelsus's view of poisons, which have a richness that has not been captured in previous scholarship. Most scholars only touched on the subject of poison and did not fully reflect on the complexity of its meaning. Consequently, I have decided to explore Paracelsus's ideas and bring together the various connotations he conferred to the term 'poison'. For the purpose of this chapter, I have chosen a methodology that would take account of the timing of Paracelsus's writings as well as their relevance to the subject at hand. I have consequently decided to take a treatise-based approach that would not only focus on works that have a particular emphasis on the topic of poison, but also reflect, to the best extent possible, the chronology of these treatises. The chapter is thus focussed on seven writings, although it makes references to other works where appropriate. At the end, I have tried to synthesise the views of these works and consider the question of consistency of ideas on 'poison' throughout Paracelsus's writings.

Two fundamental theories of poison in *Super Entia Quinque* (1520s)

Paracelsus's treatise *Super Entia Quinque* (*On the Five Entities*) is included in a fragmentary work called *Volumen Primum Medicinae Paramirum Theophrasti de Medica Industria*. *Super Entia Quinque* has been considered as one of Paracelsus's earliest writings by Karl Sudhoff, who dated it from the (early) 1520s and described it as incomplete (*Brüchstücke des Buches von den fünf Entien*).[3] This view has not been contested, but the question remains as to why this treatise was included in the *Volumen Paramirum*, whose title connects it to Paracelsus's mature Paramiran writings (1531).[4] Moreover, its reference to the famous treatise *Archidoxis* (c. 1525–6) suggests it may not have been such an early work after all.[5]

In this treatise, Paracelsus attributes disease to five entities: the entity of stars (*ens astrale*), of poison (*ens veneni*), of nature (*ens naturale*), of spirit (*ens spirituale*) and of God (*ens Dei*). Andrew Weeks has argued that these five types are inspired by theories of plague causation found in medieval treatises.[6] The entity, *ens*, is described as 'a cause or a thing which has the ability to govern the body',[7] meaning that it is a force that rules matter. For the purpose of this analysis, I will focus on the first and second entities, the *ens astrale* and the *ens veneni*, which put forth two important theories of poison.

Poison as vapour: the theory of ens astrale

In the first chapter on the *ens astrale*, the term 'poison' (*Gifft*) represents a power causing disease. Thus, Paracelsus states that 'poison is the origin of every disease, and all diseases are brought on by poison, be they of the body or a wound, nothing excluded'.[8] He argues that poisons originate from five metals and minerals: arsenic, salts, mercury, realgar and sulphur.[9] There is no one-to-one correspondence between a type of poison and a disease; a poison can, in fact, result in many separate diseases. Consequently, Paracelsus argues that it is more important for a physician to uncover the cause out of which a disease springs, rather than the reasons of its development. We can detect here a clear bias for identifying the fundamental 'causes' rather than the 'effects' of a phenomenon, because it is more efficient to tackle the former rather than the latter.[10]

Paracelsus explains how people become afflicted by disease originating from the *ens astrale*. First, he postulates that all life in things is sustained by a medium he mysteriously calls 'M.' or 'M. magnum'. This 'M.' is a vital substratum that permeates all things and supports all creatures both in heaven and on earth.[11] When M. becomes poisoned, it in turn affects the life of the beings it sustains.

The medium of M. also transmits and captures the influences of the stars to earth. Stars, we are told, are 'just like people on earth'; they have personalities, and when they are badly disposed, 'their wickedness comes to the fore'.[12] Negative influences are materialised in the form of poisonous invisible vapours or odours. These vapours of poison pollute the air, and more importantly the life-medium 'M', which weakens and thus allows living things to become diseased.[13] Astral poisons affect an entire ecosystem: they corrupt water, earth and air in specific areas, poisoning all its living inhabitants, from fish to human beings and fruit.[14] In the human body, astral poison manifests itself in various ways. It can affect the skin, the internal organs, the blood or the entire body. The type of disease and location within the body depends on the underlying chemical that causes it: mercury, for instance, affects the head, but realgar only the blood.[15]

Not everyone who is exposed to the poisonous vapours becomes ill. Paracelsus argues that only those antagonistic or incompatible with it are infected. Persons whose nature is 'compatible' to the vapours and those who can overcome poison by medical preparation or by 'the refined nature of blood' remain healthy.

This theory of the *ens astrale* is essential to the understanding of Paracelsus's view of poison as a type of invisible vapour or air that insinuates itself in the human body and causes disease. This view seems to draw on the Galenic theory of the plague as a poisonous vapour.[16] Here, the vapours originate from the stars, but in other works, Paracelsus extends the ability to emanate vapours to earthly bodies as well.

The poison in all things: the theory of ens veneni

In the chapter on *ens astrale*, Paracelsus taught that all diseases are caused by poison and that some diseases originate from the ill-disposition of the stars. In the next chapter, he went further to explain that disease was also caused by *ens veneni*, the entity of poison. Paracelsus ties *ens veneni* with a theory of universal poison; according to him, everything that we ingest contains some poison in it.[17] This may seem like a straightforward dualistic view of the universe, but Paracelsus immediately complicates it. Beings are not poisonous in themselves; in fact, God created all things perfect and good.[18] However, in respect to others, creatures are poisonous: none can be ingested as such. As Paracelsus points out in respect to the ox, '[h]ad he been created merely on man's account and not also for his own sake, he would need neither horns, bones, nor hoofs. For these do not constitute food'.[19] The existence of indigestible parts is the proof that God made beings for their own sake, not for consumption by others.

Paracelsus hence distinguishes between beings-in-themselves and beings in relationship with others. To clarify his point, he does not engage in a complex philosophical discussion; rather, he, in a typical move, offers two illustrative examples. The first example is very simple. Grass is not poisonous in itself, but it contains poison when ingested by cattle. The second example is much more elaborate and is based on a political analogy. A ruling Prince and his servants are 'perfect' in themselves. Yet they are not so in relationship with the other. The Prince needs his servants to rule, while the servants need to be compensated for their work on behalf of the Prince. This symbiotic relationship means that the Prince and the servants are both imperfect in their dependency towards each other. Seen from the Prince's point of view, a servant is both a gain and a loss.[20]

These two analogies are important in understanding Paracelsus's thinking. In the first, the example refers to straightforward ingestion. The Swiss physician claims that the act of consumption is incomplete, as beings can never completely digest food. The second example does not refer to digestion in itself; nevertheless, one can easily recognise the expansion of the act of consumption to a universal process. Digestion, it suggests, is an act of hierarchy: the superior creature consumes the inferior one. In the first example, grass is hierarchically subordinate to cattle. In the second, the Prince is superior to the servant.

We can recognise in this hierarchical view of nature both Aristotelian and Christian views; indeed, Paracelsus's discussion seems to draw on the Scholastic distinction between *ens* (being) and *esse* (existence), famously developed by Thomas Aquinas.[21] The Swiss physician accepts the basic idea that human beings stand at the top of both the ladder of being and of the food chain. On the downside, this means that they are also the most likely to be poisoned of all creatures.

Thankfully, this bleak view of a world in which poison is universal is balanced by the idea that God has gifted a way of eliminating poison from food. The method by which this is done is 'alchemy' (*Alchimey*). To understand this, we must first quickly examine what Paracelsus meant by 'alchemy'. He explains it in the following way: '[i]t divides the evil from the good, changes the good into a tincture, conditions the body so it will live, attunes the subject to nature, conditions nature so she becomes flesh and blood'.[22] This definition implies that alchemy is not simply an art invented by man but a natural process that takes place on a universal scale, which alchemists copy in the laboratory. Indeed, Paracelsus posits that an 'alchemist of nature' resides in all beings and is in charge with the separation of the good and evil in food. Paracelsus defines the good as 'essence' (*Essentia*)[23] and evil as 'poison' (*Venenum*). The *Essentia* sustains, while *Venenum* causes disease.[24]

Paracelsus further posits that the inner 'alchemist', like the exterior one, is an artisan (*Künstler*) that possesses knowledge (*Erkantnuss*) given by God.[25] It contains 'virtue, strength and art'[26] whereby the nourishment is taken into the body, while the residue is expelled. The degree of the inner alchemist's ability differs across the natural world. For instance, Paracelsus posits that the peacock's inner alchemist is superior to that of any other animal as it can consume poisonous snakes and lizards, while the pig's is better than that of man since it can digest excrements.

According to Paracelsus's view, the inner alchemist works continuously at separating the useful from the harmful. Unsurprisingly, the alchemist is found in the stomach, and his separation is a form of digestion whereby food is synthesised in products necessary for the body. Yet the process of digestion is not complete: some impurity always remains, which must be expelled via an assigned emunctory channel. For instance, mucus is described as the poison that the brain has eliminated.[27] This process is not always successful; when proper digestion fails, undigested matter accumulates in the organs and putrefies. This putrefaction leads to corruption, which gives rise to disease. Hence, disease fundamentally arises from the inner alchemist's failure to properly incorporate nourishment and expel what is harmful.[28]

Putrefaction can occur in two locations: in the organs the *Essentia* is destined for (but for failure of alchemy some *Venenum* passes through), or in the organs assigned for elimination of waste. The skin eliminates the 'mercury' of the *Venenum*; the nose, eyes and anus the 'sulphur'; the ears the 'arsenic'; and the urinary tract the 'salt'.[29] The implication is that when an organ fails or malfunctions due to the accumulation of *Venenum*, a disease of these four kinds arises in the body.

To conclude the analysis of *Super Entia Quinque*, we should observe that Paracelsus uses the term 'poison' in two fundamental ways. First, in the chapter on *ens astrale*, he describes poison as a spiritual vapour, which can be transmitted to the stars and then infect the earth and cause disease. Second, in the chapter on *ens veneni*, poison denotes a destructive essence in all types of food, which must be eliminated by the inner 'alchemist of nature' in the act of digestion. These two views of poison remained consistent in Paracelsus's later works, which expand their meaning without fundamentally denying their validity.

Theory of tartar in *Opus Paramirum* (1531)

The *Opus Paramirum* (1531) has been praised as one of the most influential mature treatises of Paracelsus, not least because it outlines very clearly the theory of the *tria prima*, the three principles.[30] According to this doctrine, the three principles of salt, mercury and sulphur are the basic building blocks of all things; together, they form everything that exists.

Opus Paramirum also outlines Paracelsus's theory of a disease called 'tartar', which is later expanded on in several treatises. The concept of 'tartar' disease had a strong afterlife amongst Paracelsian physicians. Its demise was at least partially brought about by the Flemish medical alchemist Van Helmont, who derided the notion of such a disease.[31]

In *Opus Paramirum*, Paracelsus argues that human beings swallow things that are not in conformity with themselves. These form a residue, alternatively called *stercus* or *excrementum*, which lies in opposition with nourishment, *nutrimentum*.[32] The dualism *nutrimentum–stercus* parallels that of *Essentia–Venenum* in *Super Entia Quinque*, except for the fact here *stercus* and *nutrimentum* represent physical and tangible products.

The *stercora* are described as stony residues or coagulations. According to *Opus Paramirum*, 'that which never coagulates is *nutrimentum*; that which does coagulate is *stercus*'.[33] Accumulated *stercus* in the body yields tartar.[34] Consequently, Paracelsus defines tartar as

> merely *excrementum* of the nutrition and of the drink, in and of themselves, which, in the human being, are then coagulated by the immanent *spiritus* ...Thus we eat and drink the *tartarus*...Out of this, many diseases result in many ways.[35]

As scholars have pointed out, the concept of tartar is related to the residue left by wine in casks.[36] Indeed, Paracelsus himself also refers to tartar as the stone of wine (*Weinstein*). At the same time, the word 'tartar' may also recall medieval fears of the non-Christian outsider, who was sometimes blamed for bringing epidemics to Europe.[37]

Opus Paramirum divides tartar into four types: *calculus* (stone), *arena* (sand), *bolus* (clay) and *viscus* (lute or glue). Generally, Paracelsus describes the viscose matter that results from digestion as tartar.[38] Consequently, he argues that the gluten or gum of legumes and the clay of meats are the source of disease in the human body. This is presumably so because of their sticky quality that adheres to the walls of organs just like tartar adheres to wine casks.

Tartar can form in any part of the body where digestion occurs. By comparison with *Super Entia Quinque*, Paracelsus now postulates that digestion occurs throughout the digestive tract. Thus, he maintains that the first digestion happens in the mouth, where tartar may form in the throat, on the tongue, or on the gums.[39] Next, tartar can form at the orifice of the stomach, where it manifests itself through heartburn and *paroxysmus calculi*. Finally, tartar can also form in the stomach and the lower organs, such as the intestines, liver, kidneys, bladder and others.[40] The result is symptoms such as cramps, vomiting and fevers, and diseases like hepatitis, dropsy and kidney stones.

Up to this point, Paracelsus has described tartar as a disease affecting the digestive system. Yet he is tempted to go further. He now affirms that each part of the body has its own 'stomach' that retains what it needs and rejects the rest. Thus, the brain takes nutriment and expels the excrement via the nose; the lungs take in the air and expunge the excrement in the same way.[41] In this sense, tartar can affect all organs and cause a wide range of life-threatening diseases like asthma, phthisis, consumption, mania, madness, cardiac diseases and others.

If we compare *Opus Paramirum* on tartar and *Super Entia Quinque* on *ens veneni*, it is clear that the two treatises belong to the same conceptual system. In both cases, disease is due to faulty digestion. The view of tartar fits the *Super Entia Quinque*'s theory of the nourishment-poison dualism of an ingested being. Moreover, *Opus Paramirum*'s extension of tartar from the digestive system to the entire body develops *Super Entia Quinque*'s statement that poison is expunged not only from purely digestive organs, but also from others such as the brain. Although *Super Entia Quinque* fails to mention that 'stomachs' exist everywhere in the body, it generally offers a much stronger theoretical view of disease and poison than *Opus Paramirum*. Clearly, the sophisticated view of beings containing both poison and nourishment is at the root of the more modest concept of tartar in *Opus Paramirum*. This implicitly confirms that *Super Entia Quinque* was written earlier than the *Opus*, but it also indicates that they should be read in conjunction.

Poisoned imagination in Paracelsus's pest treatises

The theory of the *ens astrale* was based on the notion that heaven infected human beings with poison. As we have seen, this action was due to a vague concept of the ill-disposition of the stars.[42] Yet in Paracelsus's first plague treatise (*Zwey Bucher von der Pestilenz* – the Nördlingen tract, dated 1529/1530), a major shift of perspective occurs. According to it, heaven continues to be the direct cause of the plague, but it is not its first fundamental cause; rather, the disease is produced by human beings themselves, who project it unto the heaven as unto a mirror. Heaven then reflects it back to us.[43] *Von der Pestilenz* classifies the plague as a 'supernatural' disease that is caused by human beings.[44]

This is a radical conceptual reversal. Where the power of the *ens astrale* was attributed to heaven in *Super Entia Quinque*, Paracelsus now chiefly blames man himself for this force, at least as far as the plague is concerned.[45] In this sense, heaven acts as a passive *medium* between the generator of the plague and its recipients. A clear association is hence made between the generation of plague and magical action, which traditionally needs a *medium*.[46] The intermediary is the imagination, as Paracelsus himself puts it. He suggests that the stars are poisoned by our corrupt imagination and then impress this poison on earth: '[s]o it is that magical imagination proceeds from us to [heaven], and from them again back to us'.[47] The idea that the imagination could cause illness or monstrous births was a familiar trope in Renaissance medicine, although physicians disagreed on whether it could work transitively (outside the body) or only within it.[48]

Heavenly infection has two main causes. One is *libido* or concupiscence; the other is witchcraft. These 'irritate' heaven.[49] Paracelsus points out that the ancient prophets understood the process since they warned people that their libidinous actions have angered their 'father', who would send back the plague.[50] By 'father', Paracelsus understands heaven, the macrocosmic counterpart of man.

Further on, *Von der Pestilenz* affirms that the plague is caused by the principle of sulphur.[51] By this, Paracelsus obviously means the fiery component of the *tria prima* out of which all bodies are made.[52] The sulphur that causes the plague lies hidden in three minerals: antimony, arsenic and marcasite. Each of these minerals affects a certain part of the body: thus, antimonial sulphur affects the groin, the arsenical one the chest and the marcasite the ears. Further, Paracelsus maintains that the sulphur is the corporeal counterpart of the astral spirit of Mars. In a rather unclear passage, he compares the process of the creation of pestilence with the engendering of a Basilisk (a mythical creature that had the power to poison at a distance) by the father alone. In a similar way, the planet Mars, infected by human imagination, can engender a pestilential 'Basilisk' and project the plague on earth by its gaze.[53]

The process of plague causation is more alluded to than explained in *Von der Pestilenz*.[54] More enlightening is the fragmentary and repetitive *De Peste Libri Tres*, dating from around 1535.[55] This treatise reaffirms the close kinship between the macrocosmic heaven and the microcosmic man.[56] It postulates the alliance between human beings and heaven in the production of the plague: 'the planet and man are one thing, not two, just as fire and wood are one'.[57] According to *De Peste*, heaven is the father of the human being and will not inflict disease on him unless it is enraged by man's behaviour, particularly envy, avarice, wars, lies and hate.[58] Indeed, Paracelsus clearly states that the birth of poison should be sought within ourselves, rather than in benevolent and pure heaven.[59] This statement confirms the change in Paracelsus's thought on heaven, already implied in *Von der Pestilenz*: while in *Super Entia Quinque*, the heaven contains and expels poison based on its own mysterious whim, here it is clearly described as a munificent being. Does this mean that we should now understand all diseases caused by the *ens astrale*, not just the plague, as actually inflicted by man's imagination? Logic would dictate it so.

Once again, we are told that the infection of heaven is done by the power of the imagination, which is described as an expulsive power.[60] Corrupt imagination ascends to heaven where it breeds the pest. We are once more referred to the Basilisk as a metaphor for how it is done, but this time the process is much clearer: human beings engender a 'heavenly Basilisk' (*Basiliscum coeli*) in heaven, which then projects it by means of its light rays unto the earth.[61] These plague rays are deemed extremely powerful; they are compared to swords that cause 'wounds', to sparks out of stone or to thunderclaps.[62]

The mechanism of pestilence is further detailed in *De Pestilitate*, a treatise that was deemed spurious by Sudhoff,[63] but is consistent with *Von der Pestilenz* and *De Peste* on the subject of the plague. It is also much more articulate on the mechanism of poisonous imagination.

Like the previous plague treatises, *De Pestilitate*'s logic is based on the macrocosm-microcosm parallel that is present throughout Paracelsus's work. First, the treatise maintains that in the universe, everything corporeal is generated by a heavenly seed that impregnates the matrix of water. Heaven, however, can also carry the seed of human imagination, which is a spiritual force. It does so because, *De Pestilitate* says, nature 'apes' man. Tradition had man 'aping' nature, but here the influence is the other way around. In fact, heaven copies what human beings do; the macrocosm follows the microcosm.[64] The sky reproduces the seed of human imagination, which it then implants into the waters, giving it life and corporeality.

In line with *De Peste*, *De Pestilitate* sees poison as a type of an 'occult sulphur' lying 'under the skin'.[65] This sulphur can be projected onto the stars. The sulphur in the stars is described as being of three kinds: 'arsenical', 'antimonial' and 'realgaric'. These sulphurs are transferred back to earth by means of the celestial rays, which infect the water and the earth, and subsequently human beings.

De Pestilitate further asserts that heaven is only one way of transmitting the plague. Contagion is also caused by human eyes.[66] According to the author, the eyes of human beings act like those of the mythical Basilisk, which was reputed to kill with its regard.[67] Here, *De Pestilitate* seems to transcend the context of *Von der Pestilenz* and *De Peste* since it bypasses heaven as a means of causing epidemic. This is complemented by a heightened emphasis on the role of witchcraft in the plague. In this sense, it elaborates on *Von der Pestilenz*'s implied association between the production of the plague and magic. The treatise proceeds to describe the figure of the *venefica*, the witch who poisons by using her evil imagination. This is in turn aroused by Satan.[68] In fact, *De Pestilitate* fully accepts the contemporary belief that witches contribute to the spread of the plague by manipulating putrefied reproductive matter.[69]

Clearly, then, Paracelsus's pest treatises reflect an increased emphasis on human agency in disease. Poison is a chemical substance, but in the case of the plague, it is found in the human body itself. From it, by the mechanism of the imagination, it is projected into the macrocosm. This reflects it as a mirror back unto other human beings, activating and propagating it in the form of epidemic.

Von der Bersucht (c. 1533/4, but probably earlier): continuity and change

Von der Bersucht und anderen Bergkrankheiten (*On the Miners' Sickness*) is a brilliant example of how Paracelsus applied and expanded on *Super Entia Quinque*'s twin theories of *ens veneni* and *ens astrale*. Sudhoff has proposed the tentative date of 1533 or 1534 for the authorship of the work. Nevertheless, there is scope to question this, as *Von der Bersucht* displays the *Super Entia Quinque*'s view of heaven rather than that of the pest treatises (of which the first is dated *c.* 1529/1530). An earlier dating of this work is also supported by the analysis of *Von der Bersucht* by Edwin Rosner.[70]

Expanding on ens astrale and ens veneni: poisonous vapours in minerals

According to *Von der Bersucht*, diseases of the element 'air', including the plague, are caused by the power of the stars.[71] The mechanism reflects the theory of the *ens astrale*: stars act by infecting a medium (no longer called 'M.' but 'chaos') with poisonous exhalations. Yet the attention of Paracelsus now shifts from the upper heaven and stars to subterranean earth. The treatise suddenly postulates that the upper heaven has a correspondent, inner heaven, inside the earth. As Paracelsus puts it, 'heaven and earth are two similar heavens, and the minerals and the stars are two similar stars'.[72] Thus within the earth, another 'chaos' can be found with its own 'stars': these are the minerals.

This was not the first time that Paracelsus has made the argument of the existence of other 'heavens' than the upper one. Indeed, in the chapter on *ens naturale* of *Super Entia Quinque*, he maintained that '[s]imilarly as the heavens are in themselves with their entire firmament and constellations, excepting nothing, so is man constellated mightily in and by himself'.[73] Here, the principle is the familiar one of the microcosm-macrocosm correspondence.[74] Yet by positing an upper and lower heaven, Paracelsus seems to draw here on the Hermetic-alchemical notion of 'as above so below', as well as the parallel notion of alchemy as lower astronomy present, for instance, in pseudo-Aristotle's *De perfecto magisterio*.

By positing this correspondence, Paracelsus can now extend the theory of the *ens astrale* and its poison to illness caused by metals and minerals in mines. He argues that, just like stars, minerals have their own area of 'influence' and act by emanating spirits.[75] A natural philosopher must know the characteristics of the earthly stars just as the astronomer must know those of the heavenly ones.

The emphasis, as in *ens astrale*, is on vapours and exhalations. However, Paracelsus now has to account for the possibility of ingesting the actual body of a mineral 'star'. He observes that eating a poisonous mineral like arsenic has a quicker impact than breathing in its vapours: 'whatever the body accomplishes in ten hours, the spiritus does in ten years'.[76]

The fact that the body of arsenic is such a strong poison might suggest that it should be cast away altogether as inimical to health. However, Paracelsus perseveres in his belief expressed in *Super Entia Quinque* (*ens veneni*) that everything has a good and an evil side. In fact, he now extends this view to argue on behalf of a special view of the 'like for like' cure. Thus, gold ore containing arsenic causes disease, but the same gold ore also hides the medicine for that disease, the *Arcanum*.[77] Thus, Paracelsus's 'like for like' principle should better be understood as a principle of complementarity: the same chemical that causes illness also contains the cure for it. The separation of the medicine from the poison is, of course, done by the art of alchemy.

Going further, Paracelsus observes that when a mineral is put in fire, it separates into a 'fixed' and a 'transient' body. The 'transient' body is its poisonous part. According to the *tria prima* theory, Paracelsus divides this transient body into the three principles of salt, mercury and sulphur. The sulphur (the 'fire') and the mercury (the 'smoke') cause diseases, as they mix with air and are breathed into the lungs. The 'adulterated' air dries up the walls of the lungs and then precipitates itself on them, causing various kinds of putrefactions.[78]

By comparison, Paracelsus seems to think that salt, whether in the transient body or as a whole substance, is generally good for health. Yet this affirmation becomes problematic when he names vitriol and alum amongst the salts. According to him, vitriol air 'has the same properties as salt in the brain, lungs and stomach'[79]; that is, it purges the internal organs of diseases. Even more, it contains *Arcana* against serious diseases like jaundice or overflow of the bile. It is surprising that Paracelsus does not address the obvious fact that ingesting vitriol is poisonous; instead, he only perceives the impure ores of salts as being so. Even then, the poison only affects human bodies externally, not internally.[80]

Poison as imperfect metals, minerals and gems

Up to this point, *Von der Bersucht* is based on the *Super Entia Quinque* framework of the *ens astrale* and *ens veneni*. Yet the third book of the treatise adds a new dimension to the discussion of poisons: a theory that originates, like *ens veneni*, from alchemy. Thus, Paracelsus maintains that metals that have not yet reached their 'perfection' contain poison.

The Swiss physician chooses to focus on mercury (quicksilver) as the archetypal poison. He argues that mercury's poisonous quality is due to the fact that it has not reached metallic perfection, that is, 'coagulation'.[81] In line with traditional alchemical theory, all metallic bodies have a preformed fluid state that precedes solidifying into the actual metal. Thus, Paracelsus explains, '[e]very coagulated metal has in it the type of mercurius'. We recognise here the medieval alchemical theory of mercury and sulphur as the origin of all metals. The conclusion is unescapable: 'every metal can arise from the *argentum vivum* by means of the vulcanic fire, as it is found and seen in its origins'.[82] Clearly, Paracelsus evokes here the theory of metallic transmutation, to which he gives a characteristically medical spin. While they are in their fluid state, metals are inherently poisonous. Once they become coagulated, they lose not only the poison, but also, paradoxically, their 'life': for instance, Paracelsus describes gold as a type of mercury that has been coagulated and is now 'dead'. The only metal that escapes this destiny is quicksilver, which remains fluid, alive and poisonous. The 'reason' for this anomaly seems to be a type of divine predestination since of all metals, it is easiest to prepare medicine out of quicksilver.[83]

Further, Paracelsus expands the theory of poisonous fluidity to stones and gems as well. They too have a liquid state that is dangerous to human health; indeed, he wonders rhetorically, 'if they were not coagulated, who would remain on the earth without an evil? That is, without disease?'[84] Human beings can only survive unharmed because most metals, gems and minerals can be found in a coagulated state.

Since quicksilver is the paradigm of his new theory, Paracelsus proceeds to analyse the poison that exists in this metal, and by extension, in all fluid metallic states. He argues that the essence of mercury is a certain coldness, or 'winter' that is opposed to the warmth of human bodies. Hence, its poison manifests itself by the shivering and chattering of the teeth.[85] The coldness of mercury drives the heat of the human body inward; hence, the heat becomes concentrated in central organs, where it triggers putrefaction. The result is serious disease: ulcers, consumption, paralysis, apoplexy, madness and others, depending on which organ the heat concentrates in. Paracelsus here observes that it 'would therefore be good if the mercurial physicians who prescribe mercurial medicines in the form of salves, fumes, precipitate, corrosive water and the like, would be better instructed concerning the nature of mercurius and would reflect upon it'.[86] The criticism of these physicians is implicit, but Paracelsus avoids polemics here. Instead, he focusses on medicinal recipes for mercurial diseases. The treatise is unfortunately unfinished; some fragments survived but do not add anything important to the discussion.

The theory of the liquid state of metals as being poisonous appears to move beyond the *Super Entia Quinque* framework. Still, it is interesting to note that there is some foreshadowing in the latter treatise. In the chapter on *ens naturale*, Paracelsus states that the humour of the *liquor vitae* in human bodies 'is an *Ens* in its own right and is the power which produces ores in the soil and in the body'.[87] In light of *Von der Bersucht*, this rather obscure statement suggests that Paracelsus already believed in the pre-metallic fluid state, which he associated with a living state, though at this time he did not necessarily deem it poisonous.

The liquid state theory represents a step towards accounting for the fact that the bodies of certain substances like quicksilver or arsenic are fundamentally poisonous. As we recall, in *Super Entia Quinque* and the pest treatises, Paracelsus defined poison idiosyncratically, as a subtle vapour that harms the human being. Yet he, of course, knew that some substances, like arsenic or mercury, are more harmful to man than others. His *ens veneni* theory does not really account for substantial poison since it considers all things as containing poison to some degree.

Consequently, Paracelsus moves towards a new theory of poison, which fuses the *ens veneni* theory with the concept of poisonous substances. Combining the two ideas results in something that can be called the 'potent poison' theory, according to which substances that have stronger poisons than others, like arsenic, also contain more potential for medicine. Indeed, in *Von der Bersucht*, Paracelsus expresses his belief that quicksilver contains within the key of a great art 'which expels both its own malady and other evils'.[88] Yet this view remains underdeveloped in this work and is better explained in his later treatises, particularly *Sieben Defensiones* (1538).

Curing with poison in *Sieben Defensiones* (1538)

Let us now review the *Sieben Defensiones* statement, the essay began with 'All things are poison, and nothing is without poison'. Clearly, this is a reaffirmation of the views expressed in *Super Entia Quinque* (*ens veneni*). That 'nothing is without poison' confirms the central theory of the *ens veneni*, according to which alchemy is the key to eliminating the poisonous part of substances. By 'all things are poison', Paracelsus also restates his theory of the imperfection of beings in relation with others, although he does so in a much more polemical and stark fashion than in *Super Entia Quinque*.

To this declaration, however, Paracelsus adds the following sentence: 'the *Dosis* alone makes a thing not poison'. This statement has been celebrated, rightly or wrongly, as the beginning of the modern science of toxicology.[89] Yet the concept of *Dosis* does not come into play in *Super Entia Quinque*, where the poison within all things should be fully eliminated, not dosed.[90]

In this sentence, Paracelsus is clearly no longer referring to the poison within things (the *ens veneni*), but to poisonous substances: 'I admit that poison is poison', he says.[91] Yet, as he puts it, 'every food and every drink, if taken beyond its Dose, is poison'. This affirmation suggests that he is trying to apply the *Super Entia Quinque* principle of 'all things are poison in relation with others' to dietary use. He maintains that, in some sense, the consumption of substances that we deem nutritive can become poisonous. We are not told why this happens, but we can speculate it is so because the 'alchemist of nature' in the stomach, is not strong enough to separate and eliminate the poison if too much of a substance is ingested. We may recall that, in *Super Entia Quinque*, the failure of the inner alchemist's digestion is given as a reason for disease; however, here this failure is much more clearly linked with the quantity of the food or medicine being consumed.

Intertwined with this discussion of *Dosis* is the 'potent poison' theory, only vaguely expressed in *Von der Bersucht*. In *Sieben Defensiones*,

Paracelsus is obliged to defend his medical use of poisons, so becomes more eloquent about this principle. What ordinary physicians deemed 'poison' he sees as potential medicine. Precisely because a dangerous substance is eminently capable of hurting health, it must be wondrously capable of restoring the human body as well: the power resident in the substance can be harnessed to good rather than evil. As Paracelsus puts it,

> Behold the toad, how poisonous indeed and detestable a creature it is: behold also the great *Mysterium* which is in it concerning the pestilence... For the *Arcanum* which is in the poison is so blessed, that the poison detracts nothing from it, nor harms it.[92]

The teaching is simple: poison is harnessed into medicine if alchemy is applied to it. The principle is still that of the *ens veneni*, adjusted to account for potent poisons.

Paracelsus further contends that Galenic physicians already know the close relationship between medicine and poison when they prescribe doses to patients.[93] Indeed, the logical implication of dosage is that if the dose is too high, poisoning occurs: this phenomenon Paracelsus interprets as a vindication of his theories of *ens veneni* and of potent poison. Overdosing reveals the poisons that lie hid within apparently inoffensive medicines. Paracelsus also points out that physicians already use small quantities of poison in their recipes. The eminent example is the *theriac*, a medicine that had been praised by Galen himself. An essential component of *theriac* was serpent venom, which acted as antidote to the venom present in the patient's body.[94]

On the other hand, the Galenic physicians are blamed as being inconsistent with their dosing principle. Paracelsus uses this opportunity to criticise once again the supporters of indiscriminate use of mercury, which 'know not the correction of mercury, nor its *Dosin*'.[95] As in *Von der Bersucht*, Paracelsus argues against understanding the principle of 'like cures like' simplistically, as 'poison cures poison'. One does not cure mercury poisoning by applying more untreated mercury to it. Poison that is not alchemically treated harms the body.[96]

Moreover, even when properly employed, the Galenic employment of dosage to 'correct' poisons is inferior to alchemy, which is solely able to eliminate them. Alchemy allows a physician to use powerful poisons like arsenic and vitriol and turn them into *Arcana* where no poison remains.[97] Arsenic, for instance, when treated with salt nitre loses its poisoning quality. An alchemist can similarly eliminate the poison in vitriol so only its sweetness, *Dulcedine* remains; this is the medical power hidden in the mineral.[98]

Conclusions

This analysis of several key treatises of Paracelsus (*Super Entia Quinque*, *Opus Paramirum*, the pest treatises, *Von der Bersucht* and *Sieben*

Defensiones) sought to show that the Swiss physician created complex and idiosyncratic philosophical theories around the notion of poison. The first, and most enduring theory, is that of the *ens veneni*, the universal poison in all things, first introduced in *Super Entia Quinque*. According to it, all beings are good in their essence but are not perfect in relationship with other beings. More specifically, a being contains both *Essentia* (good and nourishing) and *Venenum* (evil and poisonous). Paracelsus posited the existence of an agent, here called 'the alchemist of nature', and later *Archeus*, which separates the *Essentia* from the *Venenum*.

This theory remains a mainstay in the works of Paracelsus. In *Opus Paramirum*, it informs the theory of tartar disease as failed alchemical separation in the stomach. In other works, like *Von der Bersucht, Grosse Wundartzney* (1536) and *Sieben Defensiones*, the theory leads Paracelsus to reject a simple 'poison cures poison' principle in favour of careful segregation of the medical *Arcanum* from a poisonous substance. The 'potent poison' theory, where Paracelsus acknowledges the power resident in specific substances, does not diminish the explanative force of the *ens veneni*. On the contrary, it serves to heighten the importance of alchemy as the supreme key to unlocking powerful remedies.

Another important theory is that of the poison that resides within human beings. This poison is generated by negative emotions and manifested by a corrupt imagination. For Paracelsus, this inner poison hidden in the human spirit bears no redeeming quality. In fact, *De Pestilitate* puts this evil imagination in the context of Adam's Original Sin, which is described as a type of 'hereditary poison' that causes incurable diseases and cannot be eliminated by any physician except by Christ himself. The pest treatises' view of poison is highly anthropocentric since it shifts attention of medicine from natural factors to man-made ones. The Swiss physician's insistence on the ability of human beings to poison themselves and their environment would not be ignored by later medical practitioners.

We must acknowledge the fact that Paracelsus's view of poison fundamentally differs from our own. For Paracelsus, poison is chiefly a spiritual power or an active principle that is harmful towards human health. As he points out in *Sieben Defensiones*, '[p]oison is alone what turns out to the harm of man, what is not of service to him but injurious'.[99] True poison is not visible: it is a force visible only by its negative effects. Even when seen in substantial terms, it is perceived as a fluid or volatile being, such as a vapour, an exhalation or a liquid.

The present review of Paracelsus's poison theories can aid us to refine our view of the Swiss physician's philosophy. For instance, it furthers the current scholarly view that Paracelsus was keen on basing his natural philosophical system on Christian concerns.[100] Paracelsus's notion of poison reveals a specifically Christian approach to Renaissance thought. The first characteristic of this was an emphasis on the power of divine agency over the heavenly one; although, for instance, Paracelsus recognised both the *ens astrale* and the *ens Dei* as causes of disease, the power of the physician could only extend to the former. The second characteristic is the emphasis on human ability to cause widespread disease. This view, strongly affirmed in the pest treatises, describes human beings as eminently capable of infecting others and even the natural environment. The poison in human beings is evidently tied with the notion of the Original Sin. Consequently, the importance of piety, religious faith and the right use of imagination became highly important to Paracelsus's medical views and those of his followers. Finally, the recognition of the existence of poison in all things is combined with an insistence on God having made everything good and perfect in its essence. This should give food for thought to those that present Paracelsus as fundamentally a Gnostic.[101]

Another aspect that arises from the analysis of Paracelsus's poison theories is the depth and importance of alchemy in framing his medical and philosophical views. It is, of course, a well-known fact that Paracelsus was influenced by alchemy, but recent scholarship has highlighted the role played by other disciplines in the formation of his thought, particularly religion and magic.[102] Even Charles Webster, otherwise supporter of the importance of alchemy in Paracelsus's thought, has derived Paracelsus's 'homeopathic' principle ('like cures like') from his mining experience revealed in *Von der Bersucht*, maintaining that 'he was struck by the existence of beneficial and harmful substances in close proximity'.[103] From this, Paracelsus would have extended this insight to chemistry and medicine. In reality, as I have shown, *Von der Bersucht* is posterior and tributary to *Super Entia Quinque*, which expresses Paracelsus's theory of the dual existence of poison in all things in unmistakably alchemical terms. In turn, the homeopathic principle emerges as a system of complementarity between *Venenum* and *Essentia*. Moreover, his adoption of the homeopathic principle was conditioned by his alchemical experience, and as such was far more nuanced than it appears at first glance. As Paracelsus pointed out time and again, one does not simply cure poison with more poison; instead, the poison must first be treated alchemically to yield its medicine.

In the category of myths that should be completely eliminated stands the idea that Paracelsus advocated the indiscriminate use of mercury in medicine. This image of him emerged due to his involvement in the syphilis controversy, supporting mercury over guaiacum as the more effective cure for the disease. Yet in the syphilis treatises, he upheld a very mild use of mercury in comparison with the harsh prescriptions of his day; moreover, he was certainly not the introducer of mercury as treatment for syphilis![104] Instead, he recognised mercury as a powerful and harmful poison that was responsible for many diseases, and condemned those physicians who did not understand its nature. Paracelsus's advocacy of mercury as medicine was in turn deeply linked with alchemical practice: he viewed mercury as a potentially powerful medicine only after its 'Essence' was separated from its 'Poison' by alchemical means.

The general picture that emerges from the analysis of the poison theories is that Paracelsus's thought was highly complex and informed. Paracelsus is sometimes portrayed as an unlearned empiric, but the analysis does not support this view. *Super Entia Quinque*, which is after all one of the earliest Paracelsian treatises, shows that he treated the subject of poisons from a profoundly philosophical standpoint. He betrays familiarity with Scholastic philosophical distinctions and employs them to preserve the benevolence of God in the face of the empirical evidence of widespread poison. Similarly, in the pest treatises, he clearly reflects on the problems of the *ens astrale*, which not only presents heaven as unjustified originator of disease, but also sets too much weight on the role of stars in illness. His solution is to pass the blame of disease on human beings; in doing so, he manages to preserve the idea that nature is essentially good while accentuating the Christian nature of his philosophy. Such aspects confirm Paracelsus as a reflective, learned and subtle thinker.

Notes

1 Theophrastus von Hohenheim called Paracelsus, 'Seven Defensiones, the Reply to Certain Calumniations of His Enemies', trans. C. Lilian Temkin, in Henry E. Sigerist (ed.), *Four Treatises*, Baltimore: Johns Hopkins University Press, 1941, p. 22.

2 There was hardly any medical authority that Paracelsus left uncriticised; see, for instance, his attack on Galen, Avicenna, Pliny and Aristotle in Theophrastus Bombastus von Hohenheim, Paracelsus (1493–1541), 'Paragranum', in Andrew Weeks (ed.), *Essential Theoretical Writings*, Leiden: Brill, 2008, pp. 74–81. See Charles Webster, *Paracelsus: Magic and Mission at the End of Time*, New Haven: Yale University Press, 2008, pp. 113–117. Paracelsus famously burnt Avicenna's books in the public square at Basel, leading to his exile from the city.

3 Karl Sudhoff, 'Vorwort', in Theophrast von Hohenheim, gen. Paracelsus, *Sämtliche Werke*, 14 vols, I:1, Munich: R. Oldenbourg, 1929, pp. XXXIX–XLIV.

4 Andrew Weeks remarked this incongruity but did not challenge Sudhoff's dating; see *Paracelsus: Speculative Theory and the Crisis of the Early Reformation*, New York: State University of New York Press, 1997, p. 60.

5 Philippus Theophrastus Bombast von Hohenheim, Paracelsus gennant, *Der Bücher und Schrifften*, ed. Johannes Huser, 9 vols, I, Basel, 1589, pp. 60, 63.

6 Weeks, *Paracelsus*, pp. 68–69; Paracelsus does mention the five types of pestilence in his introductory remarks.

7 Theophrastus von Hohenheim called Paracelsus, 'Volumen Medicinae Paramirum', trans. Kurt F. Leidecker, in Owsei Temkin (ed.), *Supplements to the Bulletin of the History of Medicine*, Baltimore: John Hopkins University Press, 1949, p. 8, *Der Bücher und Schrifften*, I, 8: 'Ens ist ein ursprung oder ein ding / welchs gewalt hatt den leib zu regiren'.

8 Paracelsus, 'Volumen Medicinae Paramirum', 21, *Der Bücher und Schrifften*, I, p. 20: 'Dann / Gifft ist einer jedlichen krankheit angfang / und durch diese gifft werden alle kranckheiten / Leib unnd Wundt / nichts entschlossen'.

9 Paracelsus, 'Volumen Medicinae Paramirum', p. 21; *Der Bücher und Schrifften*, I, pp. 20–21. Walter Pagel, *Paracelsus: An Introduction to Philosophical*

Medicine in the Era of the Renaissance, 2nd edition, Basel: S. Karger, 1982, pp. 174–177, has maintained that Paracelsus's theory of the chemical origin of disease may have been influenced by Marsilio Ficino's work on pestilence.

10 Paracelsus, 'Volumen Medicinae Paramirum', p. 21; *Der Bücher und Schrifften,* I, p. 21: 'wissen / das ihr vergebens erfarend einer iedlichen krankheit sein sonderen ursprung / dieweil Ein ding sovil krankheiten macht'.

11 Paracelsus, 'Volumen Medicinae Paramirum', pp. 18–19, *Der Bücher und Schrifften,* I, p. 18.

12 Paracelsus, 'Volumen Medicinae Paramirum', p. 20; *Der Bücher und Schrifften,* I, p. 19: 'Die Astra haben ihr natur / und ihr mancherley eigenschafft: wie dann auff Erden die Menschen'.

13 Paracelsus, 'Volumen Medicinae Paramirum', p. 20; *Der Bücher und Schrifften,* I, pp. 19–20.

14 Paracelsus, 'Volumen Medicinae Paramirum', p. 22; *Der Bücher und Schrifften,* I, pp. 21–22.

15 Paracelsus, 'Volumen Medicinae Paramirum', p. 23; *Der Bücher und Schrifften,* I, p. 22.

16 Pagel, *Paracelsus,* pp. 174–177.

17 Paracelsus, 'Volumen Medicinae Paramirum', p. 24; *Der Bücher und Schrifften,* I, p. 24.

18 Paracelsus, 'Volumen Medicinae Paramirum', p. 25; *Der Bücher und Schrifften,* I, p. 24.

19 Paracelsus, 'Volumen Medicinae Paramirum', p. 33; *Der Bücher und Schrifften,* I, pp. 33–34: 'wer er allein beschaffen von wegen des menschen / und nit sein selbst auch / so bedörfft er der hörner nit / noch der bein / noch der flawen: wann darinn ist kein nahrung'.

20 Paracelsus, 'Volumen Medicinae Paramirum', pp. 25–26; *Der Bücher und Schrifften,* I, p. 25.

21 The classical treatment on the subject is by Etienne Gilson, *The Christian Philosophy of St Thomas Aquinas,* New York: Random House, 1956, pp. 29–45.

22 Paracelsus, 'Volumen Medicinae Paramirum', p. 29; *Der Bücher und Schrifften,* I, p. 28: 'Er scheidet diese böß vom gutten / Er verwandlet das gutt in ein Tinctur / Er tingirt den leib zu seim leben / Er ordinirt der Natur das subiect in ihr / Er tingirt sie / das sie zu Blutt und Fleisch wirdt'.

23 Paracelsus, *Der Bücher und Schrifften,* I, p. 24, also calls this essence 'the great nature' (*die gross Natur*). This terminology is repeated in *Sieben Defensiones,* where 'nature' is the force opposite to 'poison'.

24 Paracelsus, 'Volumen Medicinae Paramirum', p. 29; *Der Bücher und Schrifften,* I, p. 29: 'Essentia ist das / dass den menschen auffenthalt: Venenum das / dass ihm kranckheit zufügt'.

25 Paracelsus, 'Volumen Medicinae Paramirum', p. 29; *Der Bücher und Schrifften,* I, p. 25.

26 Paracelsus, *Der Bücher und Schrifften,* I, p. 26: 'Tugent, krafft / und kunst'. Leidecker has this as 'quality, ability and dexterity', which is less forceful; 'Volumen Medicinae Paramirum', p. 26.

27 Paracelsus, 'Volumen Medicinae Paramirum', p. 17; *Der Bücher und Schrifften,* I, p. 30.

28 Paracelsus, 'Volumen Medicinae Paramirum', p. 16; *Der Bücher und Schrifften,* I, p. 29.

29 Paracelsus, 'Volumen Medicinae Paramirum', p. 33; *Der Bücher und Schrifften,* I, p. 33.

30 This was not the first time the three principles made an appearance in Paracelsus's treatises; as Webster pointed out, they also appear in the *Elf Tractat, Von der natürlichen dingen, Von den ersten dreien principiis,* and *De mineralibus; Paracelsus: Magic and Mission,* 140–142. Yet it is *Opus Paramirum* that articulates the theory in its full and comprehensive form.

31 For a good analysis of the tartar theory, as well as Van Helmont's rejection of it, see Pagel, *Paracelsus,* 153–165.

32 Theophrastus Bombastus von Hohenheim, Paracelsus (1493–1541), 'Opus Paramirum', in *Essential Theoretical Writings,* ed. Andrew Weeks, Leiden: Brill, 2008, p. 517.

33 Paracelsus, 'Opus Paramirum', p. 517.

34 The process of formation of the *stercus* is described analogically as 'wood yields ashes; ash yields salt; salt yields the lapis [stone]; Paracelsus, 'Opus Paramirum', p. 519.

35 Paracelsus, 'Opus Paramirum', pp. 519, 521.

36 Paracelsus, 'Opus Paramirum', p. 525.

37 For instance, the 'Tatars' were blamed for spreading the Black Death; see, for instance, Ole J. Benedictow, *The Black Death, 1346–1353: The Complete History,* Woodbridge: Boydell Press, 2004.

38 Paracelsus, 'Opus Paramirum', p. 527.

39 Paracelsus, 'Opus Paramirum', p. 533.

40 Paracelsus, 'Opus Paramirum', p. 539.

41 Paracelsus, 'Opus Paramirum', p. 559.

42 This was also upheld in the foundational treatise 'Paragranum', in *Essential Theoretical Writings,* ed. Andrew Weeks, Leiden: Brill, 2008, p. 177: 'It must be understood that the human being does not poison the external [world], but vice-versa'.

43 Paracelsus, 'Zwey Bücher von der Pestilenz unnd Ihren Zufellen', in *Der Bücher und Schrifften,* III, 134: 'Im Himmel ist nie kein Pestis gewesen: Alle die ubernatürlichen kranckheiten entspringen in uns/ und seind ohne würckung eindringend durch den Himmel / in demselben generirt es sich / und falt auss demselbigen wider auff uns'.

44 Paracelsus, 'Von der Pestilenz', p. 134.

45 This was not a completely original view; as Anna Montgomery Campbell points out, some plague treatises attributed the epidemic to 'accidents of the soul' caused by intemperate emotions; *The Black Plague and Men of Learning,* New York: AMS Press, 1966, p. 77. See also Karl Sudhoff, 'Pestschriften', *Archiv für die Geschichte der Medizin* 7:2 (1913): pp. 96, 98.

46 Paracelsus, 'Von der Pestilenz', pp. 134–135. On this subject, see D.P. Walker, *Spiritual and Demonic Magic from Ficino to Campanella,* London: Warburg, 1958, p. 76.

47 Paracelsus, 'Von der Pestilenz', p. 135: 'Darum so gehet *Magica Imaginatio* von uns in ihn / von ihm wider auff uns'.

48 See, for instance, the excellent discussion of these views in Guido Giglioni, *Immaginazione e Malattia,* Milan: Franco Angeli, 2000, pp. 58–67.

49 Paracelsus, 'Von der Pestilenz', pp. 147–148.

50 Paracelsus, 'Von der Pestilenz', pp. 135–136.

51 Paracelsus, 'Von der Pestilenz', p. 136.

52 Paracelsus, 'Von der Pestilenz', p. 136.

53 Paracelsus, 'Von der Pestilenz', p. 138.

54 I am not focussing on *Von den Pestilenz ein Büchlein: Beschrieben an die Statt Sterzingen* (written around 1534), as this work mainly contains recipes for curing the plague.

55 Or could this treatise be simply another version of *Von der Pestilenz*, thus written around the same time?

56 Paracelsus, 'De Peste Libri Tres, cum quibusdam ipsius Autoris Additionibus', in *Der Bücher und Schrifften*, III, p. 153.

57 Paracelsus, 'De Peste Libri Tres', p. 154: 'Der Planet und der Mensch ist Ein ding / nicht zwey / gleich als Fewr und Holz ein ding ist'.

58 Paracelsus, 'De Peste Libri Tres', p. 156.

59 Paracelsus, 'De Peste Libri Tres', p. 162: 'Nuhn der Himmel ob uns / ist nit wider uns / sondern mit uns: Aber so wir den vergifften / so schütt er diese Gifft uber uns auß. Der anfang ist in uns / und alle falschen tücken in uns / und Untugend'.

60 Paracelsus, 'De Peste Libri Tres', p. 159.

61 Paracelsus, 'De Peste Libri Tres', pp. 163–164.

62 Paracelsus, 'De Peste Libri Tres', pp. 165, 169, 170.

63 Karl Sudhoff, 'Vorwort', XIV, p. XXXIII.

64 (Pseudo-)Paracelsus, 'De Pestilitate, Das ist / vom Ursprung unnd Herkommen Pestis', in *Der Bücher und Schrifften*, III, p. 47.

65 Pseudo-Paracelsus, 'De Pestilitate', p. 75.

66 Similarly, Paracelsus states that stars, particularly the Sun, and the Moon are the eyes of the macrocosm, and they too can infect the world below.

67 Pseudo-Paracelsus, 'De Pestilitate', pp. 76, 77.

68 Pseudo-Paracelsus, 'De Pestilitate', pp. 91–94.

69 Pseudo-Paracelsus, 'De Pestilitate', p. 92:

> Es ist auch zu Sanct Veyt und zu Villach erfaren / das solche Heren haben genommen die Erden unnd Staub vonn den Gräbern der Todten in der zeit der Pestilenz / und die zugericht mit ihrer Zauberkunst / unnd eine hefftige Pestilenz damit angerichtet / dardurch viel 1000. Menschen Inficirt und gestorben seindt.

70 Edwin Rosner, 'Hohenheims Bergsuchtmonographie', in Rosemarie Dilg-Frank (ed.), *Kreatur und Kosmos: International Beitrage zur Paracelsusforschung*, Stuttgart: Gustav Fischer Verlag, 1993, pp. 20–52.

71 Theophrastus von Hohenheim called Paracelsus, 'On the Miners' Sickness and Other Miners' Diseases', trans. George Rosen, in Henry E. Sigerist (ed.), *Four Treatises*, Baltimore, 1941, pp. 58, 59, *Der Bücher und Schrifften*, V, pp. 3–5.

72 Paracelsus, 'On the Miners' Sickness', p. 66, *Der Bücher und Schrifften*, V, p. 12: 'Himmel und Erden seindt zwey gleich Himmel / und die Miner und das Sydus seind zwey gleiche Sydera'.

73 Paracelsus, 'Volumen Medicinae Paramirum', p. 35; *Der Bücher und Schrifften*, I, p. 36.

74 On this topic, see Pagel, *Paracelsus*, pp. 55–56.

75 Paracelsus, 'On the Miners' Sickness', p. 65, *Der Bücher und Schrifften*, V, p. 11.

76 Paracelsus, 'On the Miners' Sickness', p. 69, *Der Bücher und Schrifften*, V, p. 15, 'das ist / was das Corpus zuwegen bringt in 10. Stunden / daran macht das Spiritus 10. Jahr'.

77 Paracelsus, 'On the Miners' Sickness', p. 72, *Der Bücher und Schrifften*, V, p. 18.

78 Paracelsus, 'On the Miners' Sickness', pp. 80–85; *Der Bücher und Schrifften*, V, pp. 26–31. Interestingly, there is no mention of the disease of tartar in this treatise.

79 Paracelsus, 'On the Miners' Sickness', p. 93; *Der Bücher und Schrifften*, V, pp. 38–39.

80 Paracelsus, 'On the Miners' Sickness', p. 94; *Der Bücher und Schrifften*, V, p. 39.

81 Paracelsus, 'On the Miners' Sickness', p. 104; *Der Bücher und Schrifften*, V, p. 50.
82 Paracelsus, 'On the Miners' Sickness', p. 104; *Der Bücher und Schrifften*, V, p. 50.
83 Paracelsus, 'On the Miners' Sickness', p. 107; *Der Bücher und Schrifften*, V, p. 53.
84 Paracelsus, 'On the Miners' Sickness', p. 106; *Der Bücher und Schrifften*, V, p. 52.
85 Paracelsus, 'On the Miners' Sickness', p. 114; *Der Bücher und Schrifften*, V, p. 61.
86 Paracelsus, 'On the Miners' Sickness', pp. 117–118; *Der Bücher und Schrifften*, V, p. 65.
87 Paracelsus, 'Volumen Medicinae Paramirum', pp. 44–45.
88 Paracelsus, 'On the Miners' Sickness', p. 105; *Der Bücher und Schrifften*, V, p. 51.
89 On this subject, see B. Diechmann, D. Henschler, B. Holmsted and G. Keil, 'What Is There That Is Not Poison? A Study of the Third Defense by Paracelsus', *Archives of Toxicology* 58 (1986), pp. 207–2013 (212).
90 Webster thinks that dosage was of limited concern to Paracelsus in comparison to chemistry and that 'Paracelsus was only to a limited extent the anticipator of the modern dose-response relationship, or of the homeopathic principle of serial dilution', *Paracelsus: Magic and Mission*, p. 150.
91 Paracelsus, 'Seven Defensiones', p. 22.
92 Paracelsus, 'Seven Defensiones', p. 21.
93 Paracelsus, 'Seven Defensiones', p. 22.
94 See Antoine Calvet, 'A la recherche de la médecine universelle. Questions sur l'élixir et la thériaque au 14ᵉ siècle', in Chiara Crisciani and Agostino Paravici Bagliani (eds.), *Alchemia e medicina nel Medioevo*, Florence: Micrologus Library, 2003, pp. 117–216.
95 Paracelsus, 'Seven Defensiones', p. 22.
96 Paracelsus, 'Seven Defensiones', p. 22.
97 Paracelsus, 'Seven Defensiones', p. 23.
98 Paracelsus, 'Seven Defensiones', p. 23.
99 Paracelsus, 'Seven Defensiones', p. 24.
100 This is obvious in the case of the recent treatments of Paracelsus, including Webster, Weeks and Ole Peter Grell's edited collection *Paracelsus: The Man and His Reputation, His Ideas and Their Transformation*, Leiden: Brill, 1998. This scholarship has sought to correct the views of Pagel and even Allen Debus, who set aside Paracelsus's religious views.
101 Walter Pagel was particularly keen on portraying Paracelsus as a Gnostic but based most of his arguments on the probably spurious *Philosophia ad Atheniensis*, 'The Prime Matter of Paracelsus', *Ambix* 9:3 (1961): 117–136. Pagel seems to have taken the original criticism of Thomas Erastus, Paracelsus's arch-enemy, seriously. It is true that Paracelsians found it difficult to explain *ad Atheniensis* in an orthodox fashion; see my article 'The Mystery of *Mysterium Magnum*: Paracelsus's Alchemical Interpretation of Creation in 'Philosophia ad Atheniensis' and Its Early Modern Commentators', in Caroline Vander Stichele and Susanne Scholz (eds.), *Hidden Truths from Eden: Esoteric Interpretations of Genesis 1–3*, Atlanta: Society of Biblical Literature Semeia Studies, 2014, pp. 141–162.
102 Recent scholarship includes Karl Möseneder, *Paracelsus und die Bilder: Uber Glauben, Magie und Astrologie*, Tubingen: Niemeyer, 2009, the edited collection *Paracelsus im Kontext der Wissenschaften seiner Zeit*, Berlin: Niemeyer, 2010, Jean-Michel Rietsch, *Théorie du langage et exégèse biblique chez Paracelse (1493–1541)*, Bern: Peter Lang, 2002, the books of Webster and Weeks, and articles written by Urs Leo Gantenbein, Hartmut Rudolph, Ute Gause, Heinz Schott and Dane T. Daniel. In these otherwise important works,

alchemy is secondary to other frameworks deemed more important to Paracelsus's thought, or integrated within them.

103 Webster, *Paracelsus: Magic and Mission*, pp. 148–149.
104 The Science Museum website, for instance, erroneously states that 'Paracelsus introduced new chemical substances into medicine, for instance the use of the metal mercury for the treatment of syphilis'. www.sciencemuseum.org.uk/broughttolife/people/paracelsus.aspx [accessed 1 December 2015].

6 Martin Luther on the poison of sexual abstinence and the poison of the pox[1]

From Galen to Paracelsus

Ole Peter Grell

In one of his many writings on marriage and in some of his statements on prostitution, Martin Luther turned to medical opinion to further and elaborate his arguments. In both cases, Luther was concerned with the dangers of sex: the lack of it in the first instance and the wrong kind in the second, both of which he claimed could result in the body being poisoned. In what follows, I shall seek to determine what precisely Luther's arguments were and from what sources he drew his inspiration.

Martin Luther wrote extensively about sexual desire and marriage throughout his life.[2] He had no doubt that God had ordained marriage as the natural estate for humans, as opposed to celibacy, which, in his opinion, could only result in fornication and social disorder. Luther, of course, had experienced celibacy and its effects first-hand, having spent a considerable part of his life as an Augustinian friar,[3] having joined his order in 1505. He was a mature man of 33 when in 1517 he started the Reformation by posting the 95 Theses. Eight years later, at the age of 42, he married a former nun, Katharina von Bora, as if to emphasise his total rejection of celibacy. As pointed out by Heiko Oberman, what made Luther's theology so appealing was not only its rhetorical quality, but also the connection he made between the 'Word of God and corporeality'.[4] This is an aspect that has recently been further elaborated by Lyndal Roper who argues that Luther's appeal cannot be separated from his physical presence. His theological views are in her opinion closely allied to his physicality, and as such fundamental to his rejection of monasticism with its loathing of sex, eating, and drinking. Otherwise, how could Luther have written: 'If you want to reject your body because snot, pus, and filth come out of it, you should cut your head off'?[5]

Luther was convinced that after the Fall, God had implanted an uncontrollable sexual desire in humans, which could only find release in intercourse. Such acts God intended for reproduction, and according to Luther, they should take place between married couples. The continuation of the species and the channelling of the sex drive constituted for Luther the main rationale for marriage.

Luther was adamant that sexual desire was natural and created by God, and he followed Augustine in so far as he linked the origin of sexual desire to original sin, but he differed from the church father in considering marital sex as a positive good in itself; not simply because sex led to procreation, but because he considered sex a good and pleasurable thing in itself, which served to increase affection between husband and wife, thus promoting concord in domestic life.[6] Luther referred to this in his sermon on Matthew 5:27–29 when he stated:

> Some people have argued and discussed in detail about whether it is a sin to desire a wife or husband in marriage, but this is foolish and against both Scripture and nature, for why should people marry unless they have desire and love for another?[7]

Sex could and should be enjoyable within marriage and not as had previously been the case, as Luther recalled it in his *Lectures on Genesis*, 'that before these times of revival of the Gospel husbands at confession frequently deplored conjugal fun as a most serious sin'.[8] In his pamphlet, *Against the So-Called Spiritual Estate*, from 1522, Luther emphasised the necessary and healthy power of sexual desire:

> A young woman, if the high and rare grace of virginity has not been bestowed upon her, can do without a man as little as without food, drink, sleep, and other natural needs. And on the other hand: a man, too, cannot be without a woman. The reason is the following: begetting children is as deeply rooted in nature as eating and drinking. That is why God provided the body with limbs, arteries, ejaculation, and everything that goes with them. Now if someone wants to stop this and not permit what nature wants and must do, what is he doing but preventing nature from being nature, fire from burning, water from being wet, and man from either drinking, eating, or sleeping?[9]

In 1522, Martin Luther published his sermon *The Estate of Marriage*. Luther divided his sermon into three parts. In part one, he considered who might enter into marriage with each other. In part two, he discussed who could be allowed to divorce. And finally, in part three, he considered how marriage could facilitate a Christian and godly life.

In this third part, Luther concluded that people who refused to marry 'must fall into immorality'. This was, according to him, a consequence of how God had created man and woman, namely 'to produce seed and to multiply'. The only way to prevent depravity and immorality was therefore marriage. For unless a person was granted special grace by God, he/she would naturally produce seed and want to multiply. Marriage, in other words, provided the only alternative to fornication and sinfulness. Those who claimed that they could manage to remain sexually abstinent without special grace from God were doomed. The Bible did not allow for sexual abstinence. Genesis 28 clearly stated: 'Be fruitful and multiply'. Sexual restraint was, in other words, impossible faced with God's ordinance and how He had created the natural world. For this, Luther referred to the Bible in general and Genesis in particular.

Luther then went on to support his argument by drawing on medical opinion:

> Physicians are not amiss when they say: If this natural function is forcibly restrained it necessarily strikes into the flesh and blood and becomes a poison, whence the body becomes unhealthy, enervated, sweaty and foul-smelling. That which should have issued in fruitfulness and propagation has to be absorbed within the body itself. Unless there is terrific hunger or immense labour or the supreme grace, the body cannot take it; it necessarily becomes unhealthy and sickly. Hence, we see how weak and sickly barren women are. Those who are fruitful, however, are healthier, cleanlier, and happier. And even if they bear themselves weary, or ultimately bear themselves out that does not hurt. Let them bear themselves out. This is the purpose for which they exist. It is better to have a brief life with good health than a long life in ill health.[10]

Luther, in other words, argued that according to medical opinion, sexual abstinence acted as a poison on the body, which consequently became weak, perspiring, and fetid. What had been designed to propagate mankind turned poisonous when it was retained. Luther, however, did not quote any specific medical authorities or physicians for his view.

The reformer would not have been able to find any support for his views of sexual abstinence as poisonous from most ancient medical authorities. Hippocrates supported sexual restraint but cautioned against sexual abstinence. He considered many female illnesses, especially hysteria, to be rooted in the womb, which, according to him, became dry due to lack of both male and female semen. For women, in other words, sexual intercourse was necessary for their health, which might be put at risk through virginity and celibacy. Men, on the other hand, were advised to show sexual restraint. For them, semen served to energize their bodies, and if drained away through too much sex, it could prove detrimental to their well-being.[11] Another medical authority, Epicurus, was seen as an advocate of sexual abstinence for both men and women, even if recent scholarship has portrayed him as less hostile to sex.[12] Another Greek physician from the second century AD, Soranus, argued that the body was weakened by sexual intercourse. Any discharge of sperm was detrimental to the health of both men and women, and both men and women who refrained from intercourse were healthier and stronger than those who had sex.[13]

Luther may well have read Constantinus Africanus, *De Coitu*, in either an early printed edition or in one of the many manuscript editions, which would appear to have been in circulation from the later Middle Ages onwards.[14] Its popularity is evidenced by Geoffrey Chaucer who referred to *De Coitu* in 'The Merchants Tale'.[15]

In the eleventh century, Constantinus Africanus, a Benedictine monk from North Africa, had been responsible for reintroducing knowledge of Galenic medicine into Europe via the Islamic world. In *De Coitu*, Constantinus stated that sexual intercourse was essential for human well-being. Citing 'the ancients', he pointed out that 'the things which preserve health are exercise, bathing, food, drink, sleep, and intercourse'. He then went on to elaborate how intercourse could be beneficial, when it should be performed, and what happened to those who had too much sex:

> Galen, following Epicurus, said in his book on the art of medicine: no one who abstains from intercourse will be healthy. Intercourse is without doubt beneficial and an aid to health; and Galen shows to whom it will do good and to whom it will not, and how it should be performed. For he tells when it should be done and at what intervals so that no bodily harm ensues. For if a sluggish and weak person has intercourse his body will feel more sprightly afterwards and his mind will be more cheerful. There is, however, a proper hour for intercourse, when the body is in complete outward harmony i.e. neither replete nor fasting, neither cold nor hot, dry nor wet, but well-tempered.[16]

Even if Luther did read *De Coitu*, it could not have provided him with the inspiration for the above-quoted paragraph from *The Estate of Marriage*. First of all, Constantinus's work was exclusively concerned with men, and despite its view of sexual abstinence as potentially detrimental to human health, it does not allude to its effects as poisonous.

One of the consequences of the Renaissance had, of course, been the renewed interest in Galen and Greek medicine and especially the original Greek texts. Humanists argued that the Arabic and medieval Latin translations of Galen could not be trusted. Instead, a return to the Greek sources was needed. In 1531, the physician Johann Guinther von Andernach, Andreas Vesalius's teacher, who translated Galen, expressed his joy of living at a time when medicine had been 'raised from the dead and the work of Hippocrates and Galen had been resurrected'. A not unsubstantiated claim when it is borne in mind that no less than 590 different editions of Galen's works were published between 1500 and 1600. The most important step in retrieving the unadulterated and original medicine of the Greeks was undoubtedly achieved with the publication of the complete works of Galen in Greek by the Aldine Press in Venice in 1525.[17] This, however, would have been published too late for Luther to consult when he was writing his sermon *The Estate of Marriage* some time before 1522.

Luther's view of sexual abstinence as poisonous for the human body had its inspiration from one of Galen's later works, *De locis affectis* (On the Affected Parts). Bearing in mind Luther's theological dependence on

Augustine and Augustine's view that semen had become poisoned at the Fall and served as the root of human sin,[18] Luther would undoubtedly have been attracted to Galen's view expressed in *De locis affectis*, where he sought to place the therapy of internal diseases on a rational footing by formulating a topographical diagnosis. Chapter 5, in the last of the six books which comprise this work, is of particular significance. It is noteworthy that this work by Galen was not among the required readings by medical students in the Middle Ages. It became popular in the sixteenth century, and no less than 25 separate editions were published during that century.[19] Luther is likely to have read it in one of the two known Paris editions which were published in 1513 and 1520, respectively.[20]

Galen concludes in book six, Chapter 5, that there is a clear link between female hysteria and the retention of female semen, and male melancholia and the withholding of male semen. The retention of semen proved a burden to women, whereas the situation for men was different. Some men, even when young, were 'enfeebled' by intercourse, while others who lacked regular sexual intercourse 'felt heavy in the head, become nauseated and feverish, have a poor appetite and bad digestion'. Citing Plato, Galen compared them with trees burdened with fruit. Galen personally knew a man who refrained from sex while grieving over the loss of his wife. He became unwell, lost his appetite and proved unable to hold down his food, and suffered from severe depression. He only recovered when he took up his earlier habit of frequent intercourse. Galen concluded:

> Scrutinizing these [observations] it appeared to me that the retention of semen does greater harm to the body than the suppression of the menstrual flow, [especially] in persons who have an abundance of poorly conditioned humors, who lead a lazy life, and who initially had indulged quite frequently in sexual relations but suddenly stopped their previous habit. I realized that in these patients their physical desire for seminal discharge was the cause [of the disorder], because all people of this type must ejaculate their abundant semen.[21]

Galen concludes that badly composed semen could seriously damage the body. He then refers to physicians who disagree with him on the dangers of the retention of semen, and who deny that 'a small quantity of humor in an isolated part of the body causes severe symptoms'. Galen dismisses them by pointing to the violent effects on people who have been stung by venomous spiders or scorpions despite the small amounts of poisons involved, and he concludes:

> Since it is evident that some substances have a very strong power, it is left to us to investigate whether an effect destructive for the organism can become so extensive that it attains a quality resembling the poison of a wild animal. Did not the physicians already offer an answer, when

they asked the single question whether or not typical signs exist for each poison?

Those who seem to have made the best analysis of this problem admit that identical signs arise by administration of a deadly poison as by disturbance [of the humors] of the body; also that those who took a poison were indistinguishable from others who failed to do so. When a person who had a healthy nature and led a normal mode of life dies suddenly, as it occurs by ingestion of a dangerous drug, and subsequently the body turns livid, dark and mottled, or the patient has diarrhea or acquires an annoying smell of putrefaction, then the physicians say a poison took hold of him. When, however, an affection involving our body originates inside and resembles the effect of the administration of a dangerous poison, then it is not astonishing that an abnormally composed semen or an equally abnormal menstrual discharge produces serious symptoms by stagnation or putrefaction in persons susceptible to such diseases.[22]

Comparing the above extracts from *On the Affected Parts* by Galen with that from *The Estate of Marriage* by Luther, the similarities are obvious even when bearing in mind the much shorter and generalised form they are expressed in by Luther. Luther only refers to this view as having been expressed by physicians without any direct reference to Galen or his *De locis affectis*; however, considering how the poisonous effects of sexual abstinence are described in both texts, it is difficult to imagine any other inspiration for Luther than this, then newly published, work by Galen. Likewise, Galen describes some men who did not have regular intercourse and consequently suffered from nausea, fever, and poor appetite, claiming with Plato that they were similar to trees overburdened with fruit. This comparison is embraced by Luther in *The Estate of Marriage* specifically when he refers to that which should result in 'fruitfulness and propagation', but being retained causes failing health and illness poisoning the body from within.

This, however, does not answer the question why Luther in his work on *The Estate of Marriage* included this paragraph drawn from the recently published text by Galen? Evidently, Luther was convinced that learned medical opinion added further valuable ammunition to his argument that marriage and sex was part of the divine creation and the 'divine ordinance' 'to be fruitful and multiply'. Furthermore, Luther remained convinced that health and sex were closely connected. In 1526, he referred to the case of woman he knew who had perished due to the lack of sexual intercourse. Accordingly, when his colleague and friend Justus Jonas was widowed in December 1542, Luther wrote to him a month later recommending him to remarry quickly to satisfy his sexual desire. Justus Jonas appear to have taken his advice remarrying four months later.[23]

Luther's emphasis on the value of marriage as the proper estate which God intended for most humans naturally caused him to condemn brothels and prostitutes in the strongest terms. From the late Middle Ages, most major cities in Europe had either dedicated brothels or areas of the cities where prostitution was permitted. City councils justified the existence of areas where sex could be procured for money by claiming that they served to protect honourable maids from the uncontrollable lust of young, unmarried men. This was an argument which could draw on the support of Augustine who had argued that if you did away with prostitutes, 'the world would be convulsed with lust' (*De Ordine*, II, 4). By 1500, the open toleration of prostitution was, however, already on the wane and restrictions on the clothing and mobility of prostitutes had begun to be introduced in most cities.

Thus, when it came to prostitution, Luther disagreed vehemently with Augustine, whom he otherwise admired. In his lectures on Genesis 19:9, published in 1539, he stated that existing brothels in larger cities should not be tolerated, because their presence was against the Law of God. The city councillors who publicly tolerated them should be considered heathens. He then proceeded to refute Augustine's argument for tolerating them by pointing out that licentiousness and fornication would not be reduced through prostitution. In fact, according to Luther, young men who frequented prostitutes were more, rather than less, likely to harass married women and virgins. Prostitution, in other words, served to make a community less safe for respectable women. Instead, Luther emphasised that God had provided better remedies for the sexual lust of young men, namely marriage. A godly government was therefore obliged to do its utmost to prevent prostitution, even if Luther admitted that despite consistent efforts on the part of the authorities to stop prostitution, it could probably never be completely abolished.[24] Together with other Protestant reformers, Luther's campaign against 'legalised' prostitution and brothels was increasingly successful during the sixteenth century. An early victory for the reformers proved to be the closure of the brothel run by the city council in Augsburg in 1532.[25]

Luther discussed the danger prostitution presented to young university students, in particular in one of his table talks:

> Against the whores and greasy students. Out of special hatred for our faith the devil has sent some whores to destroy our poor young men. Against this, dear children, I give you my fatherly request, as an old and faithful preacher, that you will certainly believe that the evil spirit has sent such whores here, who are scabby, scratchy, stinking, nasty and *infected by the pox*, as one can unfortunately discover every day. If only a good young man would warn his mates! For such a *pox infected* whore can poison ten, twenty, thirty or more of the children of good people, and thus is to be considered as a murderer, or worse, as a poisoner. Everyone should help those who are in such a poisonous dung-heap with true advice and warnings, as you wish would be done for you![26]

After commending the Elector of Saxony for his efforts to rid Wittenberg of prostitution, Luther added:

> And I must speak plainly. If I were a judge, I would have such a poisonous *pox infected* whore tortured by being broken on the wheel and having her veins lacerated, for it is not to be denied what damage such a filthy whore does to young blood, so that it is unspeakably damaged before it is even fully grown and destroyed in the blood [poisoned]. The young fools think that they must not hold out; as soon as they feel lust, a whore should be there![27]

By the beginning of the sixteenth century, the pox was a disease of epidemic proportions engulfing all of Europe. Initially known as the French disease (after the French soldiers who brought it to Italy), or just the pox, it later, in the nineteenth century, became known as syphilis after the title of a poem by Girolamo Fracastoro which was published in 1531 and gained widespread popularity.[28]

The disease quickly spread from Italy into northern Europe, and by the summer of 1496, it had reached the German Imperial cities of Frankfurt and Nuremberg. The Diet of Worms in that year declared the pox to be God's punishment brought about by contemporary blasphemy.[29] Despite the severe impact of the disease, both urban and territorial authorities proved remarkably reluctant to act. The disease was early on associated with sex and prostitution. In 1500, the Papal physician, Gaspar Torrella, concluded that the authorities 'should send matrons to investigate the disease, especially among prostitutes'. His view was confirmed by the Pisan chronicler Giovanni Portoveneri who was adamant that the disease 'spread through having sex with women who have these sicknesses and especially with prostitutes'. Many popular pamphlets were published which linked the disease with prostitution. However, this was not the only way contemporaries saw the disease as spreading. Many adhered to the 'contagion theory', while others saw the disease as rooted in corruption of the air which, among other things, affected people though poor diet, and yet others took the moral view of the disease as God's punishment for sins.[30]

Initially, university-trained physicians considered the pox to have been caused by everything from divine punishment, corrupt air, harmful stars, to bad life regime, either separately or in combination. Some physicians, however, conceded that the pox could be transmitted through contagion by contact, especially through sexual intercourse.[31] Others emphasised similarities to the spread of plague, pointing to the corruption of the air as a main factor. The professor of medicine at the University of Ferrara, Sebastiano dall'Aquila adhered to this theory, but accepted that the French disease could also spread through contagion, especially through sexual contact, persistent sleeping, or nursing.[32] There was, in other words, a wide variety of causations for the pox, which simultaneously demonstrates the openness of Latin Galenism as claimed by Jon Arrizabalaga, but also perhaps the desperate search for a better understanding of what caused the disease.[33]

Sexual transmission was one among a number of possible causes, and learned physicians offered a variety of reasons why the disease more often than not started in the genitals. Astrology played a significant role in connecting the disease with sex and some physicians linked the first outbreak of the pox to the conjunction of 1483 which took place under the sign of Scorpio. The Modena physician, Antonio Scanaroli, argued that the French disease only began in parts other than genitals in less than 3 per cent of cases. He was convinced that the disease was connected to the sexual organs, but not necessarily to sexual intercourse, pointing out that many 'virgin' children and old people who never copulated caught the disease in their genitals. However, a number of physicians considered the genital symptoms of the pox to be linked to sexual intercourse, but even so the issue remained in doubt. A variety of explanations for the French disease continued to coexist during the early sixteenth century, while the possible sexual nature of the new disease remained unresolved.[34]

The main preventative measures suggested by most Galenic physicians continued to involve the prescription of a regimen suitable for the patient's complexion in order to maintain the humoral balance. Some physicians who considered the pox an epidemic disease suggested ways to improve air and environment, but they also argued for sexual intercourse to be regulated. This in turn provides us with information about to what extent the French pox was perceived as venereal at the turn of the sixteenth century.[35]

Drawing on Arabic medical sources, many Galenist university physicians took the view that sexual intercourse was not only necessary for staying healthy and avoiding the pox, but that regular sex was absolutely essential as a therapeutic remedy against the disease. They considered the therapeutic benefits of sexual intercourse to be best in the morning. These benefits, however, were limited to the young, while the elderly were told to avoid intercourse altogether. Too much sex, however, might prove harmful and dangerous even for the young, especially when the air was corrupted. Thus, many university-educated physicians considered the regulation of sexual intercourse to be among the useful remedies against the French pox, even if some like Sebastiano dall'Aquila advised everyone to abstain from having sex to avoid catching the disease. This was mistaken and highly dangerous advice according to Natale Montesauro, professor of medicine at the University of Bologna. He advised that if men who were having sex regularly suddenly stopped, they imperilled their health and risked catching the pox, because the retained sperm might become poisonous and rot their genitals.

Some early modern learned physicians recommended their patients to maintain an active, but regulated, sex life, which they considered a central part of their therapeutic regimen for the pox. Even after they had caught the pox, they counselled them to continue to have sex. Others, however, underlined the risk of catching the pox by contagion, especially through sexual intercourse. Thus, the papal physician Gaspar Torrella admonished men to avoid having sex with pox-infected women, because he claimed that men were more likely than women to catch the pox by contagion. By contrast, the Tübingen professor of medicine Johann Widmann told men to avoid having sex with 'women covered with sores', and healthy women who had recently been involved with 'men covered with sores', or prostitutes.[36]

Even if early modern physicians linked the pox to sex, irrespectively of whether they considered the disease to be epidemic or contagious in nature, they failed to reach a consensus. Among those physicians who favoured contagion by contact, some warned against having sex with those already infected with the pox or suspected of it, while the significance attached to the value of regular, but moderate, sex caused others to advise patients who had caught the pox to continue having intercourse. Evidently physicians, despite linking the pox with sex, failed to reach any consensus on its causes, and as a result, a range of debatable and often contradictory medical advice was made available.[37]

The failure of learned physicians to come up with a cure for the French disease, which spread with epidemic speed across Europe, led others to suggest possible cures. Most famously, there was the German Protestant knight and scholar Ulrich von Hutten, who himself suffered from the disease for years and eventually died of it. Hutten wrote a tract about the pox, *De Guaiaci Medicina et Morbo Gallico* (On the Medicine of Guaiaci and the French Disease), published in 1519, describing the symptoms of the disease and its treatment with guaiacum wood. The wood of this tree grew in the West Indies, where the disease was supposed to have originated. There was no clear medical understanding about how it worked, but the fact that it was found geographically next to where the disease was thought to have originated made it seem appropriate even to some learned physicians. Hutten's pamphlet proved popular and was quickly translated into a number of European languages. Hutten himself vouched for the effectiveness of guaiacum and provided detailed advice for how it should be prepared before use. His decoction of guaiacum was not only an effective remedy for the disease, but could also be applied without the involvement of learned physicians who for years had failed to identify both the cause and the cure of the disease. In fact, Hutten's rejection of the authority of learned medicine was paralleled by his rejection of the authority of the Catholic Church in the religious domain.

Ulrich von Hutten's advice was quickly overruled by another outsider to learned medicine, Paracelsus, who not only rejected the use of guaiacum against the French pox, but also claimed it to be part of a conspiracy to fill the coffers of the wealthy merchant house of the Fuggers in Augsburg, who held a monopoly on the import of guaiacum. Paracelsus, however, was also opposed to all learned physicians and medicine, and rejected their claim to a monopoly. Real physicians, according to Paracelsus, were not produced by the universities with their reliance on books by heathen authors such as Hippocrates and Galen; instead, they were given a talent for medicine by God, thus making it possible for them to identify the remedies against different diseases which God had made available in the created world. That included not only the essences of plants which an alchemist like Paracelsus believed could be extracted though distillation, but chemicals too. In the case of the French pox, this meant the use of mercury. Mercury was already used externally for skin conditions by surgeons and alchemists, but to use it internally as recommended by Paracelsus as a remedy against the pox was novel. Paracelsus was aware that mercury was dangerous and potentially poisonous, but advocated its use in combinations and dilutions which made it less risky.[38]

Paracelsus had arrived in Nuremberg during 1528 after having fallen out with the medical establishment in Basle where he had briefly served as town physician. While in Nuremberg, he published a treatise on the French pox, *Von der franzosischen Krankheit* (On the French Disease) in 1529 and wrote no less than another eight works on the same topic.[39] He was, however, prevented from publishing these works by the authorities in Nuremberg, on the advice of learned physicians who wanted to bring a halt to his activities.

Paracelsus's medicine relied on a God-guided empiricism impervious to what he considered the sterile academic logic of university medicine. This was a Christian medicine, as opposed to learned medicine which drew on pagan authors such as Galen and Hippocrates. For Paracelsus, diseases had their own characteristics. He argued that the pox was a poison which occurred in connection with incontinence, promiscuity, and exuberance, which in his opinion had been endemic towards the last decades of the fifteenth century. People who were indulgent and permissive were particularly exposed to the dangers of the pox which, he pointed out, tended to develop on the back of other diseases, changing their symptoms in the process.[40]

There can be no doubt when reading the table talk by Luther cited above, that the reformer was advocating a Paracelsian view of the French pox as poison. The idea that whores afflicted by the pox spread the disease to young students by poisoning their blood was a Paracelsian interpretation of the disease and its origin. We can only speculate on how Luther encountered these ideas. He may, of course, have read Paracelsus's tract *Von der franzosischen Krankheit* (On the French Disease) or encountered such Paracelsian views through other sources. The fact that the reformer embraced Paracelsus's idea of the pox as poison is in this context of greater significance than how he encountered it. The fact that Luther and Paracelsus had both grown up within mining communities and consequently shared an instinctive hostility towards wealthy merchant-banking houses such as the Fuggers, who through their domination of the capital markets were able to control the mining communities, is significant.[41] Bearing this affinity in mind, we should not be surprised that Paracelsus, who was labelled 'Luther medicorum' by contemporaries, and who emphasised the similarities between his reforms of medicine and Luther's of religion, should have been able to shape Luther's view of the pox.

Luther's knowledge of and attraction to Paracelsian ideas would undoubtedly have been further facilitated by his interest in alchemy. Thus, Luther declared that he was attracted to alchemy, because it was the philosophy of the Ancients. He praised its economic value through melting metals and extracting and distilling herbs, but he was also drawn to its religious significance. It served him 'as an allegory and secret significance' of the Last Days. Like the fire of the alchemist's furnace which served to separate the dregs from the distilled substance, so God on the Day of Judgement would separate the ungodly from the godly with fire.[42]

It is noteworthy that Luther clearly found it unproblematic to deploy medical arguments from two very different and opposed medical systems, drawing freely on authorities such as Galen and Paracelsus to provide support for his religious and moral views.

Acknowledgements

I would like to thank my colleagues Helen King and Jon Arrizabalaga for their advice.

Notes

1 I have used the sixteenth-century term pox or French disease here rather than the term syphilis which only became commonly used for venereal disease in the nineteenth century; see J. Arrizabalaga, 'Syphilis' in K. F. Kiple (ed.) *The Cambridge World History of Human Disease*, Cambridge 1993, 1025–33; see also C. Stein, *Negotiating the French Pox in Early Modern Germany*, Aldershot 2009, 3–14.

2 See Martin Brecht, *Martin Luther. Shaping and Defining the Reformation 1521–1532*, Fortress Press, Minneapolis 1990, 90–95 and Martin Brecht, *Martin Luther. The Preservation of the Church, 1532–1546*, Fortress Press, Minneapolis 1993, 236.

3 Luther was a friar, not a monk as is often stated. As such, he was attached to an order, not a monastery, and was ordained to serve the Church in the secular world; see K. Hagen, 'Was Luther a 'Monk'?' *Lutheran Quarterly*, LXXIV, vol. 2 (2010), 183–85.

4 Heiko A. Oberman, *Luther. Man between God and the Devil*, New Haven 1989, 274.

5 Lyndal Roper, 'Martin Luther's Body: The 'Stout Doctor' and His Biographers', *American Historical Review*, (April 2010), 379–84.

6 See the chapters on marriage and the family and sexuality in Susan C. Karant-Nunn and Merry E. Wiesner-Hanks (eds.), *Luther on Women. A Sourcebook*, Cambridge University Press, 2003, especially 88–89 and 137–39. See also M. E. Wiesner-Hanks, *Christianity and Sexuality in the Early Modern World. Regulating Desire, Reforming Practice*, London 2000, 60–93.

7 Karant-Nunn and Wiesner-Hanks, *Luther on Women*, 145.

8 Ibid., 147.

9 Cited in Oberman, *Luther*, 275–76.
10 The Estate of Marriage, 1522, in Walther Brandt (ed.), *Luther's Works*, vol. 45, Fortress Press, Philadelphia 1962, 45.
11 Alaine Rouselle, *Porneia. On Desire and the Body in Antiquity*, Oxford 1988, 71 and Elizabeth Abbott, *A History of Celibacy*, Cambridge 1998, 198–99.
12 Jacqeline Murray, 'Hiding Behind the Universal Man. Male sexuality in the Middle Ages', in V. L. Bullough and J. A. Brundage (eds.), *Handbook of Medieval Sexuality*, Garland Press, New York 1996, 127 and Tad Brennan, 'Epicurus on Sex, Marriage, and Children', *Classical Philology*, vol. 91, no.4 (1996), 346.
13 Rouselle, *Porneia*, 72–73.
14 Monika H. Green, 'Constantinus Africanus and the Conflict between Religion and Science', in G. R. Dunstan (ed.), *The Human Embryo. Aristotle and the Arabic Traditions*, Exeter 1990, 68 note 64.
15 See J. Murray, 'Hiding Behind the Universal Man', 138.
16 Paul Delany, 'Constantinus Africanus' De Coitu: A Translation', *Chaucer Review*, vol. 4, no. 1 (1970), 59.
17 Andrew Wear, 'Medicine in Early Modern Europe, 1500–1700', in Lawrence I. Conrad, Michael Neve, Vivian Nutton, Roy Porter, and Andrew Wear (eds.), *The Western Medical Tradition 800 BC to AD 1800*, CUP, 1995, 250–56.
18 E. Abbott, *A History of Celibacy*, Cambridge 2001, 199.
19 Rudolph E. Siegel, *Galen on the Affected Parts. Translation from the Greek Text with Explanatory Notes*, Basel 1976, Preface.
20 R. J. Durling, 'A Chronological Census of Renaissance Editions and Translations of Galen', *Journal of Warburg and Cortauld Institutes*, vol. 24 (1961), 252.
21 Siegel, *Galen on the Affected Parts*, 184.
22 Ibid., 186.
23 Lyndal Roper, *Martin Luther. Renegade and Prophet*, London 2016, 297.
24 Lectures on Genesis 19:9 in Jaroslav Pelikan (ed.), *Luther's Works*, vol. 3, Fortress Press, Philadelphia 1968, 259.
25 Lyndal Roper, *The Holy Household: Women and Morals in Reformation Augsburg*, Oxford 1987, 89–97. Significantly Roper argues that the closure of the brothel in Augsburg was not related to any ambition to halt the spread of pox/syphilis.
26 Table Talk no. 4857 in Karant-Nunn and Wiesner-Hanks, *Luther on Women*, 157. I have replaced 'syphilitic' with *infected by the pox* in this translation.
27 Ibid., 158. I have replaced 'syphilitic' with *infected by the pox* in this translation.
28 Jon Arrizabalaga, John Henderson, and R.K. French, *The Great Pox. The French Disease in Renaissance Europe*, Yale University Press, 1997, 245–51; Andrew Cunningham and Ole Peter Grell, *The Four Horsemen of the Apocalypse: Religion, War, Famine and Death in Reformation Europe*, Cambridge 2000, Chapter 5, 'The Pale Horse: Disease, Disaster and Death'.
29 P. A. Russell, 'Syphilis, God's Scourge or Nature's Vengeance? The German Printed Response to a Public Problem in the Early Sixteenth Century', *Archive for Reformation History*, vol. 80 (1989), 286–307.
30 Arrizabalaga, *The Great Pox*, 34–36.
31 In what follows, I have been guided by the excellent article by Jon Arrizabalaga, 'Medical Responses to the 'French Disease' in Europe at the Turn of the Sixteenth Century', in Kevin P. Siena (ed.), *Sins of the Flesh. Responding to Sexual Disease in Early Modern Europe*, Toronto 2005, 33–55.
32 Ibid., 39.
33 Ibid., 42.
34 Ibid., 42–45.
35 Ibid., 45

36 Ibid., 45–49.
37 Ibid., 53.
38 *Arrizabalaga, The Great Pox*, 101–2. See also W. Pagel, *Paracelsus. An Intro-duction to Philosophical Medicine in the Era of the Renaissance*, New York 1958, 24.
39 C. Webster, *Paracelsus. Medicine, Magic and Mission at the End of Time*, Yale University Press, 2008, 14.
40 Pagel, *Paracelsus*, 139 and Arrizabalaga, *The Great Pox*, 104.
41 For Paracelsus see Stein, *Negotiating the French Pox*, 102; for Luther, see Roper, *Martin Luther*, 30 and 160.
42 See Tara Nummedal, '*Alchemy and Religion in Christian Europe*', Ambix, vol. 60, no. 4 (November 2013), 311.

7 Poisoning as politics
The Italian Renaissance courts

Alessandro Pastore

According to a traditional and long-accepted representation, the political framework created by the end of the balance among the Italian states in the late fifteenth century and the involvement of France and the Holy Roman Empire in the Italian Wars was the ideal breeding ground for a web of plots and conspiracies in which poison played a crucial role. The humanist Francesco Patrizi of Siena (1413–1492) wrote in his treatise *De regno et regis institutione* that discord and corruption are born from human greed and 'from this arise plots and conspiracies, murders, destruction, poisonings and those black plagues, which are wont to undermine all public and private establishments'.[1] Therefore, two of the causes of death considered by historians of medicine of the Early Modern Age – the plague and poison – were seen at the time as factors that altered and weakened the civil and political order of states and cities.

In the early nineteenth century, Marie-Henri Beyle (Stendhal) described the role of poison several times in his accounts of Renaissance life, above all with reference to papal Rome. In *Promenades dans Rome* (Walks in Rome), he recounts his lively discussions with Agostino Manni, an accomplished qualified chemist, about the poisoning techniques used by the Roman nobility in the Renaissance. They were most often adopted in cases of love-related jealousy, using *bagues de mort* (sharp poisoned rings, which took effect instantly) or other toxic substances that acted slowly but relentlessly.

As we know, Stendhal was fascinated by Italy as a land of great passions, and the subject of death inspired by love was certainly a fitting one for him. However, the chronological thread is lost among the interweaving of historically documented episodes and stories from the oral tradition that make up the *Promenades*. Indeed, the pinnacle of the practice of poisoning is variously given as the sixteenth and mid-seventeenth centuries. In any case, although detailed knowledge of poisons was still widespread in the mid-eighteenth century, the art was no longer practised in the top echelons of society at the time of Stendhal's stay in Rome and was only documented in episodes of common criminality.[2] The pivotal element in his account was the emphasis on the contrast in Renaissance Italy between the 'highly refined civilizations' and the regularity of 'atrocious crimes, merciless vendettas [...] repugnant vices'. Stendhal was not able to explain this combination in a convincing way, but it formed part of his notion, applied equally to the present and past, of the 'Italian soul' and the decadence of the peninsula, which were reflected in the 'image of a bloodthirsty and immoral society in Rome'.[3]

Thirty years or so later, Jacob Burckhardt's fascinating writings bequeathed a similar impression: a muddled picture of a phase of Italian history packed with plots and conspiracies aimed at eliminating opponents, sometimes quite openly and sometimes in hidden ways. Together with the dagger, poison was the favourite instrument of death, and the main targets were political exiles who were hostile to the power of the princes.[4] The papal court was once again at the heart of many of these plots in the fifteenth and sixteenth centuries: as Burckhardt wrote, 'those whom the Borgias could not assail with open violence fell victims to their poison'.[5]

The plentiful case records of the time also mentioned the presumed death of Alexander VI, the Borgia Pope, from arsenic, which was emphatically defined as 'the prince of poisons, the poison of princes'.[6] We shall take the rumours surrounding Alexander VI's demise as our starting point. What is available to us is not the reality of the facts, but the circulation of gossip and beliefs that did not necessarily have any foundation. Indeed, medical analysis of the symptoms documented in sources at the time established the causes of the pontiff's death as pathological rather than criminal, probably due to an attack of malaria complicated by heart problems.[7] The most authoritative reconstruction of the sensational event focuses above all on the range, over and above the foundation, of the rumours and opinions that spread immediately after his death and were documented in chronicles at the time. These rumours said that the Pope's son, Cesare Borgia, who had created his own state between Romagna and the Marches, had aimed to use the poison to eliminate a rich cardinal, but that the Pope ate the food or drank the wine not intended for him, either by mistake or out of greed.[8] It was therefore a two-way question; victims may also have played an active role in the use of poison or at least in the threat to use it.

The issue of poisoning and its use for political purposes forms an integral part of the focus on conspiracies and plots in recent historical literature, just as it did in the past. To this end, it is fitting to quote a passage from *Discorsi* (Discourses on Livy) by Niccolò Machiavelli, in which the author dwells on the use of poison:

> This is all that occurs to me to say on the subject of conspiracies. If I have noticed those which have been carried out with the sword rather than those wherein poison has been the instrument, it is because, generally speaking, the method of proceeding is the same in both. It is true, nevertheless, that conspiracies which are to be carried out by poison are, by reason of their uncertainty, attended by greater danger. For since fewer opportunities offer for their execution, you must have an

understanding with persons who can command opportunities. But it is dangerous to have to depend on others. Again, many causes may hinder a poisoned draught from proving mortal; as when the murderers of Commodus, on his vomiting the poison given him, had to strangle him.[9]

In this way, Machiavelli underlined the elements of weakness in poison-based conspiracies, with the risk of betrayal by the accomplices who procured the toxic substance and an uncertain outcome if the poison proved not to be lethal. Failure was also often the result of the network of accomplices being unable to fulfil their role of providing support to the leading player rather than betrayal by the suppliers of the poison.

The fact remains, however, that the history of the Italian Renaissance is full of poison conspiracies, or at least constant and repeated rumours on the matter. As the Florentine Ambassador in Rome, Francesco Vettori, said, 'it is almost always said of great men', whether laymen or clergymen, that their death was due to poison, 'especially when they die of an acute illness'.[10] One such example is the (alleged) attempt to eliminate Emperor Rupert of Bavaria by the Duke of Milan, Gian Galeazzo Visconti, in 1401, an event which was interpreted in the light of the hostile political situation between Milan and Florence. Visconti is said to have acted with the complicity of a court doctor, who intended to achieve his goal by using an enema rather than the traditional contamination of food or drink. The main source regarding this episode, a report by the Florentine Bonaccorso Pitti, underlined the author's merits in having warned the Emperor about the risks of poison. In reality, he falsely accused Visconti of intent to murder, as he wanted Rupert of Bavaria to adopt a hostile attitude towards Milan.[11]

In general, though, diplomatic correspondence and diaries of chroniclers in this period provide accounts of episodes featuring suspicions, fears and denunciations concerning poisoning. We can highlight a few episodes from these vast case records that illustrate both the rumours that were spread and the fact that they were frequently unfounded. For example, although the death of Bianca Maria Visconti, widow of Francesco Sforza, the Duke of Milan, in 1468, was attributed to poisoning by a chronicler at the beginning of the sixteenth century ('it is said that she died more from poison than natural illness'), the most reliable reconstruction, conducted on the basis of court correspondence and letters from doctors in the Duchess's service, suggests that she died simply due to her worsening health. As we know, every retrospective diagnosis is made difficult by the lack of precise indications of the symptoms, but letters from the doctors involved focus on a disease of the respiratory tract complicated by acute dysentery in the last weeks of life.[12] In keeping with the spirit of the times, there is also the news provided a few decades later by the Venetian Ambassador in Milan that King Louis XII of France harboured serious fears of death by poisoning in Milan from conspiracies by local plotters.[13] This is the beginning of the political myth of the Italian traitor and poisoner that earned a significant reputation in French culture in the Early Modern Age.

In 1498, Luca Landucci, a chronicler and apothecary, reported that two gentlemen who had planned to poison the Duke had been beheaded in Milan. In the following year, Caterina Sforza, the Lady of Forlì, was accused of having inspired an attempt to poison ('atosegare overo amorbare') Pope Alexander VI. The rumour that spread said that Cardinal Raffaele Riario was also involved in the plan. However, the alleged material authors (who were 'two soldiers dressed as peasants' who had 'different kinds of poison on their person') were stopped in Rome and imprisoned in Castel Sant'Angelo. Whether or not the accusation was founded, it is certainly true that Caterina Sforza's private recipe book of so-called 'pharmaceutical and cosmetic experiments' featured remedies against the plague and poison, including an antidote for neutralising a 'poisoned sword'; this mixture of figs and walnuts was supposed to be able to absorb the toxic substance and thus remove it from the sword.[14] Less than twenty years later, Riario made an attempt on the life of Pope Leo X, this time with the agreement of two cardinals (Alfonso Petrucci of Siena and Raffaello Sauli of Genoa). According to the rumours that reached a Florentine artisan, who recorded them in his chronicle, their aim was the good of the Church (indeed, for the supporters of the conspiracy, the death of the Pope would have benefited the 'health of all Christianity'). Their chosen weapon was a 'poisoned *trafiere*' (a pointed dagger), which Cardinal Petrucci wanted to use in person against the Medici Pope.[15] To give another example, a recent study by Elena Bonora[16] has brought to light the details of a conspiracy to assassinate Pope Pius IV, discovered in 1564. The death sentence handed down for the attempted crime of *lèse-majesté* states that the conspirators were armed with a sword and a dagger soaked in a 'poisonous juice'. Aside from the legitimacy and the reliability of these accusations (the British scholar Kate Lowe has analysed the distinction between documented conspiracies and spurious or imagined conspiracies[17]), it is significant that the detail of the poison is underlined in letters between Rome and the Italian and European courts that conveyed political information and the rumours in circulation. Furthermore, the conspiracy with the combined use of a sword and poison against Pope Pius IV fuelled the tensions and disputes within the Roman Curia and in relations between the papacy and Spain. The detailed commentaries provided in the last two examples (the preparatory stages for the murder, the plans to put it into practice and the consequences suffered by the conspirators) are an important indicator of the spread of rumours from the Curia that first circulated around Rome and then reached other Italian cities either by letter or word of mouth.[18] This means of spreading news is widely documented in numerous cases.[19]

The criminal justice files also cast significant light on the causes of the suspicious death of prominent political figures. In 1535, the court of the Governor of Rome ordered the arrest and interrogation of Giovanni

Andrea Franceschi of Borgo San Sepolcro after the dubious death of Cardinal Ippolito de' Medici, for whom he worked as a *scalco* (a kind of banquet manager).[20] In the end, Franceschi's gradual admission of guilt, which was partly obtained through the use of torture, clarified that the poisoning was not a response to the Cardinal's criticism of the work of his servant, but was linked to the plots of Duke Alessandro de' Medici,[21] who had promised to provide a helping hand up the career ladder to whoever managed to eliminate Cardinal Ippolito. Franceschi's replies show that there were actually two poisons. The first of these was a yellowish white powder, bought from an apothecary outside Rome and kept hidden by the accused in his codpiece, the item of male clothing that contained and accentuated the genitals. The other poison was greenish in colour and kept in a phial. The two substances were then mixed into a soup of broth and bread, and taken to the powerful prelate's dining hall, where it achieved its expected result, despite the successive administration of antidotes (oil and *terra sigillata*, or 'sealed earth'). Cardinal Ippolito realised the strength of the poison he had ingested when he said to the doctor who was trying to save his life: 'Give me whatever you want, but I think it'll be of little use if it comes from Florence'. He was probably alluding to the instigator of the act of poisoning and, at the same time, to the in-depth knowledge of poisons that was said to be widespread in the Tuscan city. The doctors who were present confirmed that the external signs found on the body revealed a non-natural origin. One of them, Francesco da Norcia, stated that the cause of death was to be attributed to a poison for killing mice, probably arsenic, whose appearance corresponds to the previously mentioned whitish powder. Earlier, another doctor, Giovan Battista Teodorici, had provided an accurate description of the symptoms exhibited by the prelate and suggested that they could be attributed to a poison, although he lacked any certainty with regard to the substance used.[22]

The report by the doctors selected as experts and the testimonies of witnesses state that the body was dissected. The internal organs were removed (intestine, kidneys, liver, spleen, stomach and lungs), and the abdominal cavity was filled with salt, lime, aloe and myrrh so that it could be transported to Rome. The coffin was left open in the church of San Sebastiano, but there was no further investigation into the cause of death because of the intolerable stench that emanated from the clergyman's body. It was impossible to observe the human remains with diligence, as doctors and surgeons were afraid of somehow being infected and consequently dying from the effects of the same poison. This is a significant observation, as it highlights the close connection between the conveyance of poison and contamination by the plague. It was thought that the latter was favoured by bad odours and could therefore also be fought by burning perfumed substances.[23]

As we have seen, the recurring frequency of poisonings generated a stereotype that in all probability went beyond the reality of the facts, but in any case influenced episodes associated with political plots of varying degrees of organisation. In the mid-seventeenth century, a conspiracy to kill Pope Urban VIII gave rise to a trial in which the presumed culprit confessed under torture that the means prepared to eliminate the pontiff had included a poisoned host that was going to be offered to him during Mass. It has been noted that this admission was unrealistic and connected to typical themes of the time.[24] However, it is more important to identify and analyse the reactions to what was believed to have happened than to ascertain the authenticity of such tales.[25] It is not always easy to distinguish between the two levels, also because poison and poisoning found a platform in the fables ('fole'), rumours and convictions that were in common circulation. This genuine form of 'popularis persuasio' (popular belief)[26] is substantially confirmed by a current study of trials for poisoning held in Bologna between the Late Middle Ages and the Early Modern Age.[27]

While the use of toxic substances for political as well as private purposes was undoubtedly widespread in the Italian Renaissance, there were even more frequent occasions on which rivals falsely accused each other of poisoning. We therefore need to proceed with extreme caution on the matter, although we should stop short of believing that the use of poison for murder was only part of the imaginary realm. As a late-nineteenth-century scholar wrote about a case of poisoning in the early fifteenth century, 'in a corrupt age, the attribution to others of a crime that many are capable of becomes much more credible'.[28] The English traveller Fynes Moryson expressed this awareness that criminal cases in which death was obtained or sought using secret techniques were not only the subject of public interest, but also contributed to the construction of the myth of poison and poisoning. When visiting Italian cities at the end of the sixteenth century, he left the following succinct comment:

> Historyes pleasant to reade, and of good use to observe, but I will not inlarge them here, because in this worke I have formerly related the last of them falling in our age, and both are otherwise famously knowne in historyes and the mouthes of living men.[29]

These 'historyes' and 'mouthes', or written statements and popular hearsay, are the two channels that helped to form and consolidate the reputation and stereotype of poison conspiracies.

The combination of the closely interrelated verbal and written information processes emerges in the story of the illness and death of the English cardinal Christopher Bainbridge in 1514, after five years at the Roman Curia of first Julius II and then Leo X. The reconstruction of the event highlighted the fact that even the official correspondence gave importance to the rumours ('it is thought', 'some say that it was poison', etc.) that attributed the Cardinal's death in suspicious circumstances to toxic effects, as well as the death of other members of the Roman Curia too. In the case in question, the time calculated between the supposed ingestion of the poison in a soup and the time of death was not convincing. However, the supposed material perpetrator of the murder (a priest from Modena) committed suicide 'with a small kniff that he had secrett', revealing to the surgeon who helped him that he had acted by order of another prelate. In the end, the complex material interests linked to the archbishopric of York, of which Bainbridge was the title-holder, prevented the Cardinal's loyal secretary from formulating a concrete charge against the suspected proponent of the crime.[30]

In addition to the secret agreements to organise poisonings and the methods established by those in power to identify the material authors of the crimes and strike back at their instigators, there is a third important element that we have to consider to complete the picture: the knowledge and study of toxic substances and, at the same time, the antidotes that could counter their effects. At the beginning of the sixteenth century, a leading prelate in the Roman ecclesiastical hierarchy, Cardinal Ferdinando Ponzetto, published a treatise on poison. He wrote that he had consulted books of medicine to learn the necessary methods and remedies to combat the effects of different poisons, also in relation to the difficulties, pitfalls and dangers of public and private life at the time. In terms of prevention, the prelate suggests checking the colour of food and drink which might have been tampered with by the addition of toxic substances (for example, a white colour can be attributed to the presence of arsenic or a green colour to the addition of monkshood or oleander). Knowledge of poisons was therefore an instrument of effective caution against their effects at a time when those in power were often considered to be at risk of death.[31]

The network and exchange of information was duly designated to the knowledge of experts. For example, in 1472, the doctor Battista Massa gave Ercole d'Este a copy of his treatise, *De venenis*, so that the Duke of Ferrara could learn how to look out for dangerous substances.[32] The attention that courts devoted to the issue of poison is effectively documented by the experiments commissioned by princes, popes and cardinals, who entrusted their chosen doctors with condemned men before execution, so that they could be subjected first to the administration of poisons and then of the supposed antidotes. Condemned men that survived could hope to be pardoned. In this way, in 1539, Cardinal Benedetto Accolti was given a servant sentenced to hang by Ercole II d'Este to subject to his experiments, while Cosimo I de' Medici had a number of condemned men poisoned with arsenic or aconite, two of whom survived and were then pardoned.[33]

We shall now return to Jacob Burckhardt. He linked the criminal use of poisonous substances to the construction of a strong independent image of the Italian Renaissance, 'where individuality of every sort attained its highest development', and he confirmed the presence of 'absolute wickedness which delights in crimes for their own sake, and not as means to an end, or at any rate as means to ends for which our psychology has no measure'.[34] Nevertheless, Burckhardt was well aware that it was always necessary to assess historical sources with a critical eye, above all with regard to interpretations that amplified practices where the crime was hidden by poison. This emerges from one of his precise observations: 'the proportion which mineral and vegetable poisons bore to one another cannot be ascertained precisely'.[35] The German historian Ferdinand Gregorovius was also against hurried judgements that saw the Borgias as a 'pack of beasts that are ferocious by nature'; he felt that as they were princes of their time, they therefore 'used poison and the dagger ruthlessly and heinously; they wiped out everything that seemed to go against their interest'.[36]

On the other hand, although Burckhardt's perspective featured an overall moderate judgement about controlling testimonies, it was rooted in an older tradition that had been formulated in ways that were also more vivid and clear-cut. In the mid-seventeenth century, the French scholar Guy Patin, a doctor with links to Gabriel Naudé's libertine coterie, stated that Italy was still a 'country of syphilis, poisoning and atheism'.[37] These three crucial elements attributed to the character and behaviour of the Italians are connected to the spread of a negative political myth about the inhabitants of the peninsula. Therefore, according to Patin, the significant point is the link between free sexual mores, the lack of authentic religious faith and the widespread recourse to the physical suppression of counterparts using the lethal techniques of poison.

Voltaire's thinking on the subject in *Essai sur les moeurs* was more articulate and complex. In a phase of European civilisation before the high point of Louis XIV's France, the author offered an image of Renaissance Italy based on a combination of mutually contradictory characteristics (*esprit* and superstition; atheism and devotion), but which nevertheless highlights the central role played by another element, namely 'poisoning, assassination'. However, with Voltaire, the trembling indignation of the Enlightenment Age polemicist was restrained by the critical spirit of the historian. Therefore, although he recognised the reality of 'episodes of absurdity and horror' that happened in Alexander VI's Roman Curia, he was equally critical of those who exaggerated the scope of the Borgias' criminal activities.[38]

In any case, the rumours generated widespread fears, and the Early Modern Age was thus familiar with the terror of poison among its many other trepidations.[39] Fear is an emotion which provoked widespread reflection: in his *Essais*, Michel de Montaigne pondered over the impulses that trigger this 'strange passion' and mentions the opinion of physicians on fear that 'there is no other whatever that sooner dethrones our judgement from its proper seat' and generates 'terrible astonishment and confusion', even among those who normally show sangfroid.[40] While the fear of poison was widespread in almost every social class, it was above all men of state and the ruling class who suspected that they had been poisoned. Back in the Middle Ages, Pietro d'Abano noted that kings, prelates and noblemen had reason to fear poison, while Francesco Petrarca observed that poverty was the best antidote against poison. He felt that poison was the weapon of the rich and powerful who lived in luxury and used jewel-encrusted gold vases, but was not found in places where earthenware crockery was used.[41] As we have seen, testimonies in the Renaissance became more frequent and more concrete, to the point where they occupied a regular place in political as well as medical discourse. The French surgeon Ambroise Paré noted that prelates and holders of ecclesiastical benefits were most liable to fear being victims of poisoning by those who wanted to procure their sizeable revenues.[42] In Paolo Cortese's *De cardinalatu*, dedicated to Pope Julius II, a text which is comparable in literary terms to *Cortegiano* by Baldassar Castiglione, the author provides advice and rules for cardinals, including an exhortation for care and prudence against the risks of poisoning. Above all in a city like Rome, the longing for wealth and honours and the desire to take revenge for insults were a constant lurking presence. It was therefore necessary to be able to identify different types of toxic substances in order to counter their effects and also have suitable materials for 'recognising' poisons, even though the most effective protection was still to surround oneself with loyal family members and servants.[43] The main danger was in the dining hall, with food and drink that could have been tampered with shrewdly and secretly, either while it was being prepared or brought to the table of the rich and powerful man. Caution required the adoption of two possible solutions: tasters who tested food, drink and medicine on themselves before giving them to their master, and *probae*, or substances that were believed to react when placed in close proximity to poison. It was thought that certain precious stones such as emerald and coral, as well as deer antlers, teeth of various real or imaginary animals and dried snakes' tongues would change colour or generate dampness in such circumstances.[44]

The dining halls and kitchens of princes and other important figures were the places favoured by their internal or external enemies for putting their plans to eliminate them into practice. It was not only visitors to Italian courts, but also doctors from every part of Europe who exhorted people not to undervalue the danger of intoxicated food and drink concealed behind refined aromatic delicacies.[45] At the end of the sixteenth century, when dedicating his work on poisons to Cardinal Decio Azzolini, the physician Andrea Bacci mentioned not only that men of power were in danger of being exposed to a cruel death inflicted by poison, but also that they should pay due attention to the problem on official trips and during contact with foreigners.[46]

Different reasons were given to explain the use of these means that were brutal but silent, and painful but hidden, used to kill others as well as take one's own life. General categories were established that characterised each time, such as the intrinsic cruelty of the individual, or reference was made to the 'wickedness of the present times'. The Florentine historian and scholar Benedetto Varchi used the latter explanation to account for the decision to terminate the life of Luisa Strozzi with a dose of 'corrosive poison' in 1534. The choice was made by the woman's relatives, who suspected her of having amorous relations with Duke Alessandro de' Medici, who was hostile towards the Strozzis. In Varchi's opinion, this was a 'barbarous and cruel' act, both because it was only fuelled by suspicions devoid of any conclusive evidence and because the poisoning involved the ignominious act of staining hands with family blood.[47] In any case, the ease with which princes, cardinals and men of court adopted secret methods to eliminate personal enemies and public opponents remained a characteristic element of the representation of life in the Italian Renaissance, in accordance with the interpretation put forward in 1860 by Jacob Burckhardt in *The Civilisation of the Renaissance in Italy*. It has recently been underlined that this secrecy was in keeping with the 'décor ostentatoire' ('ostentatious setting') that strongly characterised the forms and rituals of power and which conspirators were sometimes also inspired by.[48]

The nefarious presence of Italians was blamed for the export and spread of the use of poison in France, where – as Francesco Guicciardini said, even though the statement was questionable – it was previously 'almost unknown'.[49] At the end of the sixteenth century, a well-informed witness like Filippo Cavriani, an agent and informer for the Grand Duke of Tuscany in France, as well as a physician in the service of Caterina de' Medici, wrote that 'the use of poisons, which were already familiar to Italian princes, has now moved into France, so that we will no longer be blamed for the crime of poisoning'.[50] In reality, the previous decades of French history had made a decisive contribution to the negative image of Italy: extremely disparate sources (such as the *cahiers des doléances* presented at the States-General in Blois, anonymous *placards* and booklets, and treatises on trade practices) warned against the danger represented by men from the states and courts of the Italian peninsula. It was an economic and moral risk that helped weaken the Valois monarchy, on which the Wars of Religion had taken their toll; both Catholics and Huguenots attributed Italians who were present at court or involved in negotiations with the worst characteristics, ranging from treachery and treason to sodomy, atheism and the practice of magic and necromancy, even stretching to accusations of killing children to procure blood for therapeutic purposes, made at the same time as those against Jewish communities.[51]

The insistence on the political use of poisoning also contributed to fuelling an out-and-out 'black legend', projected over a wide time span, about the practice of 'state' murder by poison in the Republic of Venice. To this end, in-depth documentary research was conducted in the Venetian archives in the late nineteenth century, triggering a heated debate involving French scholars, Russian historians and Italian abbots in a crescendo of agitated accusations and indignant statements regarding the drastic methods devised and implemented by the Council of Ten.[52] This story ran and ran, and even as late as the mid-eighteenth century, the Inquisitors of State issued an order to put away the toxic materials (or 'poisonous things') that were available to the court and were scattered around in various archive cupboards. As a result of this order, the substances in question had to be placed in a special box, together with a book illustrating its contents and explaining the methods for administering the poisons, for the benefit of future Venetian magistrates.[53] This is a story that could be interpreted as a symbol of the decline of the Serenissima in the eighteenth century. However, it might be more valid to chronicle the episode of the 'black legend' of the history of Venice which, in the course of the nineteenth century, set French scholars against their Venetian counterparts. The former were keen to reveal 'macabre incidents' for the 'sometimes morbid curiosity' of readers, while the latter wanted to defend the reputation, honour and traditions of their city. It is interesting for us to observe that a crucial point of the dispute is the role played by secret crimes supposedly carried out by the Council of Ten and the Inquisitors of State, sometimes with the aid of toxic substances.[54]

Finally, alongside the violent disputes in the political struggle between Italian states and the harsh confessional conflicts in sixteenth-century Europe, there was a third significant aspect of the image of plots and conspiracies at an international level regarding the threat of contaminated wells. Returning to papal Rome, a city chronicle provides a detailed account of the terrible violent execution suffered by a nobleman from the Marches, Cristoforo Castagna, known as Macrino, in March 1490. After being forcefully dispossessed of his feudal property by a protonotary apostolic, he plotted his revenge while taking refuge in Constantinople. Sultan Bayezid II provided him with numerous gifts and money, but also a phial of poison. When Castagna reached Rome, he intended to pour its contents (an unspecified substance that would only take effect after five days) into the spring used by men serving the pontiff, as well as Bayezid's brother Cem, who had been defeated in the struggle for the succession to Mehmed II and was in the custody of Pope Innocent VIII at the time.[55] The Roman chronicler's account dwells on the sumptuous gifts (large sums of money, gold brocade clothing and precious stones) and the Sultan's extravagant promises (rule over a city, command of a fleet of two hundred ships), leaving the reader with a sense of wonder and amazement at the Turkish ruler's boundless wealth, which was naturally being used to serve a plan that was hostile and lethal towards the Christian world. However, under the surface, we can see that in the courtly world there was latent fear and constant suspicion of poison-based traitorous attacks. Indeed, it is mentioned that the well in question was defended and protected by walls and windows fitted with shutters, so that it could not be polluted with toxic substances. Furthermore, Castagna did not act alone: he could count on help from a Dominican friar, whose name is omitted. As the nineteenth-century scholar notes, at this point of the manuscript, 'the other words have been carefully erased' in order to blot out the memory of the name of the friar and the other accomplices in the poisoning. The news reached Ferrara by means of 'letters from Rome', confirming the extent of the circulation of information from Rome to the other Italian courts.[56]

I shall now draw to a close. The emphasis that both qualified historians and popularisers of history have placed on poisoning as an effective
weapon in the struggle for power in Italian Renaissance courts has to
be considered alongside other aspects of the question. Franck Collard's
book, *Le crime de poison au Moyen Âge*, had the merit of showing that in
reality, there were already many accusations of poisoning in the political
sphere in the last centuries of the Middle Ages, thus suggesting a perspective of continuity rather than one of interruption.[57] Equally, we can now
question the idea that the criminal use of poison was the exclusive prerog-
ative of the world of the courts. This is confirmed by two widely differing
sources such as criminal justice proceedings and the accounts that chroniclers dedicated to spheres of everyday social life in Italian cities between
the late fifteenth and the mid-sixteenth centuries.[58] These sources document the fact that men and women from mercantile, artisanal and popular classes in Italian cities in the Renaissance were familiar with toxic
and lethal substances, but it would go beyond the objectives and scope
of this chapter to consider such aspects of social and judicial life in the
Early Modern Age. Nevertheless, sources verify the strong presence of the
practice, and even more so of the issue of poison, as a political weapon in
Renaissance Italy.

Notes

1 Francesco Patrizi, *Enneas de regno et regis institutione* (Paris, 1531), 158 (see
   David Herlihy, 'Some Psychological and Social Roots of Violence in the Tuscan
   Cities', in Lauro Martines (ed), *Violence and Civil Disorder in Italian Cities,
   1200–1500* (Berkeley, Los Angeles, and London, 1972), 132). It is strange
   that the mention of 'veneficia et pestes' was removed from the 1547 Italian
   translation dedicated to Cosimo I de' Medici by the Tuscan Giovanni Fabrini
   (Venice, 1547, c. 82v). On the general question, see the papers in the special
   dossier 'Congiure e complotti' of *Roma moderna e contemporanea*, 11, n° 1–2
   (2003), in particular Marina Caffiero and Maria Antonietta Visceglia, 'Congiure romane e cultura politica europea: riflessioni introduttive', 7–27, and
   Andrea Gardi, 'Congiure contro i papi in età moderna. Per un'interpretazione
   generale', 29–51.
2 Stendhal (Marie-Henri Beyle), *Promenades dans Rome* (Paris, 1858), vol. I,
   266–268, 345–346; vol. II, 167–169.
3 Francesco Novati, *Stendhal e l'anima italiana* (Milan, 1915), 106–107; Irene
   Fosi, *La giustizia del papa. Sudditi e tribunali nello Stato Pontificio in età
   moderna* (Rome and Bari, 2007), 218. See also Giulio Bollati, 'L'italiano', in
   Storia d'Italia, vol. I, *I caratteri originali* (Turin, 1972), 952.
4 The passage taken from *Reflections of World History* by Jacob Burckhardt
   is quoted by Karl Löwith, *Jacob Burckhardt. L'uomo nel mezzo della storia*
   [1936] (Rome and Bari, 2004), 109.
5 Jacob Burckhardt, *The Civilization of the Renaissance in Italy* (New York,
   2010), 73.
6 Francesco Mari and Elisabetta Bertol, *Veleni. Intrighi e delitti nei secoli* (Florence, 2001), 19. For a different perspective, see Alessandro Pastore, *Veleno.
   Credenze, crimini, saperi nell'Italia moderna* (Bologna, 2010).

7 According to the qualified opinion of Anna Celli, widow of the famous malariologist Angelo and herself also a doctor: Anna Celli, 'La morte di Alessandro VI', *Ricerche religiose*, 5 (1929): 435–439.

8 Ottavia Niccoli, *Rinascimento anticlericale. Infamia, propaganda e satira in Italia tra Quattro e Cinquecento* (Rome and Bari, 2005), 64–69.

9 Niccolò Machiavelli, *Discourses on Livy*, III.6.41 (thanks to Filippo de Vivo for indicating this passage from *Discourses*). On this question, see the essay by Elena Fasano Guarini, 'Congiure 'contro alla patria' e congiure 'contro a uno principe' nell'opera di Niccolò Machiavelli', in Yves-Marie Bercé and Elena Fasano Guarini (eds), *Complots et conjurations dans l'Europe moderne* (Rome, 1996), 9–53.

10 Quoted in Niccoli, *Rinascimento anticlericale*, 65.

11 Giacinto Romano, 'Giangaleazzo Visconti avvelenatore. Un episodio della spedizione italiana di Ruperto di Baviera', *Archivio storico lombardo*, 21 (1894): 309–360, and 336 for the quotation; Bonaccorso Pitti, *Cronica [...] con annotazioni*, ed. by Alberto Bacchi della Lega (Bologna, 1905), 116–122.

12 Marilyn Nicoud, 'Expériences de la maladie et échange épistolaire. Les derniers moments de Bianca Maria Visconti (mai - octobre 1468)', *Mélanges de l'École française de Rome – Moyen Âge*, 112 (2000): 311–458, in particular 331, 332, 335, 439.

13 'Sans soupçon ou crainte de poison, de fer, de feu ou de mort, l'esprit joyeux, tu t'en vas en public et en privé, à tout heure et en tout temps, par ta ville': M.H. Smith, 'Complots, révoltes et tempéraments nationaux: français et italiens au XVIe siècle', in *Complots et conjurations dans l'Europe moderne*, 97, 98.

14 Pier Desiderio Pasolini, *Caterina Sforza* (Rome, 1893), vol. III, 406–410, 672–673, 765.

15 *Ricordanze di Bartolomeo Masi calderaio fiorentino dal 1478 al 1526*, ed. by Giuseppe Odoardo Corazzini (Florence, 1906), 223–227. The most recent essay on the matter is by K.J.P. Lowe, 'An Alternative Account of the Alleged Cardinals' Conspiracy of 1517 Against Pope Leo X', in *Congiure e complotti*, 53–78.

16 Elena Bonora, *Roma 1564. La congiura contro il papa* (Rome and Bari, 2011).

17 K.J.P. Lowe, *The Political Crime of Conspiracy in the Italian Renaissance*, in Trevor Dean and K.J.P. Lowe (eds), *Crime, Society, and the Law in Renaissance Italy* (Cambridge, 1994), 184–203.

18 Regarding the methods and times for the circulation of information, see Mario Infelise, *Prima dei giornali. Alle origini della pubblica informazione (secoli XVI–XVII)* (Rome and Bari, 2002), and, above all, Filippo de Vivo, *Information and Communication in Venice. Rethinking Early Modern Politics* (Oxford, 2007).

19 See, for example, regarding the fact that news about Luther was not widespread in Italy: Ottavia Niccoli, *Il mostro di Sassonia. Conoscenza e non conoscenza di Lutero in Italia nel Cinquecento (1520–1530 ca.)*, in Lorenzo Perrone (ed), *Lutero in Italia. Studi storici nel V centenario della nascita* (Casale 1983), 5–25.

20 Archivio di Stato di Roma, *Tribunale del Governatore*, Processi, 10, fasc. 3. Regarding this magistrature, see Fosi, *La giustizia del papa*, 23–24.

21 Regarding the assassination of Duke Alessandro de' Medici by his cousin Lorenzino, see Stefano Dall'Aglio, *L'assassino del duca. Asilio e morte di Lorenzino de' Medici* (Florence, 2011).

22 Archivio di Stato di Roma, *Tribunale del Governatore*, Processi, 10, fasc. 3, c. 16r–v.

23 Ibid., c. 78v.

24 Maria Antonietta Visceglia, 'Attentare al corpo del papa: sortilegi e complotti politici durante il pontificato di Urbano VIII', in Vincenzo Lavenia and

Giovanna Paolin (eds), *Riti di passaggio, storie di giustizia. Per Adriano Prosperi* (Pisa, 2011), 243, 245.

25 Rudolf Wittkower and Margot Wittkower, *La figura dell'artista dall'Antichità alla Rivoluzione francese* (Turin, 1968), 203.

26 Christian Gottfried Stentzel, *Toxicologia pathologico-medica, sive de venenis libri tres* (Wittenberg and Leipzig, 1733), 10.

27 I am referring to the doctoral thesis by Margaux Buyck, *Crimes de poison dans la Bologne médiévale et moderne (XIV–XVIIe siècles)*, in preparation at the Universities of Nanterre and Verona.

28 Romano, *Giangaleazzo Visconti avvelenatore*, 316; Augustin Cabanès and Lucien Nass, *Poisons et sortilèges. Les Césars, envoûteurs et sorciers, les Borgia* (Paris, 1903), IV.

29 *Shakespeare's Europe. Unpublished Chapters of Fynes Moryson's Itinerary, Being a Survey of the Condition of Europe at the End of the 16th Century*, ed. by Charles Hugues (London, 1903), 407.

30 David S. Chambers, *Cardinal Bainbridge in the Court of Rome 1509 to 1514* (Oxford, 1965), 131–140, in particular 134, 136, 138 for the quotations.

31 'Dum a veneficis praecavere studemus, aliquos latenter instruere videamur', Ferdinando Ponzetto, *Libellus de venenis*, in the appendix of Sante Arduini, *De venenis* (Basilea, 1563), dedication to Agostino Nifo; the second quotation, ibid., 530.

32 Franck Collard, *Le crime de poison au Moyen Âge* (Paris, 2003), 47–48.

33 For further information, see Alfonso Corradi, 'Gli esperimenti tossicologici in anima nobili nel Cinquecento', *Memorie del R. Istituto Lombardo*, classe di scienze matematiche e naturali, (1886): 31–51.

34 Burckhardt, *The Civilization of the Renaissance*, 278.

35 Ibid., 277.

36 Ferdinand Gregorovius, *Lucrezia Borgia secondo documenti e carteggi del tempo* (Florence, 1874), 89.

37 Guy Patin, *Lettres*, ed. by J.H. Reveille-Parise, vol. III (Paris, 1846), 80. The letter is not dated, but is placed between two letters of June 1657 and March 1658.

38 Voltaire, *Essai sur les moeurs et l'esprit des nations et sur les principaux faits de l'histoire depuis Charlemagne jusqu'à Louis XIII*, ed. by René Pomeau, vol. II (Paris, 1963), 69, 222; Furio Diaz, *Voltaire storico* (Turin, 1958), 207.

39 Jean Delumeau, *La paura in Occidente (secoli XIV–XVIII). La città assediata* (Turin, 1979), 36–37. See, more specifically, David Gentilcore, *Healers and Healing in Early Modern Italy* (Manchester, 1998), 101–106, and Ibid., 'The Fear of Disease and the Disease of the Fear', in William G. Naphy and Penny Roberts (eds), *Fear in Early Modern Society* (Manchester and New York, 1997), 184–208.

40 Montaigne, *Essays*, I, XVII.

41 Smith, 'Complots, révoltes et tempéraments nationaux', 96. Regarding Pietro d'Abano, see P. Morpurgo, 'I veleni nella letteratura e nell'iconografia al tempo di Pietro d'Abano', *Medicina nei secoli. Arte e scienza*, 20 (2008): 525–545. The passage from Petrarch is in *De remediis utriusque fortunae*, II, 116.

42 Ambroise Paré, *Le vingt-troisiéme livre, traitant des venins et morsures des chiens enragés, et autres morsures et piqueures de bestes vénéneuses*, in Ibid., *Oeuvres complètes*, ed. by Joseph-François Malgaigne (Paris, 1841), t. III, 293.

43 Paolo Cortesi, *De cardinalatu libri secundi oeconomici* ('in Castro Cortesio', 1510), cc. LXVIIv–LXVIIIv.

44 [Nicola Bertrucci] *Nusquam antea impressum collectorium totius fere medicine Bertrucij Bononinensis in quo infrascripta continentur [...] Quinto de*

venenis, [Lyon, 1509], c. CCXXXVIIIr.; Paul Freedman, *Out of the East. Spices and the Medical Imagination* (New Haven and London, 2008), 32.

45 'Intoxicationes et venenata pocula timenda, quae sub exquisitissimis epulis et fragrantissimis unguentis saepe latere solent' (Hendrik van Bra, *De curandis venenis per medicamenta simplicia et facile parabilia libri duo* [Arnhemii, 1603], c. [*7] *v*).

46 Andrea Bacci, *De venenis et antidotis seu communia Προλεγομενά praecepta ad humanam vitam tuendam saluberrima* (Rome, 1586), c. + 2r–v.

47 Benedetto Varchi, *Storia fiorentina*, ed. by Gaetano Milanesi, vol. III (Florence, 1858), 74–75.

48 Bercé, 'Introduction', in *Complots et conjurations dans l'Europe moderne*, 2.

49 Smith, 'Complots, révoltes et tempéraments nationaux', 95–99; Collard, *Le crime de poison au Moyen Age*, 93.

50 Smith, 'Complots, révoltes et tempéraments nationaux', 99, note 25, for the reference to a passage from Guicciardini's *Storia d'Italia*.

51 See above all Henry Heller, *Anti-Italianism in Sixteenth-Century France* (Toronto, Buffalo, and London, 2003), in particular VII, 80–81, 120, 181. But see also Vincenzo Lavenia, *La fides e l'eretico. Una discussione cinquecentesca*, in Paolo Prodi (ed), *La fiducia secondo i linguaggi del potere* (Bologna, 2007), 204–205.

52 Vladimir Lamansky, *Secrets d'état de Vénise. Documents extraits, notices et études servant à eclaircir les rapports de la seigneurie avec les Grecs, les Slaves et la Porte Ottomaine à la fin du XVe et au XVIe siècle* (Saint-Pétersbourg, 1884); [Louis de] Mas Latrie, 'De l'empoisonnement politique dans la République de Vénise', *Mém. de l'Inst. Nat. de France. Académie des Inscrip. et Belles Lettres*, 34, 2° (1895): 197–259; Rinaldo Fulin, 'Errori vecchi e documenti nuovi. A proposito di una recente pubblicazione del co. Luigi di Mas Latrie', *Atti del R. Istituto Veneto di scienze, lettere ed arti*, series 5, 8 (1881–1882): 133–150, 1065–1207. But see also Paolo Preto, *I servizi segreti di Venezia* (Milan, 1994), 329.

53 Lamansky, *Secrets d'état de Vénise*, 151–152; Preto, *I servizi segreti di Venezia*, 361–374.

54 See Mario Infelise, *Venezia e il suo passato. Storie, miti, 'fole'*, in Mario Isnenghi and Stuart Woolf (eds), *Storia di Venezia. L'Ottocento e il Novecento* (Rome, 2002), 967–988, in particular 977–978.

55 Stefano Infessura, *Diario della città di Roma* (Rome, 1890), 253–255.

56 Giovanni Ricci, *Ossessione turca. In una retrovia cristiana dell'Europa moderna* (Bologna, 2002), 34.

57 Collard, *Le crime de poison au Moyen Âge*, 247.

58 Ibid., 281; Pastore, *Veleno*.

8 Gender, poison, and antidotes in early modern Europe

Alisha Rankin

In December 1580, the German countess Anna of Hohenlohe acquired a promising new poison antidote, a clay known as Silesian terra sigillata. Named after an ancient Greek antidote prized by Galen and resurgent in the Renaissance, the terra sigillata from Silesia became a sought-after remedy in the western part of the Holy Roman Empire in the 1580s, thanks to the efforts of a salesman named Andreas Berthold.[1] Countess Anna caught wind of the promising new antidote in the wake of an extensive – and ostensibly successful – trial on dogs conducted by Landgrave Wilhelm IV of Hesse-Kassel. According to the Hohenlohe councilor Jörg Söffler, the countess bought a quantity of the Silesian terra sigillata from Berthold after reading the 'Hessian Certificate,' almost certainly a reference to a handwritten report of the trial that circulated several German courts. Anna may have been shown the certificate by her close friend Elisabeth of Pfalz-Lautern, who owned a copy, or she may have received her own copy directly from Wilhelm's wife Sabine, with whom she corresponded about medical matters.[2] In any case, her interest brought the terra sigillata to the court of her son, Count Wolfgang II of Hohenlohe, at his castle in Langenburg.

Thus was set in motion a rather extraordinary event. Apparently with the encouragement of his mother, Count Wolfgang proposed a test of the antidote on a recently condemned criminal in order, as Söffler put it, 'to see if it also works on people against poison the same way as it work on animals.'[3] He asked for his councilors' advice on the wisdom of this trial. In consultation with the Countess Anna on the proper way to take the antidote, Söffler first tested it on himself to try to cure the buzzing in his ears, with inconclusive results. He agreed that a test using poison on a human might be useful. Countess Anna's name later appeared, alongside those of her sons, on the official documents enabling the court to pronounce the death sentence of the criminal, a horse thief named Wendel Thumbler.[4] In the following days, Thumbler agreed to participate in a trial of the poison antidote – which ended up working in his favour, as he survived the poisoning and his sentence was commuted to banishment in thanks.

The trial to which Thumbler submitted himself became the last of a trio of poison trials mentioned in Berthold's book on the Silesian terra sigillata, published in 1583 and translated into English in 1587.[5] The role of Countess Anna in the archival documentation of Thumbler's case, however, is noteworthy, as she is completely absent from the print record. In her son's official testimonial letter certifying the success of the trial, Count Wolfgang stated that *he* had bought the antidote from Berthold. In describing the poison trial itself, Wolfgang noted that it took place 'in the presence of our selfe, and our wellbeloved Cosin the Countie George Friderick of Hohenloe ... and in the presence of all our Nobilitie and Commons,' with no specific mention of his mother.[6] While this elision may be a product of the tense relationship Wolfgang had with his mother, who had the reputation of being rather overbearing, there is potentially a broader significance that has to do with the gendering of poison antidotes in early modern Europe.[7] As has become increasingly clear over the last two decades, elite women became widely known as healers across early modern Europe. Their signature remedies tended to be multipurpose distillates, especially in France and Germany, as well as remedies for pregnancy, childbirth, and the care of small children.[8] Rarely, however, did they become widely known for their antidotes to poison.

When one reads about the connection between women and poison in early modern Europe, the link tends to be in terms of *causing* poisoning rather than *curing* it. Poisoning frequently was depicted as a crime of women in early modern documents, as a number of historians have noted.[9] This perception was closely connected to the factors that made women known as healers: their access to kitchens, food, and the household medicine chest.[10] Poison masked itself as nourishment or medicine and was a much more feasible murder weapon for women than blunt force. As Ulinka Rublack has noted, poison was seen as the most convenient way for a woman to get rid of an undesirable or abusive husband.[11] While some of the best-known poison plots in early modern Europe were actually contrived by men, women were more likely to be portrayed as poisoners in historical documents, especially in sensationalized printed pamphlets depicting prominent murders.[12]

Did this connection between women and poisoning prevent women from being seen as likely candidates to cure poison? On the one hand, there is evidence to suggest that there was a public perception of poison antidotes as part of a male domain. There were a number of well-known proprietary poison antidotes in early modern Europe – that is, antidotes attached to a specific person's name. Nearly all of the antidotes that circulated widely and appeared in printed works were tied to men, including empirics, charlatans, a few physicians, and a number of prominent princes.[13] In terms of the public depiction in print, the healing of poison appears to have been gendered male, whereas writings about poisoning were heavily weighted toward discussions of women.[14]

Yet as usual, a much more interesting and nuanced situation can be seen in medical manuscripts. In particular, if one examines handwritten medical recipes for antidotes, one finds quite a number of sixteenth-century women authors, owners, and compilers.[15] Contemporary letters similarly depict elite women who, like Countess Anna, were actively involved in acquiring antidotes for their courts.[16] Moreover, remedies for poison went far beyond a narrow concern for poisoning. For most people, an important use of poison antidotes was in the curing of plague and other poisonous diseases, and women were involved with these kinds of remedies as well. This essay examines the relationship between gender, poison, and antidote, including both the cause and the cure of poison. It demonstrates that some consistent gender differences can indeed be seen in both the manuscript and print records. Nevertheless, it argues that there were no firm distinctions, particularly in manuscript sources. If one casts a wide net and looks at the variety of remedies that involved poison, one finds ample evidence of women's medical interests, a finding that should come as no surprise given the wealth of information on women's medical activities in recent scholarship.[17] More revealing, however, is the heavy correlation between highly elite princes and certain kinds of poison and plague cures – a connection, I argue, that was related more to the public role of the prince than to specific gender expectations.

Women as poisoners

Poisoning was frequently depicted as a female crime in early modern Europe. Indeed, Collard sees a long tradition of casting women as poisoners, lasting from Roman antiquity through the modern period. There were, he argues, deliberate attempts in the Middle Ages to connect women with poison, both in their use of poisonous substances and the poisonous nature of their own bodies, namely menstrual blood.[18] That association remained strong in the early modern period. In his *Discoverie of Witchcraft* (1584), Reginald Scot cited various Greek, Roman, and early Christian authorities in claiming that 'women were the first inventers and practisers of the art of poisoning,' while Italian physician Giovanni Battista Codronchi stated in 1595 that for one *veneficus*, one finds 50 *veneficae*.[19] As Garthine Walker notes, poisoning was typically a domestic crime perpetrated on those closely connected with the alleged criminal, and it belonged to the female domains of food and medicine.[20] Arsenic was regularly found in homes as a means against household pests such as rats and lice and was easily accessible. In the fascinating diary kept by the Nuremberg executioner Franz Schmidt from 1573 to 1617, he recorded three cases of attempted murder by 'insect powder,' all perpetrated by women.[21] Similarly, Randall Martin notes that the ambiguous boundaries between medicine, food, and poison left women open to accusations regarding the cause of sudden death of people in their households.[22]

Poisoning was seen as a particularly vile crime because of its duplicitous, secretive nature, intimately related both to early modern understandings of negative female characteristics and to witchcraft.[23] In western Europe, witchcraft and poisoning had been connected since antiquity, both conceptually and semantically. The words *pharmakeia* in Greek and *veneficium* in Latin could denote either poisoning or witchcraft (and in Greek had the initial meaning of medicines).[24] The crimes of poison and magic were closely linked in the Middle Ages, and although this connection faded somewhat in the sixteenth and seventeenth centuries, numerous early modern authors retained the association, most prominently French demonologist Jean Bodin.[25] Lutheran theologian Ludwig Milichius (1530–1575) included a chapter on poison magic in his demonological treatise, while English writer Henry Goodcole mentioned the dual meaning of *veneficium* in his 1635 pamphlet on a woman who had poisoned her husband.[26] Dutch physician Johan Wier (or Johann Weyer) argued against the conflation between 'witches' and 'poisoners' in his famous criticism of witch persecutions, *De praestigiis daemonum ac Incantationibus et Veneficiis* (*On the Illusions of Demons and on Incantations and Poisons*, 1563). Nevertheless, he portrayed – and did not contradict – a longstanding tradition of women poisoners.[27]

Poisoning was by no means seen as an exclusively female crime – Jews, Muslims, lepers, and foreigners were also portrayed as typical poisoners, leading Collard to term poisoning 'a crime of the other'.[28] Moreover, we should not assume that the early modern trope of women as poisoners means that they actually *were* poisoners. Walker's careful study of poisoning cases in the city of Cheshire suggests that although poisoning was by far the most common female homicidal crime, absolute numbers of poisoning cases show little gender difference. (Men simply committed more homicides, especially more violent homicides.)[29] Wolfgang Behringer has noted that accusations of poison magic in the heyday of the Bavarian witch trials tended to fall especially on tavern keepers, butchers, bakers, and apothecaries – that is, professions with access to food, drink, and medicine.[30] Despite the continual fear of poison, moreover, it appears to have been a fairly rare crime in comparison with others. Of the 299 people who the hangman Schmidt executed in Nuremberg over his long career, only four had allegedly attempted poison – the three women accused of using 'insect powder' and one man specifically accused of using poison (*Gift*).[31] None of the poisoning victims died. Likewise, Martin notes the relative rarity of poisoning cases in his study of the sensationalist English pamphlet literature on murders, although those that did appear were described in especially dramatic terms.[32] Studies of crime in early modern Germany mention poison only as an aside, although Behringer's work on Bavaria suggests that accusations of poisoning against women increased in the late seventeenth century.[33] While both the incidence of poisoning cases and the representation of women as poisoners may have been overstated, the *idea* of women as quintessential poisoners was widespread across early modern Europe.

Gender and poison antidotes

Despite this well-documented association between women and the crime of poisoning, there is no reason automatically to assume that they should therefore *not* be associated with poison antidotes. In fact, one might assume that the same connection to food and medicine that made them open to accusations of poisoning would also give them access to curing poison. However, there were a number of independent factors that potentially explain why women tended not to be associated publically with poison antidotes. While there were hundreds of different kinds of poison antidotes in early modern Europe, the most sought-after tended to be exotic materials and/or ancient remedies. Among the most popular antidotes were animal objects such as unicorn (narwhal) horn and bezoar stone; precious gems, especially emeralds; clays such as terra sigillata and Armenian bole; and the electuaries theriac and mithridatium. The first three categories were all exotic objects and prized commodities.[34] The last were complex compounds that in theory needed to be purchased from an apothecary's shop.[35] All of them involved the intervention of vendors – merchants, traders, drug sellers, pharmacists – who would have been almost exclusively male.[36] Indeed, apothecary Euricus Cordus criticized the presence of women and other empirics in the theriac trade, insisting on the primacy of apothecaries to sell the storied drug.[37]

Cordus' criticisms notwithstanding proprietary poison antidotes – that is, antidotes attached to a particular person – became extraordinarily popular. Many empirics, such as the *Theriakkrämer* (theriac hawkers) in Germany or the snake handlers in Italy, specialized in selling antidotes in public spaces.[38] In his study of Italian charlatans, David Gentilcore notes that poison antidotes, especially electuaries and 'earths,' were extremely common among charlatans' proprietary medicines. The marketing of these drugs often involved a dramatic show. Snakehandlers, among the first to market antidotes in the late fifteenth century, would allow themselves to be bitten by poisonous snakes in order to prove the efficacy of their remedies. Later charlatans would similarly swallow poison and then take the antidote.[39] Theriac hawkers in Germany also demonstrated their wares in the marketplace from at least the fourteenth century, both in snakebite demonstrations on themselves and by feeding theriac to supposedly poisonous animals such as turtles and snakes, who then died (on the theory that antidotes were poison to poisonous creatures). The large yearly markets in cities such as Frankfurt and Leipzig served as focal points for these demonstrations.[40]

Some of the most prominent new antidotes were created by licensed physicians and surgeons. Italian physician Pietro Andrea Mattioli described the success of a poison antidote oil created by his mentor, the surgeon Gregorio Caravita.[41] Mattioli also touted his own scorpion oil as a marvelous antidote and remedy, just as he disparaged the antidotes sold in the marketplace by charlatans.[42] German physician Caspar Kegler became famous for an electuary against plague and poison, one of the first truly widespread proprietary remedies in Germany and highly regarded from the 1520s into the seventeenth century. As Erik Heinrichs has shown, Kegler printed vernacular pamphlets describing his electuary and dropping hints about its content (unicorn horn, theriac, and mithridatium, for starters), while keeping the recipes secret.[43] In the later sixteenth century, a number of German empirics like Berthold began to market new antidotes, mimicking the language and authority of physicians.[44]

All of these cases highlight the impressive commercial potential for poison antidotes. Although many drugs had commercial value, antidotes were particularly sought-after commodities owing to a number of factors: the great fear of poisoning (both malicious and accidental) among all classes, the close relationship between poison antidotes and plague cures, and the use of many poison antidotes as cure-alls. The significance of antidotes as important commodities in the medical marketplace can also be seen in the rampant trade in exotic counter-poisons such as the highly expensive bezoar stone. As Peter Borschberg has shown, it became popular for princes and commoners alike to own at least one – and preferably multiple – bezoars, which led to a trading frenzy.[45] In his 1598 treatise in praise of the bezoar, partially drawn from his own travels in Portuguese India, Constance city physician Christoph Hyeble (or Hieblin) described both the high prices bezoars commanded at the marketplaces in Goa and Kochi as well as the fraud he had seen perpetrated by unscrupulous salesmen.[46] This hyper-commoditization of prized antidotes did not make for an environment friendly to women participants. As I have argued elsewhere, women tended to be most prominent and respected in pharmacy when they avoided the commercial marketplace.[47] While it is likely that women operated in the background as helpmeets for their merchant, physician, and apothecary husbands and sons, they did not appear as major actors in the international drug trade.

Not all proprietary poison antidotes were linked to monetary gain, however. Numerous prominent princes became known for their antidotes, which they used in the context of early modern courtly patronage and gift exchange. The tradition of prince-as-antidote-creator reached all the way back to antiquity and the famous antidote mithridatium, named after King Mithridates VI Eupator of Pontus (120–63 BCE), and it was revived with fervor in the sixteenth century.[48] Dozens of German princes had 'poison powders' (*Giftpulver*) that circulated under their names, with the most prominent being from Elector Moritz of Saxony, Elector August of Saxony, Archduke Ferdinand II of Tyrol, and Emperor Maximilian II. Italian princes similarly became interested in creating effective antidotes, although they preferred oils over powders. Jo Wheeler has noted that Cosimo de'Medici perfected a counter-poison oil, which he passed on to his son, Duke Francesco de'Medici, who personally helped refine it in the ducal *fonderia* or laboratory. Cosimo's oil appears to have been a modified version of the surgeon Caravita's antidote mentioned by Mattioli.[49]

The princes did not only create antidotes; they also conducted tests to ascertain the effectiveness of both traditional and new antidotes. Under the direction of powerful princes, including Pope Clement VII, Emperor Ferdinand I, Cosimo I de'Medici, and King Charles IX of France, as well as Count Wolfgang II of Hohenlohe, court physicians conducted a series of high-profile trials on condemned criminals, with the majority of the tests occurring between 1524 and 1581. The trials all proceeded similarly: a prominent prince wished to test a particular antidote, whether a time-honored remedy such as bezoar or a new antidote such as Caravita's oil, Silesian terra sigillata, or Archduke Ferdinand's poison powder. A condemned criminal was found and voluntarily agreed to subject himself to the trial, usually in exchange for a pardon should the trial succeed. The poison was administered to the criminal by a court apothecary, and progression of the trial was carefully recorded by physicians. In many cases, a record of the trial appeared in print as part of a larger medical treatise, including both general medical works such as Mattioli's *Discorsi* (1544) and more targeted drug treatises like Berthold's *Terrae sigillatae* (1583).[50]

This princely practice of testing antidotes on criminals was a learned tradition, not a tradition of empirics, as Alessandro Pastore has noted.[51] Physicians directed all of these trials, with the exception of a trial on bezoar conducted by prominent French surgeon Ambroise Paré, and they communicated the results with careful observations. The emphasis on the learned nature of these tests likely acted as a means to distinguish princely poison trials from the marketplace antics of charlatans and other empirics. Instead of taking place in the market plaza for all to see, most princely tests occurred in a prison cell – and accounts of the trials frequently emphasized that the prisoner welcomed the private nature of this death, should it come to that.[52] Yet the emphasis on the learned nature of these trials made it less likely that women – even noblewomen – would appear as participants in the printed record. Even in cases in which women were centrally involved, as in Countess Anna's encouragement of the trial in Langenburg, their presence did not make it into the printed record.

Interestingly, this association of princes with the testing of antidotes left *them* open to the charge of being poisoners. One traveler to Italy in the 1590s, an Englishman named Fynes Moryson, noted in his remembrances of his journey that

> In our tyme, it seems the Art of Poysoning is reputed in Italy worthy of Princes practice. For I could name a Prince among them, who having composed an exquisite poison and counterpoyson, made proofe of them both upon condemned men giving the poison to all, and the Counterpoyson only to some condemned for lesse Crymes, till he had found out the working of both to a minute of tyme, upon divers complections and ages of men.[53]

Moryson's claims portrayed Italian princes as intent not only on creating and testing new poison antidotes but also (and primarily) poisons. This caricature had some basis in actual practices. There was at least one case, described by Mattioli, of a prisoner given a poison but no antidote as a control.[54] In another instance, the anatomist Gabriele Falloppio allegedly engaged in an eventually fatal experiment of opium dosages on a condemned criminal given to him by Cosimo I de' Medici.[55] For the most part, however, poison trials appear to have been aimed at testing antidotes, not poisons, and they were relatively rare. Nevertheless, Moryson's satire suggests that princes were in danger of being seen not as benevolent purveyors of counter-poisons but, rather, poisoners in their own right. If princes, who did not have existing gender stereotypes to contend with, walked this fine line, it is small wonder that princesses remained absent from the public record of these sorts of trials. The elision of Anna of Hohenlohe from the printed account of the poison trial may have been for her benefit as much as for Count Wolfgang's. Whatever the case may be, princes in early modern Europe were publically associated with poison antidotes in a way that their female consorts were not.

Overall, then, discussions around poison antidotes appear to have occurred mainly in social and economic spaces dominated by men. Nevertheless, there are a number of caveats that should caution us against assuming that poison antidotes were seen as a 'masculine' drug. The vast majority of antidotes listed in written documents were not 'gendered' at all. Despite the prevalence of proprietary counter-poisons, most antidotes were not attached to any particular name. Exotic objects and proprietary drugs were also not the only remedies for poison – herbal antidotes were also highly regarded, including common herbs such as gentian, sage, veronica, and perforata. Hieronymus Bock listed nearly 50 herbs that could drive out poison and contended that gentian was so effective that unscrupulous drug peddlers simply mixed it together with honey and sold it as theriac.[56] There were too many varieties of antidotes to make any claims about gender based on the accounts in a few printed sources.

It is also difficult to neatly divide 'male' and 'female' spheres of medicine: women frequently engaged in practices that mirrored the work of empirics, and they also made remedies that technically should be compounded in the apothecary's shop. Noblewomen certainly did not shy away from exotic and expensive ingredients, and they participated in the antidote trade as purchasers, if not as purveyors. Anna of Hohenlohe's acquisition of some Silesian terra sigillata began the chain of events that led to the trial in Langenburg, and she was not the only princess interested in poison trials. Pastore calls attention to a letter from Cardinal Benedetto Accolti to the Marchesa Margherita of Mantua in 1539, in which Accolti described an antidote test he had conducted on a prisoner he had received from Duke Ercole II of Ferrara.[57] *The Secrets of Isabella Cortese* (1565), a popular Italian book of secrets, opened with a recipe for the poison antidote oil tested on a condemned criminal by Pope Clement VII's physicians (although it remains unclear whether Cortese's book was written by a man or a woman).[58] While these trials may have been conducted publicly by princes and medical men, they certainly interested women behind the scenes.

Antidotes in manuscript

In medicinal recipe manuscripts, moreover, there is ample evidence of women's interest in poison antidotes. Recipe books generally do not contain substantial numbers of recipes for countering poison, but most contain a few, a pattern that is consistent across collections compiled by both women and men. Indeed, many recipe collections were collaborative documents that involved both sexes.[59] Despite the infrequency of antidote recipes, the way they were included in recipe collections underscores a perceived importance that reveals very little gender differentiation. Countess Dorothea of Mansfeld (1493–1578), for example, began her recipe collection in her own hand with recipes for eye pain, in a typical head-to-toe format. On the back side of the third page, however, another hand began a long regimen on how to cure malicious poisoning: 'It is known that many people are fearful of all poison coming in drink and look for a way to preserve themselves against it.'[60] The tone of the entry suggests a learned physician, as it references Latin texts and learned concepts and gives recommendations that allude to the supposed occult qualities of poison. Much of the material was drawn from the treatise on poison by medieval physician Pietro d'Abano (1257–1316), such as the advice that a snake's tongue would sweat in the presence of the poisons napellus or leopard's gall and that a stone called prassius, known as the 'matrix' or 'palace' of emeralds, would darken when poison was nearby.[61] These magical and occult elements in conjunction with poison were common in learned treatises, as Luke Demaitre has noted.[62] The physician's advice was followed by recommendations for curing poison, including seven helpful herbs and the ubiquitous antidote and cure-all theriac. The entry concluded with a section on specific poisons and their effects on the body, each followed by a suggested cure.[63]

The regimen is significant not merely for its content, which is lengthy and thorough, but also in its placement. After the entry concluded, Dorothea continued on with her recipes for eye complaints. One can surmise that an opportunity arose to have the antidote regimen copied – likely owing to a physician's visit – and Dorothea deemed it worthy enough to interrupt her head-to-toe format. This transfer of information would have been in keeping with her general interest in exchanging ideas with learned physicians, which she did frequently.[64] There are also other signs that Dorothea prized poison antidotes. A recipe in her hand toward the end of the manuscript, a distilled water for use against all poisons, stretches over 18 folio pages and calls for hundreds of herbs, numerous precious gems, and a smattering of tried-and-true poison antidotes such as theriac, unicorn horn, and

Armenian bole. The recipe is heavily abbreviated in places and contains few instructions on what to do with the ingredients at each stage. The only directives are occasional schematic notations to crush herbs or distill ingredients. This brevity of instructions suggests that Dorothea wrote the recipe down for her own use or for someone familiar with the process.[65] These two antidote entries comprised two of the longest contributions to her recipe book.

An even clearer sign of noblewomen's interest in antidotes appears in the medicinal recipe collection Cod. Pal. germ. 287, which was entirely dedicated to poison antidotes and plague cures. The manuscript, likely compiled by Countess Palatinate Elisabeth of Saxony (1552–1590), ended up among the numerous recipe collections in the princely Palatine library (Biblioteca Palatina).[66] It is organized into sections by the type of medicament, including chapters for pills and electuaries (including theriac), powders, distilled waters, oils, salves, and a final section on very simple drinks and 'arts' (*Künste*), with space after each section to add additional recipes. All recipes were aimed at treating plague, poison, or both, with a few cures for animal bites. Out of the 149 recipes in the manuscript, 60 contain attributions. The recipes in the sections on electuaries and powders contain a particularly large proportion of attributed recipes, while the final section on 'arts' has very few. Overall, there is only a small gender differentiation in these attributions, with 27 recipes attributed to women and 33 to men. Noteworthy, moreover, is the number of repeat attributions, led by Doctor Plaussin (5), the Lady of Neuhof (4), and the Countess of Stolberg (4). Several doctors and noblewomen have three attributions each. Women, then, appear frequently as authors of antidote recipes in this manuscript, a trend that is consistent with other recipe manuscripts in the Biblioteca Palatina, which generally have attributions to both women and men.[67] The large number of noblewomen and doctors is also in keeping with other manuscripts.

If one looks more closely at the specific breakdown in the types of recipes, however, a significant gender differentiation becomes apparent: the large number of poison and plague powders attributed to men. Overall, the number of powders is skewed significantly toward men (14 men to nine women), and that gap becomes particularly pronounced if one excludes the powders against animal bites and rabies and focuses solely on powders specifically for plague, poison, or both (12 men to five women). More significant than these bare numbers is the profile of the men to whom the poison and plague powders are attributed. A few of the male contributors (three) are physicians, as is common in the rest of the manuscript. There are, moreover, a significant number of recipes (six) attributed to men from the upper nobility, including Elector Moritz (of Saxony), Elector Friedrich (III of the Palatinate), Count Wolf of Barby, the Prince of Henneberg, the Prince of Anhalt, and the Margrave of Baden. In other sections, attributions to noblemen are rarer, although Moritz of Saxony is also cited as the author of a theriac recipe, and another plague electuary is attributed to Emperor Ferdinand. A long recipe for an aqua vitae against plague and poison is attributed to Emperor Maximilian.[68] Overall, then noblemen are cited mainly as authors of poison/plague powders or of lengthy and grand recipes for electuaries (including theriac), aqua vitae, and potions. They are almost entirely absent from attributions for more quotidian remedies like animal bites or external remedies such as salves and oils. This convention was not absolute: the final section on drinks and 'arts' contains two very simple recipes attributed to the 'King of France,' a modest plaster for plague buboes and a drink to protect against plague and bad air.[69] Nevertheless, the recipes in Elisabeth's manuscript confirm the connection between prominent noblemen and poison antidotes discussed earlier in this essay, and it confirms as well the preference for poison powders among German noblemen in particular.

The presence of a disproportionate number of men does not, however, coincide with an absence of women. Along with poison and plague powders attributed to noblemen are a fair few attributed to noblewomen, including the Lady of Neuhof, the Old Duchess of Barby, the Countess of Stolberg, and the Countess of Falckenstein. Moreover, several recipes are attributed to men and women with unclear status and prominence: plague powders attributed to men named Kosswitz and Ketzler, and a 'powder for all poison' attributed to 'Mrs Wurm' (*der Wurmin*).[70] While remedies for poison – especially powders – appear to have had some association with German noblemen, as with most remedies there are too many exceptions to form strict rules. Combined with the evidence from poison trials related in print, the correlation between princes and poison antidotes is striking, but by no means exclusive.

Poison, plague, and disease

The combined focus on poison and plague in Elisabeth's manuscript points to another important factor to consider in discussing gender and poison antidotes. Although the crime of poisoning was a grave concern in early modern Europe, especially in courtly spheres, antidotes had far broader uses than merely to prevent or combat malicious poisoning. As the essay in this volume by Jon Arrizabalaga shows, poison and plague were linked from the earliest onset of the Black Death in the Middle Ages, and the link between poison and disease in general expanded greatly in the following two centuries. The close tie between plague and poison can be seen clearly in Cod. Pal. germ. 287, which contained a number of recipes that aimed to cure both ailments, including 'the Duchess's electuary or Golden Egg for the pestilence and all poison,' 'Mrs. Salhaus's (*der Saulhaussin*) electuary for pestilence and poison,' and 'Emperor Maximilian's aqua vitae for pestilence and evil air, also for whoever fears poison.' Other recipes called attention to the poisonous nature of plague, such as 'The Lady of Neuhof's salve for pestilence buboes, and [it] draws out all the poison.' Conversely, some recipes primarily aimed at poison noted the poisonous nature of many diseases, as in 'Mrs. Haubelt Pflug's theriac for poison and all evil poisonous diseases' or 'Duke Moritz of Saxony's theriac to use for poison and all poisonous fevers and other poisonous diseases.'[71] Poison, plague, and disease in general were thus intimately intertwined by the late sixteenth century.

This connection between poison and disease, especially plague and the continual public health threat it brought with every epidemic, further cemented the tie between prominent princes and antidotes/plague cures. Many of the poison antidote trials mentioned at the beginning of this essay had plague as a backdrop. The trials in Hesse and Hohenlohe that tested the efficacy of Silesian terra sigillata on poison, for example, occurred during a plague epidemic in 1580, during which time Landgrave Wilhelm of Hesse-Kassel was keeping careful track of remedies administered to residents of many Hessian towns. Indeed, his trial of the terra sigillata on dogs occurred during a time of concern about a lack of effective remedies.[72] We can only assume that Wilhelm would have been attracted to the antidote's purported efficacy in 'resist[ing] the most cruell and horrible infection of the Pestilence, not onely in preserving such as use it, but also in speedie curing and calling to life, such as are infected, and halfe dead.'[73] A motive of broader usefulness than simply protecting a prince from poison tended to be given for conducting the poison trials; in the Hohenlohe trial, for example, a potential benefit to 'all of Christendom' was mentioned many times in both the archival and the print documentation. This assertion was almost certainly a reference to its potential usefulness against plague.[74]

Yet this indisputable connection between princes and plague cures also did not occur to the exclusion of women. A recipe book compiled by the Italian noblewoman Caterina Sforza in the first decade of the sixteenth century, for example, included three recipes that specifically claimed to combat poison (*veleno*), three aimed at plague and poison (*peste et veleno*), and at least 20 aimed at plague.[75] Fifteen plague remedies are attributed to women in the plague and poison manuscript from the Biblioteca Palatina. As we have already seen, Countess Anna of Hohenlohe obtained a sample of the Silesian terra sigillata in late 1580, during which time the antidote was so much in demand that the Archbishop of Cologne was unable to get his hands on any.[76] Her concern for plague may well have been a primary motivator for her interest in the antidote. While her name does not appear in conjunction with recipes for poison antidotes, she is listed in several manuscripts as the author of recipes for plague; indeed, one manuscript in the Biblioteca Palatina contains four different plague recipes attributed to her.[77] Most of these recipes also mention poison, as in

> The Countess of Hohenlohe's first water and medicine to use at the beginning of plague and also against any kind of poison, very useful so that nothing unclean is left in the stomach, but instead lifts and expels it through vomiting.[78]

For early modern men and women alike, the concern about poison was subsumed into the omnipresent fear of plague.

Nevertheless, one gender difference does come to the forefront when plague is added to the conversation, at least in German sources: the prominence of learned physicians as authors of plague remedies. In the manuscript Cod. Pal. germ. 287, nearly all contributions from learned physicians are plague remedies (11), with a small number of recipes for animal bites (3), one for poisonous diseases in general, and only one recipe specifically couched as an antidote to ingested poison. This unevenness suggests that, at least in the estimation of the female compiler, physicians remained authority figures for combatting plague – or, potentially, that physicians themselves preferred to be known for their plague remedies. The prominence of physicians makes for a significant overall gender imbalance in plague remedies (23 to 15). If one removes physicians from the equation, women outnumber men in plague recipe attributions 15 to 12, in remedies described as useful for both plague and poison four to one, and in remedies for poisonous animal bites four to zero. Only in recipes specifically described as poison antidotes do attributions to laymen outnumber those to women, a further confirmation of the tie between princes and antidote powders mentioned earlier. Importantly, women are prominent as authors in all four of these categories.

Conclusion

What broader conclusions can we draw from this evidence? First, there is no doubt that there was a close connection between elite princes and poison antidotes, a tie that comes through strongly in printed sources and in vernacular collections of medicinal recipes alike. As I have argued in previous work, noblemen generally tended to be less closely tied to pharmaceutical practice than noblewomen, although princes were also well represented in recipes for alchemical medicines and in remedies for wounds received in battle.[79] In short, highly elite men show up most commonly as authors of grand remedies befitting a powerful prince. Poison antidotes clearly fell into that category, valuable both in their perceived use for protecting against the scourges of poisoning and plague and in their epistemological connection to other exotic and highly prized antidotes.

Likewise, these sources highlight the connection between poison antidotes and cures for plague, an area that tended most commonly to be depicted as the realm of physicians, princes, and public health officials in early modern Europe.[80] The institutions and infrastructures that determined and delivered plague cures over a broad population mainly involved male officials, as evidenced by Wilhelm of Hesse-Kassel's attempts to deliver remedies to his plague-stricken towns.[81] To some extent, medicinal recipes reinforce this connection. As in the case of recipes described primarily as poison antidotes, plague cures included numerous remedies attributed to highly elite men, as well as a large number of remedies attributed to learned physicians – in theory exactly the authority figures to whom populations looked for help.

Despite this connection between princes, physicians, antidotes, and plague cures, strong gender differences quickly evaporate when one looks at medicinal recipes. There are a few tantalizing correlations, such as the connection between elite German princes and counter-poison powders or the connection between physicians and plague remedies, but none of them are absolute. Women appear as authors of recipes in all areas, and their names appear alongside names of prominent princes with no apparent differentiation, as was common in recipe collections. As evidenced in Giulia Calvi's work on plague in early modern Florence, behind the façade of officialdom lay a vast network of women and men trying to get through plague epidemics.[82] Similarly, women were unsurprisingly just as concerned about poison as their male counterparts. There was a wide range of ways that female healers, especially noblewomen such as Caterina Sforza or Anna of Hohenlohe, created and circulated antidotes for both poison and plague. While it is safe to say that poison antidotes were publicly much more connected with men, especially princes and physicians, women were very prominent indeed as authors of antidote recipes, and they clearly sought new antidotes with great interest. There is certainly no evidence whatsoever that the longstanding connection of the female sex, in general, with the crime of poisoning had any bearing on any given woman's perceived ability to cure it.

Returning to the case of Countess Anna of Hohenlohe and the trial of the Silesian terra sigillata, we cannot know for certain why her son, Count Wolfgang II, erased her role as the purchaser of the terra sigillata in the printed account. Was it to simplify the narrative presented in the official account? Was it to heighten Count Wolfgang's own role in the successful poison trial? Was it to protect his mother from potential slander? Was it to better match the Hohenlohe trial with previous poison trial descriptions? Any (or all) of these options are possible. The account may well have been altered to fit into an existing genre of poison trial accounts that was centered in learned spheres – a genre that highlighted the combined efforts of a prince and his physicians rather than the broader circle of interested parties, male and female, contributing to the trial. Yet despite their relative exclusion from official accounts, women had a great interest and involvement in poison antidotes, even in high-profile poison trials. Whatever the reason behind Countess Anna of Hohenlohe's disappearance from her son's account of his poison trial, she certainly had a lot to say about poison and plague in other arenas.

Acknowledgments

My thanks to the organizers and participants of the Medicine and Poisons conference for the helpful feedback they provided on this topic and to Tara Nummedal for reading a draft of this chapter.

Notes

1 The terra sigillata allegedly was discovered by a Paracelsian physician in Striga named Johannes Montanus, who appears to have partnered with Berthold, who described himself as a *Bergmeister* or mine foreman. The men published Latin descriptions of the drug together in 1583. Andreas Berthold, *Terrae sigillatae nuper in Germania repertae* (Frankfurt am Main, 1583).

2 Elisabeth's copy of the 'certificate' can be found in Universitätsbibliothek Heidelberg, Cod. Pal. germ. 177, fols. 16r–17v.

3 "vnd man also / dardurch erfarenn khöndt Ob es also bey dem menschen / der giefft halbenn *operiert* / Wie bey dem Viech." Hohenlohe Zentralachiv Neuenstein, La 5 Bü 400, Nr. 5.

4 HZA Neuenstein, La 5, Bü 400, Nr.

5 Andreas Berthold, *The Vvonderfull and Strange Effect and Vertues of a New Terra Sigillata Lately Found out in Germanie* (London, 1587), 34. See Alisha Rankin, "Anecdote, Experience, and Trial: Poison Antidotes and Drug Testing in Early Modern Europe," article under review at the *Bulletin of the History of Medicine*.

6 Berthold, *Wonderful and strange effect*, 34.

7 On Anna of Hohenlohe's "strong personality," see Jost Weyer, *Graf Wolfgang II. von Hohenlohe Und Die Alchemie: Alchemistische Studien in Schloß Weikersheim 1587–1610* (Sigmaringen: Jan Thorbecke, 1992), 23.

8 Alisha Rankin, *Panaceia's Daughters: Noblewomen as Healers in Early Modern Germany* (Chicago, IL: University of Chicago Press, 2013), introduction.

9 See, for example, Garthine Walker, *Crime, Gender and Social Order in Early Modern England* (Cambridge: Cambridge University Press, 2003), 144; Randall Martin, *Women, Murder, and Equity in Early Modern England* (New York: Routledge, 2008), chap. 4; Franck Collard, *The Crime of Poison in the Middle Ages*, trans. Deborah Nelson-Campbell (Westport, CT: Praeger Publishers, 2008), 97–100.

10 Martin, *Women, Murder, and Equity*, 123.

11 Ulinka Rublack, *The Crimes of Women in Early Modern Germany* (Oxford: Clarendon Press, 1999), 225–228.

12 Walker, *Crime, Gender and Social Order*, 143–147; Martin, *Women, Murder, and Equity*, chap. 4.

13 David Gentilcore, *Medical Charlatanism in Early Modern Italy* (Oxford: Oxford University Press, 2006), esp. 203–205.

14 On sensationalist pamphlets about women poisoners, see Martin, *Women, Murder, and Equity*, chap. 3.

15 This essay draws in particular on the recipe collections in the Codices Palatini Germanici (Cod. Pal. germ.) at the University of Heidelberg library, now digitized. http://digi.ub.uni-heidelberg.de/de/bpd/virtuelle_bibliothek/codpalgerm/index.html.

16 Nearly any collection of noblewomen's letters demonstrates this interest. In addition to the Hohenlohe citation above, see, for example, letters from Electress Anna of Saxony: Sächsische Hauptstaatsarchiv Dresden, Kop. 526, fols. 98v–99r.

17 See especially Rankin, *Panaceia's Daughters*; Elaine Leong, "Collecting Knowledge for the Family: Recipes, Gender and Practical Knowledge in the Early Modern English Household," *Centaurus* 55 (2013): 81–103; Michelle DiMeo and Sara Pennell, eds., *Reading and Writing Recipe Books, 1550–1800* (Manchester: Manchester University Press, 2013); Lynette Hunter, "Women and Domestic Medicine: Lady Experimenters 1570–1620," in *Women, Science, and Medicine: Mothers and Sisters of the Royal Society 1500–1800*, ed.

Lynette Hunter and Sarah Hutton (Phoenix Mill: Sutton Publishers, 1997), 89–107.

18 Collard, *Crime of Poison*, 97–100.

19 Reginald Scot, *The Discouerie of Witchcraft* (London: Henry Denham for William Brome, 1584), 116; Giovanni Baptista Codronchi, *De morbis veneficis ac veneficiis libri quatuor* (Venice, 1595).

20 Walker, *Crime, Gender and Social Order*, 143–148.

21 Franz Schmidt, *Das Tagebuch des Meister Franz, Scharfrichter zu Nürnberg* (Dortmond: Harenberg, 1980), 31–32, 117.

22 Martin, *Women, Murder, and Equity*, 123.

23 Esther Fischer-Homberger, *Medizin vor Gericht: Gerichtsmedizin von der Renaissance bis zur Aufklärung* (Bern: Huber, 1983), 364–374.

24 Edward Bever, "Poison," in *Encyclopedia of Witchcraft: The Western Tradition*, ed. Richard M. Golden (Santa Barbara, CA: ABC-CLIO, 2006), 906.

25 Collard, *Crime of Poison*, 141–145; Jean Bodin, *De la démonomanie des sorciers* (Paris, 1581), 222; Jean Bodin and Johann Fischart, *De magorum daemonomania: Gegen des Herrn Doctor J. Wier Buch von der Geister verführungen* (Strasbourg, 1586).

26 Ludwig Milichius, "Von Zauberey, Warsagung, Beschwehren, Segen, Aberglauben Hexerey, vnd mancherley Wercken des Teuffels," in *Theatrvm Diabolorum*, ed. Sigmund Feyerabend (Frankfurt am Main, 1569), 220–221; Henry Goodcole, *The Adultresses Funerall Day in Flaming, Scorching, and Consuming Fire, or, the Burning Downe to Ashes of Alice Clarke* (London, 1635), B3v–4v.

27 Johann Weyer, *Witches, Devils, and Doctors in the Renaissance: Johann Weyer, De Praestigiis Daemonum*, ed. George Mora and Benjamin G. Kohl, trans. John Shea (Binghamton, NY: Medieval & Renaissance Texts & Studies, 1991), 93–98 and 559–561.

28 Collard, *Crime of Poison*, 101. This otherness is also mentioned in Miranda Wilson, *Poison's Dark Works in Renaissance England* (Lanham, MD: Bucknell University Press, 2013), introduction.

29 Walker, *Crime, Gender and Social Order*, 144–145.

30 Wolfgang Behringer, *Witchcraft Persecutions in Bavaria: Popular Magic, Religious Zealotry and Reason of State in Early Modern Europe* (Cambridge: Cambridge University Press, 1997), 189.

31 Schmidt, *Das Tagebuch des Meister Franz, Scharfrichter zu Nürnberg*.

32 Martin, *Women, Murder, and Equity*, 123–129.

33 Rublack, *The Crimes of Women in Early Modern Germany*; Behringer, *Witchcraft Persecutions in Bavaria*, 189; Joy Wiltenburg, *Crime and Culture in Early Modern Germany* (Charlottesville: University of Virginia Press, 2012).

34 On the trade in exotica, see Peter Borschberg, "The Euro-Asian Trade in Bezoar Stones (approx. 1500 to 1700)," in *Artistic and Cultural Exchanges between Europe and Asia, 1400–1900*, ed. Michael North (Aldershot: Ashgate, 2010), 29–43; Marnie P. Stark, "Mounted Bezoar Stones, Seychelles Nuts, and Rhinoceros Horns: Decorative Objects as Antidotes in Early Modern Europe," *Studies in the Decorative Arts* 11 (2003): 69–94, doi:10.2307/40663065.

35 See James E. Shaw and Evelyn S. Welch, *Making and Marketing Medicine in Renaissance Florence*, vol. 89, Wellcome Series in the History of Medicine (Amsterdam: Rodopi, 2011).

36 On drugs and the apothecary's trade, see Lydia Mez-Mangold, *A History of Drugs* (Carnforth: Parthenon, 1986), 94–110; Günther Stille, *Krankheit Und Arznei: Die Geschichte Der Medikamente* (Berlin: Springer-Verlag, 1994).

37 Euricus Cordus, *Von Der Vielfaltigen Tugent Vnnd Waren Bereitung / Deß Rechten Edlen Theriacs* (Marburg, 1532).

38 Thomas Holste, *Der Theriakkrämer: Ein Beitrag zur Frühgeschichte der Arzneimittelwerbung*, vol. 5, Würzburger medizinhistorische Forschungen (Pattensen: Horst Wellm Verlag, 1976); Katharine Park, "Country Medicine in the City Marketplace: Snakehandlers as Itinerant Healers," *Renaissance Studies* 15 (2001): 104–120.

39 Gentilcore, *Medical Charlatanism in Early Modern Italy*, 176–205.

40 Holste, *Theriakkrämer*, vol. 5, 80–83.

41 Pietro Andrea Mattioli, *De i discorsi di M. Pietro Andrea Matthioli* (Venice, 1585), 1153.

42 Gentilcore, *Medical Charlatanism in Early Modern Italy*, 41; Mattioli, *Discorsi*, Book VI.

43 Erik Heinrichs, "The Plague Cures of Caspar Kegler: Print, Alchemy, and Medical Marketing in Sixteenth-Century Germany," *Sixteenth-Century Journal* 43 (2012): 417–440.

44 See Alisha Rankin, "Empirics, Physicians, and Wonder Drugs in Early Modern Germany: The Case of the 'Panacea Amwaldina,'" *Early Science and Medicine* 14 (2009): 680–710.

45 Borschberg, "The Euro-Asian Trade in Bezoar Stones (approx. 1500 to 1700)."

46 Christoph Hieblin, *Tractat Von der aller furtrefflichsten vnd kräftigsten Artzney wider allerley Gifft: welches der Stein Bezaar ist* (Konstanz am Bodensee, 1598), 23r–25v.

47 Rankin, *Panaceia's Daughters*, 53–54.

48 Laurence M.V. Totelin, "Mithradates' Antidote: A Pharmacological Ghost," *Early Science and Medicine* 9 (2004): 1–19.

49 Jo Wheeler, *Renaissance Secrets, Recipes & Formulas* (London: Victoria and Albert Museum, 2009), 76–77. Additional information can be found at http://renaissancesecrets.blogspot.com/2013/06/medici-anti-poison-oil.html.

50 Alisha Rankin, "On Anecdotes and Antidotes: Poison Trials in Early Modern Europe," *Bulletin of the History of Medicine*, 91 (forthcoming 2017).

51 Alessandro Pastore, "Médecine légale et investigation judiciaire: expérimenter le poison sur les animaux en Italie à l'époque moderne," *Revue d'Histoire des Sciences Humaines* 22 (2010): 17–35; Alessandro Pastore, *Veleno: Credenze, Crimini, Saperi nell'Italia Moderna* (Bologna: Il mulino, 2010).

52 Rankin, "Anecdote and Antidote."

53 Fynes Moryson, *Shakespeare's Europe; Unpublished Chapters of Fynes Moryson's Itinerary, Being a Survey of the Conditions of Europe at the End of the 16th Century* (London: Sherratt & Hughes, 1903), 407.

54 Mattioli, *Discorsi*, 1152.

55 Alfonso Corradi, "Degli esperimenti tossocologici in anima nobili nel cinquecento," *Annali universali di medicina e chirurgica* 277 (1886): 73; Gabriele Falloppio, *Gabrielis Falloppii ... Libelli duo: alter de ulceribus, alter de tumoribus praeter naturam ...* (Venice, 1563), 47v–48r.

56 Hieronymus Bock, *Kreüter Buch* (Strasbourg, 1546), 56r.

57 Pastore, *Veleno*, 223.

58 Isabella Cortese, *I secreti de la signora Isabella Cortese* (Venice, 1565), 3. See also Meredith K. Ray, *Daughters of Alchemy: Women and Scientific Culture in Early Modern Italy* (Cambridge, MA: Harvard University Press, 2015), chap. 2; Claire Lesage, "La litterature des 'secrets' e 'I secreti d"Isabella Cortese," *Chroniques italiennes* 36 (1993): 145–178.

59 Leong, "Collecting Knowledge for the Family."

60 Sächsische Landes- und Universitätsbibliothek Dresden (hereafter SLUB), Ms. C317, 3r.

61 Pietro d'Abano, *De Venenis Atque Eorundem Commodis Remediis* (Marburg, 1537), http://archive.org/details/clarissimipetri00sammgoog.

62 Luke E. Demaitre, *Medieval Medicine: The Art of Healing, from Head to Toe* (Santa Barbara, CA: Praeger, 2013), 71–72.

63 SLUB, Ms. C317, 4r–v.

64 Rankin, *Panaceia's Daughters*, chap. 3.

65 SLUB, Ms. C317, 172v ff.

66 UB Heidelberg, Cod. Pal. germ. 287. For information on the manuscript, see Matthias Miller's Wissenschaftliche Beschreibung at www.ub.uni-heidelberg. de/digi-pdf-katalogisate/sammlung2/werk/pdf/cpg287.pdf. See also Debra L. Stoudt, "The Medical Manuscripts of the Bibliotheca Palatina," in *Manuscript Sources of Medieval Medicine: A Book of Essays*, ed. Margaret Rose Schleissner (New York: Garland, 1995), 159–181; Rankin, *Panaceia's Daughters*, chap. 2.

67 Rankin, *Panaceia's Daughters*, chap. 2.

68 UB Heidelberg, Cod. Pal. germ. 287, fols. 79r–80r.

69 Ibid., 276r and 280r.

70 Ibid., 38r–43v.

71 Ibid., 1r–4v.

72 HStA Marburg, Best. 17I, No. 4750.

73 Berthold, *VVonderfull and Strange Effect*, 1.

74 Councilors of Hohenlohe in Neuenstein, 10 January 1581, HZA Neuenstein, La 5, Bü 400, Nr. 5.

75 Pier Desiderio Pasolini, *Caterina Sforza*, vol. 3 (Roma: E. Loescher, 1893), 617–807. See also Ray, *Daughters of Alchemy*, chap. 1.

76 Andreas Berthold's supplies of terra sigillata were in such great demand that they were completely sold out in November 1580 and did not officially become available again until the following April. HStA Marburg, Best. 4f Köln 84.

77 Cod. Pal. germ. 256, fols. 500r–502r.

78 See also Cod Pal. germ. 177.

79 Rankin, *Panaceia's Daughters*, 10–14.

80 Plague and public health.

81 HStA Marburg, Bestand 17I, Nr. 4750.

82 Giulia Calvi, *Histories of a Plague Year: The Social and the Imaginary in Baroque Florence*, University of California Press, 1989 (Italian orig. publ. 1984).

9 Mateu Orfila (1787–1853) and nineteenth-century toxicology

José Ramón Bertomeu-Sánchez

Mateu Orfila (1787–1853) is mentioned in popular accounts of the history of toxicology and legal medicine as one of the founding fathers of these disciplines. Thanks to his participation in famous trials, he became a nineteenth-century celebrity. Many biographical accounts were published when he was alive. On his death in 1853, obituaries appeared in academic journals and leaflets, reflecting his fame at that time. This literature was later added to by local historians and physicians in further commemorations of his birth or death. In contrast with this popular literature, his work barely attracted the interest of the scholars working in history of science, technology, and medicine during the twentieth century. The absence of any associated dramatic discovery and his ambiguous situation in disciplinary history (as well as in national histories of science) explains his mysterious banishment from mainstream narratives on history of science and medicine during most of the twentieth century.[1] In recent times, Orfila has been resuscitated in the context of new studies on experts, history of crime, and science and the law. The new studies have shown that Orfila was a protagonist of many developments not only in toxicology, but also in the new role of forensic physicians during the first half of the nineteenth century. His biography sheds light on many problems concerning the role of doctors in criminal courts: the sources of legitimacy and the extension of the group of experts, the tensions between scientific and legal forms of proof, the conditions of acceptability of new technologies in courts, the management of uncertainties prompted by the advancement of science, and the closure of expert controversies, among many other issues raised by recent studies.[2]

In this chapter, I will review the biography of Orfila in order to undermine two extreme and rather contrasting views on science and the law, which are popular in both academic literature and mass media. I will employ the convenient expressions "junk science in courtrooms" and "CSI-effect" to refer to them. The first image emerges from the prejudice that the adversary atmosphere of courts is a very bad context for the kind of balanced and disinterested activity ideally associated with scientific research. Science made for courts seems to involve partisan experts, selective use of available data, biased reports, counterfeit controversies, and unfair inequalities concerning access to resources for making certitude, reasonable doubts, and ignorance.[3] Many of these features can be found not only in late-twentieth-century American tort litigations, but also in nineteenth-century criminal trials and patent litigation. Even so, I will show that the most celebrated research work of Orfila, namely his studies on the absorption of poisons, could hardly be pursued without the assets provided by courts: corpses and organic samples, unique clinical cases, reports of post-mortem examinations, and refined versions of chemical tests. Moreover, the challenges faced by Orfila in courtrooms prompted new animal experiments, academic debates, and publications in medical journals. In other words, I claim that nineteenth-century toxicology was developed in close connection with poisoning trials, which inspired new original experiments and provided unique data and material resources.[4]

In contrast with the former image, the expression "CSI-effect" was coined in order to refer to the high hopes concerning science in criminal investigations, which were created by TV series and literature. Some journalists and lawyers have worried in recent times about the unwanted consequences of these effects in the administration of justice, for instance, in jurors who could be misled by these popular images, sometimes by attributing extra probatory value to scientific evidence, which is portrayed as based on unquestionable matters of fact obtained by means of sophisticated mechanical devices, free of partisan interests and biased prejudices. With this expression, I do not refer only to this very recent (real or imaginary) effect, but also to the similar technocratic dream, which is commonly conveyed in popular narratives on the history of crime and forensic science in which the replacement of traditional proofs (witness testimony and confessions) by scientific evidence is regarded as a privileged path for progress in criminal justice.[5] Like many other master narratives of technological progress, this powerful picture of uninterrupted success can be questioned by focusing on particular cases that are barely mentioned in popular accounts. I will review a group of poisoning trials from the end of the 1830s, in which Orfila introduced his new version of the Marsh test for arsenic. Even accepting that the new methods were faster and more sensitive than their predecessors, I will show that their use also led to many puzzling problems and unforeseen consequences. High sensitivity involved a larger spectrum of impurities coming from reagents, vessels, and the environment, as well as more severe chains of custody. The most confusing impurity was found inside the human body and was named "normal arsenic". At the end of the day, there were more expert controversies and additional difficulties for judges, lawyers, and jurors in evaluating scientific evidence.[6]

I will discuss the first issues through scarcely known poisoning trials in which Orfila participated when he was at the height of his career as a toxicologist. Many studies on forensic science have been focused on "causes célèbres" such as the trials of Marie Lafarge, William Palmer, or doctor Crippen.[7] The advantage of these famous cases is the large amount of documents available for historical scrutiny, but the exceptional feature of these trials is a serious difficulty in reaching general conclusions. Thus, I will review a handful of poisoning cases taking place at the end of the 1830s in France. Among the main actors are the parricide Victorine Cumon in Périgueux, the poor farmer Nicolas Mercier and his handicapped son in Dijon, the adulterous Antoine Rigal who poisoned his wife in Albi, and the infamous assassin Soufflard who committed suicide in prison by poisoning himself with arsenic. In contrast with popular images, people accused of poisoning were both men and women, many of them were poor and unknown, and the final verdicts were hardly questioned and never appealed, even less transformed into a long-term public controversy as in the cases of William Palmer, Doctor Crippen, or Marie Lafarge (although the uncertainties concerning scientific evidence were very similar, or even greater).

After a brief sketch of the biography of Orfila, I discuss how he managed to obtain the main sources needed for his toxicological work: clinical symptoms, post-mortem examinations, animal experiments, and chemical analysis. I show that the origins and uncertainties associated with each type of data were diverse and played different roles in classrooms, academies, and courts. I analyze how and why Orfila decided to give a privileged status to chemical tests as the main source of evidence in toxicology. I will focus on two key features: his training in analytical chemistry and the controversies around animal experimentation in early-nineteenth-century France. Then, I will review several poisoning cases taking place around 1839 and 1840, the crucial years in which Orfila developed his celebrated work on the absorption of poisons with a refined version of the new Marsh test for arsenic. Finally, I will review how Orfila confronted the controversy on "normal arsenic" and other uncertainties emerging from the new high-sensitivity chemical tests introduced in those years.

***

Mateu Josep Bonaventura Orfila I Rotger (1787–1853) was born in Mahon, on the island of Minorca (Spain). He moved to Valencia to study medicine, but, disappointed by the uninspiring atmosphere, he decided to travel to Barcelona and enroll on a new chemical course set up by a pharmacist, Francesc Carbonell i Bravo (1768–1837). Most of the students were surgeons, physicians, and pharmacists, so Orfila learned here the debates on the uses of new chemistry in medicine, a controversial topic that had been the main theme of the doctoral thesis of his teacher. Thanks to the recommendation of Carbonell, Orfila obtained a travel grant and he became one of the many Spanish young students (the "pensionados") who moved to Paris to learn chemistry.[8] In Paris, he enrolled as a student of the new Paris Medical Faculty, which had emerged after the French Revolution. The center attracted students from all over the world. The courses placed special emphasis on clinical observation in the hospital and on practical exercises for students.[9] Like many other students, Orfila attended many other public and private courses in Paris, notably the lectures given by Jacques Thenard (1777–1857) at the Collège de

France. Thenard became one of the most influential French chemists during the first half of the nineteenth century, thanks to his textbooks and his role in shaping scientific education. He also published one of the first books on analytical chemistry and organized a research school of students and laboratory assistants who worked on different problems around mineral analysis. Orfila also attended the courses on chemistry delivered by Nicolas Vauquelin (1763–1829) at the Museum of Natural History, another important institution created after the Revolution. Vauquelin, a pharmacist who was a close collaborator of Antoine Fourcroy (1755–1809), was famous for his research on vegetal and animal chemistry. Vauquelin and Thenard patronized the first years of the career of Orfila in Paris: they recommended him for jobs in educational institutions, wrote very positive reports about Orfila's work, and introduced him to other important Parisian scientists. Vauquelin even rescued Orfila from prison in 1808, at the beginning of the Peninsular War.[10]

In 1811, Orfila passed the required examinations at the Medical Faculty and obtained his medical degree after writing a thesis on medical chemistry and the analysis of urine.[11] While still a medical student, Orfila gave public courses attended by a substantial number of students. Private lectures and textbooks were important sources of income for the young Orfila. Moreover, the courses involved a large number of experimental demonstrations and animal vivisections, which were a key feature of his initial research on poisons. According to his autobiography, it was during one of these courses when the "Eureka moment" took place, launching his future research on toxicology. In April 1813, he was lecturing on the different chemical tests for arsenic in front of a hundred and a half students. Following the regular methods of his days, he employed different reagents for making the characteristic colored solutions and precipitates employed to detect arsenic. He wanted to show that these reactions were unaffected by the presence of organic matter (as commonly happened in forensic research), so he took a cup of coffee and poured it into the arsenical solution, but something unexpected happened:

> I prepared a mixture of this drink [coffee] and the arsenical solution. I said to my students: "You are going to be convinced about the accuracy of what I affirmed". Not at all! Lime-water, which should have caused a white precipitate, yield a purplish-gray turbidity; ammoniacal sulfate of copper yielded a black-olive precipitate, instead of a grass-green one, etc. You can imagine how embarrassed I was! I thought these results were due to the presence of colored organic materials, without being able to explain properly what had happened.[12]

After this embarrassing situation, Orfila concluded that "toxicology did not exist", because in most cases, forensic physicians worked with organic mixtures (similar to coffee) which could change the color of solution and precipitates during a chemical test. He realized that the use of regular chemical tests in criminal investigations was meaningless or, even worse, dangerously

deceitful. His reconstruction of the "Eureka moment", which is vividly described by Orfila in his autobiography, is a good example of the importance
he conceded to chemical tests in toxicological research. The quotation also
unveils Orfila's concerns regarding the uses of chemistry in medicine and the
difficulties of transporting chemical tests from laboratories into crime scenes.
The episode also shows the type of analytical tests that Orfila learned when
attending the courses of Thenard in Paris: different reagents were employed
in order to produce chemical reactions yielding colored solutions and precipitates, which were regarded as peculiar to the different chemical products.
The detection was based on the identification of specific nuances of colors,
so it required a trained eye and skills in laboratory work, two features which
could hardly be acquired without practical training.[13] Apart from colored
tests, Orfila adapted for courtrooms the form of proof typical of chemistry
lectures: experimental demonstrations. He largely employed the dramatic
effect of chemical experiments in order to offer convincing evidence about
his claims in classrooms, academies, and courts (Figure 9.1).

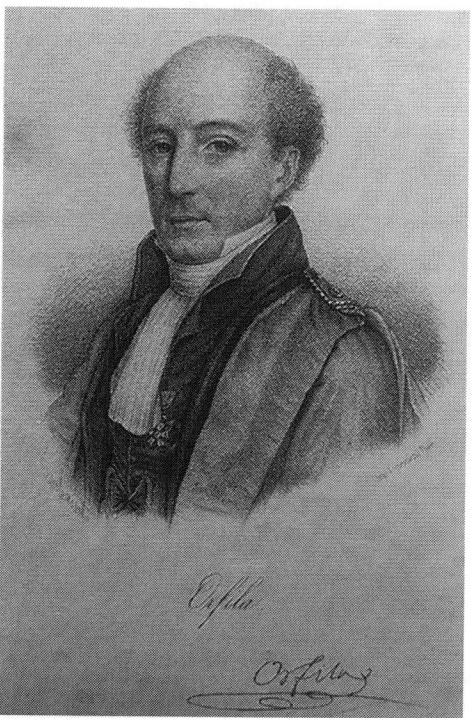

Figure 9.1 Mateu Orfila (1787–1853) when he was dean of the Paris Medical Faculty. From Mateu Orfila, *Tratado de medicina legal...* Madrid: José
María Alonso, 1847–1849, vol. I.

Courtesy of the Institute for the History of Medicine and Science "López Piñero" (University
of Valencia). Historical Library. Ref.: IHMC 1831–1900 / 6155 v.1.

Apart from Orfila's background in chemistry, another reason for favouring chemical tests was the difficulty of gathering information about the other sources of toxicological evidence. Animal experiments were expensive and time consuming, while clinical data and autopsies concerning poisoning cases were rare and difficult to access. In the first edition of his *Traité des poisons*, Orfila employed clinical data on poisoning cases obtained from medical literature or reports offered by friends and colleagues. Just in very rare examples, he employed data from his own practice as a physician (which was always very limited). The data on autopsies were even more difficult to obtain before Orfila started to participate as an expert in poisoning trials. In his first publications, Orfila could only employ reports sent by his friends or published in medical literature.[14] After gathering all the available information, Orfila wrote his famous *Traité des poisons* and signed a lucrative contract with the publisher Nicolas Crochard (who also published the famous journal *Annals de Chimie*). The book was ready to be printed at the end of November 1813, but the unstable political climate delayed the publication of the second volume until the end of 1815. The book went into several editions in France and was soon translated into English, German, Italian, and Spanish, so it became the most important reference book on poisons during the first half of the nineteenth century.[15]

***

Like other important scientific books published in France, the *Traité des poisons* was reviewed by a commission of the Paris Academy of Science. The report highlighted the value of animal experiments performed by Orfila remarking that he was compelled to spend "whole sleepless nights" doing nauseating experiments.[16] Orfila employed the data published in medical journals concerning experiments with animals and poisons, which had been more and more frequent and sophisticated since late seventeenth century.[17] However, in contrast with clinical symptoms and post-mortem examinations, most of the experiments on animals reported in the *Traité des poisons* had been performed by Orfila. In that way, he could control and selectively modify the dosage, timing, and ways of administration of poisons. One of his English students reported that Orfila included in his textbook many of the experiments performed in his private lectures:

> M. Orfila, whose character has of late become so well known, is one of these private teachers, and his Toxicologie Générale contains the materials of his very valuable course on Chemistry and Médecine Légale. He employed some hundreds of dogs during the last winter, for exhibiting the effects of poisons, which he injects into the stomach, through an opening made in the oesophagus; and afterwards, when the poison begins to shew its effects, he injects the antidote to counteract them, and save the animal.[18]

Orfila employed the data obtained from animal experiments for studying a broad range of questions: the absorption and elimination of poisons, the different dosages and their poisoning effects, the anatomical damage produced in the gastrointestinal tract and internal organs, and the value of antidotes (he wrote a popular book on this last issue). By analyzing samples of the poisoned dogs, he also refined the chemical tests available for detecting poisons. He attempted to mimic as closely as possible the situation of criminal investigations: for instance, he buried poisoned dogs, which were exhumed after several days, and then their organs were analyzed following the methods employed in real poisoning cases. The use of animal experiments in courts was, however, limited due to their contested status. Since their beginning, criticism against animal experiments was based on ethical and methodological reasons.[19] When Orfila passed away in 1853, a British medical journal remarked that he, "like his contemporary Magendie", had been "accused of an inordinate sacrifice of animal life in carrying on his experimental inquiries, and met with much censure thereupon".[20]

Antivivisectionist feelings were not so strong in France, and the criticism was focused on methodological issues: the differences between humans and animals regarding the action of drugs and poisons, and the unnatural conditions of experiments that could substantially alter the observed results and mislead the experimenter. Orfila attacked those who did not accept the "identity of the action of poisons in humans and dogs", asserting that this idea would have fateful consequences for the advancement of science.[21] One of these critics was Antoine Portal (1742–1832), a renowned anatomist and first doctor to the King during the Bourbon Restoration, who defended the idea that the study of poisons and its antidotes had to be based on "clinical observations on humans who had really been poisoned", not on "chemical decompositions and experiments with living animals". Portal criticized the specific antidotes suggested by Orfila because their efficacy had been proved only in animal experiments or in chemical test-tubes, not in humans.[22] Another group of critics, while accepting animal experiments for dealing with particular problems on human therapeutics, physiology, or toxicology, remarked that experiments placed animals in unnatural conditions of extreme pain that might produce misleading results. Vivisection caused an abnormal situation that might substantially differ from the natural state one wished to assess. For instance, the British antivivisectionist George Macilwain (1797–1882), referring to Orfila's experiments, affirmed that "one could not have imagined any conditions better calculated" for "interfering with and obscuring the processes of nature by every conceivable ingenuity".[23]

One of the most important techniques, the ligature of the esophagus, came in for particular criticism because of its occasionally dangerous side effects or even death, when it was performed by unskilled hands. This technique was important for preventing the animals from vomiting the poison (or the antidote), so the experimenter could control the dosages and timings. The surgical technique was so painful for the animals that some critics argued that the observed effects could be rather produced by this unnatural state than by the poisons or drugs studied. Orfila was compelled to perform further experiments allegedly showing that the ligature of the esophagus was both indispensable for his toxicological experiments and harmless for the dogs. However, the technique would remain controversial during the following years in medical academies.[24] Among the critics was Ambroise Tardieu (1818–1879), a colleague of Orfila at the Paris Medical Faculty, who turned out to be the most influential French toxicologists of the second half of the nineteenth century. He claimed that the ligature "modified in such an artificial way the conditions of poisoning" that the experiments furnished results that were inconclusive for medicolegal purposes. Using this example, Tardieu claimed that earlier toxicologists such as Orfila had relied excessively on animal experimentation and laboratory tests, instead of the more reliable source of information provided by "clinical observations and anatomo-pathological data" of poisoned individuals.[25]

The critical remarks from medicolegal physicians such as Tardieu highlight the fact that Orfila's chemical and experimental approach was just one of the many possible ways of dealing with toxicological issues in the nineteenth century. The relative importance of the different sources of information such as clinical symptoms and autopsies and the nature of (chemical and physiological) experiments were issues opened to discussion. Given that animal experiments were so controversial and having limited access to clinical data and post-mortem reports, Orfila was encouraged to employ chemical tests as the main reliable source of toxicological evidence. His activities in the courtrooms, which started in the 1820s, offered him a new flow of valuable data reinforcing this approach to toxicology. Moreover, as described in the next section, the advent of a new type of tests in the 1830s provided him with new tools for making conclusive proofs based on chemical analysis.

***

After the publication of the *Traité des poisons*, Orfila started a successful career in Paris that reached its apex during the 1830s, when appointed as dean of the Paris Medical Faculty and member of many commissions related to French education. The fame of Orfila grew not only due to his research on poisons, but also thanks to his talent as singer in the Parisian salons. The young physician had a remarkable voice, and it was even said that "offers have been made to him to exchange the amphitheatre and the lecture room for the boards of the opera".[26] In 1840, the *Medical Times* reported that "no other chemist can approach M. Orfila in the sweetness with which he warbles a ballad. Toxicology and *cavatinas* are equally familiar to him: he is equally successful in administering poisons and striking the guitar".[27] In the French *salons*, Orfila met many physicians, lawyers, and politicians whose support and influence would prove decisive in his career as a toxicologist. He even claimed to have "had more success" in projects relative to the improvement of medical studies and research "in *salons* than in the meetings of commissions and in government offices".[28]

With the support of this influential circle, Orfila obtained an appointment as Royal physician, and then he became professor of the Faculty of Medicine and was also elected as one of the founding members of the Paris Academy of Medicine. Thanks to the support of one powerful minister, who frequented the musical soirées organized by Orfila, he managed to obtain funding for his textbooks on toxicology and legal medicine. And, even more important, with all these influential friends, he earned the trust of important politicians who, after the revolution of 1830, became decisive members of the French administration. After being appointed as dean of the Faculty of Medicine, Orfila was requested to develop delicate missions for the French Government. For instance, he participated in the secret commission in charge of attesting the pregnancy of the Duchesse de Berry, who was the leader of the royalists groups fighting for the return of the Bourbon dynasty in the early 1830s. Orfila also played a decisive role in putting down the riots of Republican students between 1833 and 1836.[29]

Supported by his fame as a toxicologist and his connections to political and academic powers, Orfila started to be requested by judges as a forensic physician during the early 1820s. His first case took place in 1823 during a poisoning trial in Paris. Orfila employed liquid tests based on color changes for proving the existence of arsenic in the stomach of the victim. His report was contested by other experts and was not convincing enough for the jurors who delivered an absolutory verdict. The next trial in which he participated was even more deceptive for Orfila: the poisoner (a physician) apparently had employed vegetal poisons, which were very difficult to detect by chemical tests. The first group of experts based their report only on the observed clinical symptoms and, to the despair of Orfila, they did not keep the liquids from the stomach after the autopsy. In court, Orfila angrily recognized that without these materials, no conclusive proof could be provided because the *corpus delicti* was lacking.[30] Orfila confronted many similar awkward situations during the next years, when he was requested to offer his advice concerning many other aspects of legal medicine: identification of corpses, date and place of death, nature of stains (blood and sperm), etc. Sparked by these questions, Orfila performed new animal experiments, refined chemical tests, introduced new procedures for avoiding misleading results, and wrote new papers and books. One of them was about the identification of long-term buried corpses and was later incorporated in his comprehensive textbook on legal medicine.[31]

The participation of Orfila in criminal trials was more and more frequent during the 1830s, particularly in trials concerning arsenic. It was the period when new tests based on the reduction of arsenic to its metallic state were popularized. In contrast with clinical symptoms or colored reagents, the new reduction tests seemed to remove the interpretative role of experts:

metallic arsenic could now be dramatically presented in court as the *corpus delicti*, resembling something like a bloody knife in other criminal trials. Many toxicologists affirmed that "for medico-legal purposes", no other test was "at once so satisfactory, convenient, and delicate as the test of reduction".[32] The most famous test of this kind was presented in October 1836 by James Marsh (1794–1846) during a meeting at the Royal Society of Arts of London. The sample was placed in a flask with arsenic-free zinc and sulfuric acid in order to produce hydrogen. If the sample contained arsenic, arsine was produced, and this compound was then decomposed into hydrogen and arsenic, which formed a thin metallic film on the porcelain. Apart from providing this visual form of proof, the new test was so sensitive that it could detect minute amounts of arsenic, which would have remained unnoticed by using old colored tests. The famous German chemists Justus Liebig affirmed that a sensitivity (whose limits he calculated at 1/500,000 parts) was "beyond any imagination" (Figure 9.2).[33]

Mateu Orfila very soon adapted the Marsh test for his own research on two relevant and interrelated issues: the absorption of poisons and the detection of arsenic in long-buried corpses. He had been interested in the first issue since the beginning of his career, and he soon realized that the high sensitivity of the Marsh test for arsenic offered a new way to approach this elusive question, which had also attracted the attention of experimental physiologists such as François Magendie. Starting in 1838, Orfila

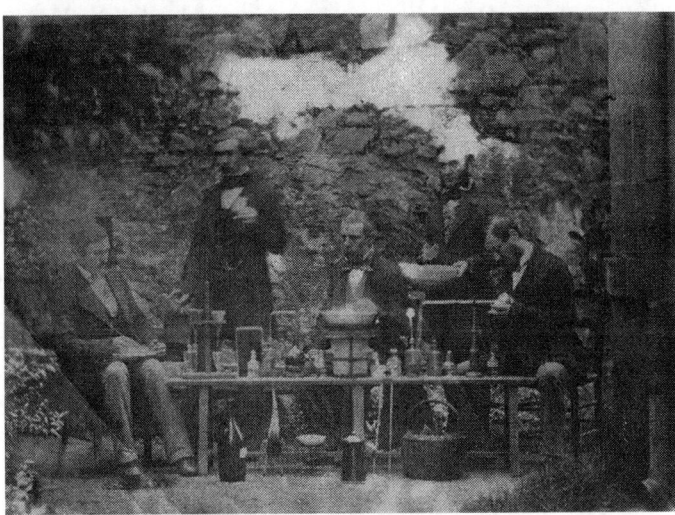

Figure 9.2 A group of experts performing the Marsh test for arsenic (right). The samples were previously treated in a large container (center) and then placed in a glass flask (right). When the test was positive, stains of metallic arsenic were collected in the small porcelain vessel which is in the hands of one of the analysts (far right). On the left side, another expert is portrayed when writing the report for the judge.

Courtesy of Archives départementales de la Corrèze (22 Fi 366).

performed numerous experiments with dogs using a modified version of the Marsh test with a bigger flask and new reagents for dissolving the organic materials to be tested. As mentioned before, Orfila acknowledged that animal experiments offered substantial but limited, and sometimes misleading, information concerning human poisoning, so he was compelled to look for available clinical data and post-mortem examinations from poisoning cases. One of them involved Soufflard, a convicted murderer who had committed suicide in March 1839 by ingesting a large amount of arsenic in prison. Just a few days later, Orfila performed several tests on Soufflard's blood in the presence of "around 1200 students" who attended his lectures at the Faculty of Medicine. He obtained a "notable proportion" of absorbed arsenic, which could be "seen and touched" by the audience.[34] During the following week, Orfila delivered a talk at the Paris Academy of Medicine, in which he described his experiences and discussed the problem of absorption. Again, he employed the dramatic power of experimental demonstrations: he showed Soufflard's stomach to his colleagues, who could also see the arsenical black stains obtained by means of the Marsh test.[35]

Orfila knew that his research on the absorption of poisons could provide important results for the advancement of the physiology and pharmacology, while opening the window for new possible medicolegal applications. If the process of absorption was identified, toxicologists could look for arsenic not only in vomit and in the gastrointestinal tract, but also in other organs and fluids such as the liver, spleen, kidneys, muscles, blood, and urine. The new method could be applied to long-buried bodies, in which the stomach or vomit were not available – a forensic problem which Orfila had recently analyzed with Octave Lesueur (his brother-in-law) in the already-mentioned book on "legal exhumations".[36] Orfila enthusiastically described the consequences of his research at the beginning of 1839. The Marsh test seemed to herald a new era in which all poisoning crimes would be successfully solved by forensic experts:

> From now on, crime will be successfully hunted down to its last refuge because, without doubt, several poisons acting by absorption will be detected in different tissues of the animal economy. This great problem of legal medicine will soon be solved by new research in that direction, founded on the work I have just read. Probably you already foresee that it will shed light on certain points of physiology and therapeutics.[37]

Orfila's enthusiasm was shared by many toxicologists and judges, who placed high hopes in the Marsh test, as it seemed likely to deter would-be murderers from using arsenic forever. He applied his new findings for the first time during a poisoning trial which took place in the small village of Villey-sur-Tille (Northwest France) during the late months of 1838. The victim was Nicolas Mercier, the mentally handicapped son of a poor farmer who was accused of performing the crime under the requests of his new wife. Local experts could not prove the existence of arsenic in the vomit

and the stomach of the victim, so Orfila was compelled to search for absorbed arsenic in the remains of a long-buried corpse, a situation which was
repeated in other trials during the following months. Another common feature of these trials was the controversy concerning Orfila's methods, which
emerged thanks to the reports prepared by other experts, particularly by
François-Vincent Raspail (1794–1878). Raspail had already questioned the
reliability of Orfila's methods employing two main arguments: substances
different from arsenic could give similar results when chemical tests were
applied, and countless sources of contamination could explain the existence
of arsenic in corpses without implying a poisoning crime. The extraordinary
sensitivity of the Marsh test made the second objection more likely. In the
case of Mercier, whose remains had been buried for several months before
being analyzed by Orfila, Raspail argued that arsenic might be passed on
to the corpse from the soil of the graveyard. Again, Orfila was compelled to
perform new animal experiments, some of them with poisoned dogs buried
for several weeks in arsenic-containing soils (mimicking somehow corpses
in graveyards). In response, his critics employed the broad range of arguments against the probatory value of laboratory and animal experiments in
legal medicine. Like in many other cases, starting from technical issues concerning chemical tests and reagents, the controversy turned into a general
discussion concerning the epistemology of medicine and the value of proofs.

***

In the midst of these debates, Orfila soon understood that the extreme
sensitivity of the Marsh test was a double-edged sword. It was true that experts
could detect very small quantities of arsenic, so they could offer convincing
visual evidence in difficult poisoning crimes. But the defense, with the help
of imaginative experts such as Raspail, could also present a broad spectrum of arguable sources of impurities which could sow doubt in the juries'
minds and render a positive test inconclusive from the legal point of view.
The criticism was even more powerful when taking into account the ample
range of uses of poisons such as arsenic in nineteenth-century France: rat
poison, pesticide, agriculture, paper-painting, drugs (Fowler liquor), etc.
The most confusing source of impurity was found inside the human body
just a few months after the introduction of the Marsh test in France, and
was subsequently named "normal arsenic", that is, the quantity of arsenic
supposed to be contained in "normal" non-poisoned human bodies. It was
a very tiny amount of poison, which could only be detected by means of
high-sensitive methods such as the Marsh test. This was a good reason for
explaining why "normal arsenic" had remained unnoticed for previous toxicologists. Orfila, who was one of its first discoverers, immediately realized
that "normal arsenic was a perturbing element", a "terrible blow" for
legal medicine, because, when arsenic was found in a corpse during a trial,
attorneys and judges could always ask whether it was part of arsenic found
in normal human bodies (instead of being a result of criminal poisoning).[38]

In order to deal with this problem, Orfila employed two strategies: the identification of the organs in which normal arsenic was concentrated (so chemical tests could be applied to the remaining organs, in which arsenic did not exist in a normal state); and the differences in chemical properties between "criminal" and "normal" arsenic, so they could be distinguished during the chemical analysis (for instance, taking into account their different solubility in boiling water). Both strategies involved new research in the laboratory (refining procedures and testing new reagents), animal experiments (analyzing and comparing samples taken from poisoned and non-poisoned dogs), and post-mortem examinations (chemical analysis of human organs from both poisoned and healthy individuals). As in previous cases, Orfila's research on normal arsenic was prompted by his participation in the trial of Mercier. "I could not have appeared in that court", he affirmed in one of his later papers, "if I had been unable to prove that the internal organs of Nicolas Mercier had presented arsenic to the Parisian experts *only because he had been poisoned* by an arsenical preparation".[39] He summarized the results of his research in September 1839 during a meeting at the Paris Academy of Medicine. Orfila claimed that "it was always possible to ascertain" in forensic medicine whether the arsenic identified by the Marsh test was normal or absorbed, provided that his instructions on reagents and chemical manipulations were strictly followed (Figure 9.3).[40]

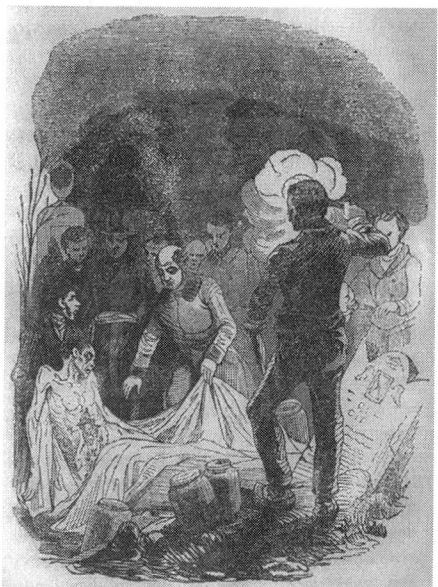

Figure 9.3 Exhumation of Charles Lafarge in September 1840. It was one of the most famous poisoning trials in which Orfila participated as expert. From *Procès de Madame Lafarge*, Paris, Bureaux de l'Audience, 1841.
Personal collection.

The issue of "normal arsenic" was raised during the trial of Mercier in Dijon at the end of 1839, but it played a minor role in regard to the debate about the arsenic found in graveyards. As long as the research on normal arsenic was more and more known, the issue became more and more important during the trials. A desperate Orfila wondered, "how can one persuade juries that the minute quantity of arsenic which has been obtained [by means of the Marsh test] was not furnished by the arsenical preparation which is naturally contained by the human body?"[41] In June 1840, he met this challenge when defending his expert report against both Raspail's skeptical arguments and the objections made by lawyers and jurors, who were surprisingly well acquainted with recent developments in research on normal arsenic. One of the jurors remarked that the test had been performed on the whole corpse of the victim, including the bones, so he asked Orfila whether "it could be possible to affirm that the arsenic yielded by means of the Marsh apparatus was in fact the normal arsenic of bones". Orfila answered this objection by using his second strategy, that is, by reminding the alleged differences in solubility of normal and absorbed arsenic:

> [Normal] arsenic cannot be extracted from bones by means of boiling water [...], strong acids are needed; so, even if the analyzed liquids were obtained by boiling the victim's bones, the liquid could never contain an atom of the normal arsenic found in bones.[42]

Just two month later, in September 1840, Orfila was requested to participate in the most famous poisoning trial of his times: the trial of Marie Lafarge in Tulle. Normal arsenic was so well known that it was mentioned by the judge when asking one of the local experts: "Has it not been acknowledged for some time that the human body in its normal state contains some arsenic?" The doctor Massénat, who had been in touch with Orfila some months before, offered a similar answer:

> It has been recognized that the bones of adult humans contain some arsenic but, in order to obtain it, the bones have to be calcinated and treated with sulfuric acid and the Marsh apparatus. It is a new discovery arising from the works of 1840, but it by no means proves that we acted incorrectly with the substances brought to us, and above all we did nothing that might have produced normal arsenic.[43]

The answer shows that the main features of normal arsenic, and the ways of dealing with it in forensic analysis, were well known by local doctors such as Massénat or even judges or jurors who participated in poisoning trials around 1840. In the trial of Marie Lafarge for having poisoned her husband, these uncertainties were expanded by the contradictory results obtained by the different groups of experts. Three different expert reports were prepared and discussed before Orfila's analysis of the exhumed organs of the victim. The first one was inconclusive but suggested a poisoning crime. The other two groups of experts, who employed the Marsh test, could not find any arsenic in the human remains of the victim. On 14 September 1840, amid great excitement, Orfila read the final report in which he affirmed that he had indeed found arsenic in Lafarge's body. He provided a likely explanation of the differences between his results and those of the three previous chemical tests. He also remarked that the arsenic detected came neither from the reagents nor from the earth of the graveyard in which the body was buried; nor did it belong to the "arsenic portion that naturally exists in the human body". In contrast with the previous trial, Orfila adopted here his first strategy, that is, the idea that normal arsenic was located only in the bones, so any arsenic detected in the internal organs would necessarily have been ingested and absorbed:

> Thanks to my experiments, which I started 18 months ago, today it is acknowledged that a very small quantity of arsenic naturally exists in the bones of humans and many other animals; but it is also acknowledged that, following the current method, not even the smallest trace of arsenic is ever obtained from the human stomach, liver, spleen, kidneys, heart or lungs. We operated not on the bones but on the internal organs. Therefore, what we removed is not normal arsenic.[44]

The controversy around the Lafarge trial sparked off an intense debate inside the Paris medical community, which soon spread to other academic and social contexts during the following months. The controversy reached its peak in 1841, when special sessions were held at the Academy of Science and the Academy of Medicine. Moreover, the debate was not confined to the scientific and medical community. Orfila prepared a group of lectures on toxicology at the Paris Medical Faculty in November 1840, which were delivered in a large amphitheater crowded with a varied audience. The lectures were fully covered by the popular press and many medical journals, even in foreign countries. Again, Orfila employed all the resources provided by experimental demonstration and the visual power of the black stains obtained by means of the Marsh test. Orfila performed many chemical analyses of different organic samples and conducted numerous animal experiments related to contentious topics, some of them suggested by members of his audience on issues raised during the trial of Lafarge.[45]

With his experimental performance in amphitheaters, also repeated in courtrooms and in academies, Orfila attempted to transform what were highly controversial issues into plain matters of fact, dramatically proved by experiments and material evidence that could be seen and sometimes touched by the audience. In spite of his pedagogical skills, academic power, and laboratory resources, he could not avoid the spreading of the controversy in the public sphere. Poisoning trials attracted the attention of the public and were usually commented in newspapers and salons. The trial of Marie Lafarge turned up to be one of the most popular topics for polite conversation during these years. On 14 September 1840, just when Orfila presented his report in court, the duchesse de Dino noted in his diary that all conversations in the salons were about the affair Lafarge: "Here, as everywhere, there are quite contrasting views on this issue", she wrote. A "war of salons" broke out in the form of passionate discussions between "Lafargistes" and "anti-Lafargistes", to such an extent that the journal *Le Siècle* announced in September 1840 that some invitations to salons included a warning: "We will not talk about the trial of [Madame] Lafarge". However, in November 1840, a Parisian pharmacist organized a soirée at which he explained in front of around twenty people, "all the experiments regarding arsenic poisoning", reconstructing the chemical analysis performed by the experts during the Lafarge trial and supporting Orfila's views on this issue. Medical, scientific, and popular journals dealt at length with the Lafarge drama, not only in France but elsewhere in Europe.[46]

At the end of the day, the advent of the Marsh test and the new research on the absorption of arsenic was not the final panacea against crimes of poisoning.[47] Jules Barse (1812–1878), a pharmacist who started his career in courts at the end of the 1830s, remembered those days as a mixture of hope and confusion: "the facts multiplied infinitely [...] arsenic was found everywhere. Soon it was found that this new method, this radiant light, merely revealed a situation of total chaos".[48] Apart from the mentioned uncertainties concerning minute quantities of arsenic, the high sensitivity of the Marsh test introduced new potential "organizational contingencies" which could produce misleading results at any point of the "chain of custody" between the crime scene and the court.[49] These almost unlimited sources of impurity, including normal arsenic, were capitalized on by defense attorneys and proved to be very damaging for the authority of Orfila and the credibility of his toxicological methods.

Paradoxically, more general criticism and fundamental doubts emerged when the new toxicological methods were employed to question previous tests whose results were until then accepted as reliable. The issue was pointed out by Raspail during the Mercier trial when he affirmed: "Gentlemen, you must doubt the omnipotence of legal chemistry because it refutes itself every six months".[50] This skeptical feeling damaged also the reliability of the results obtained by means of the Marsh test, including those related to normal arsenic. The writer George Sand, who like many others passionately followed the news of the Lafarge trial, doubted the reliability of the expert reports: "Maybe Orfila will discover in the next six months that arsenic does exist in the liver or in the brain of all corpses".[51] From the point of view of an expert in legal medicine, the young doctor Ambroise Tardieu summarized the awkward situation in the following terms:

> Concerning arsenic poisoning, it seems that we have suddenly and completely forgotten the most ordinary procedures of the philosophy

of the sciences, and even more, the most common facts regarding their history. What is the cause of all this big stir, if not that absolute certainty has always been required in matters in which the truth will be always just relative? The proof is easy: it was a real advancement in the tools [employed in toxicology] introduced the doubt about the value of these tools! It has been the Marsh test which has rendered suspicious the chemical assays longtime accepted for arsenical materials. In this one fact there is something strange enough to bring to the fore the lack of reason in these unusual requirements.[52]

Like many other forensic experts, Tardieu acknowledged that the replacement of the old chemical analysis by the new Marsh test involved a danger for the credibility of toxicological methods. In fact, as Tardieu remarked, nothing could be more damaging for the credibility of toxicologists than the sharp contrast between the great hopes of absolute certitude and the "situation of total chaos" produced by the advent of new high-sensitivity methods. The chaos described by Jules Barse was not only due to the skeptical objections lodged by Raspail and other experts. It also emerged from the new experiments performed by other chemists and physicians whose attention was attracted to this issue by the ongoing controversy. The poisoning trials, along with new research undertaken in academies and laboratories, provided a constant flow of unforeseen and embarrassing data on poisons which were obtained by means of more and more refined versions of chemical tests during the following years.

Not even Orfila could imagine that the new studies on arsenic would yield such harmful results for his authority as expert. At the end of 1840, different authors proved by new experiments that normal arsenic did not exist: it was just a mistake produced by high-sensitivity chemical tests. These surprising and embarrassing conclusions were reviewed and finally approved by a commission from the Paris Academy of Science in June 1841. And yet, prompted by these challenges, Orfila pursued his work on the absorption of poisons at the Paris Faculty of Medicine. He carried out new laboratory research and performed more animal experiments, which became the bases of new papers presented at the Paris Academy of Medicine and eventually abridged and transformed into new sections of his authoritative textbooks on legal medicine, which were employed as reference books in courts and classrooms all over Europe.[53]

***

Like DNA fingerprints at the end of the twentieth century, the Marsh test raised great expectations concerning the role of science in criminal investigations. For a while, both technologies were employed for testing other forms of evidence and produced controversies with the unforeseen result of questioning forensic science in general. However, in contrast with DNA fingerprints, the controversy on chemical tests never reached a closure by the emergence of new technologies granted with "exceptional evidentiary status".[54] Debates on the use of the Marsh test were frequent in courts even during the second half of the nineteenth century. The controversy over normal arsenic was far from being definitively closed after the report of the Academy of Science in 1841. The final consequences were damaging in terms of credibility for the kind of toxicology prompted by Orfila and based on experimental demonstrations, high-sensitivity chemical tests, and animal experiments. He finally decided in 1843 to turn his back on the courts and only sporadically did he accept requests of judges during the last ten years of his life. By the middle of the nineteenth century, many toxicologists felt that Orfila's approach has reached a dead-end. As said before, his colleague Ambroise Tardieu called for a return to more traditional sources of toxicological knowledge such as clinical observations and anatomo-pathological data of poisoned individuals.

The approach to toxicology developed by Orfila was thus contingent and emerged from a mixture of many personal and local circumstances revisited in this chapter: an exceptional training in analytical chemistry, social networks with connections to the political power, animal experiments with an eye on their uses in medicine, widespread fame and academic authority, material resources and convenient spaces provided by the Paris Faculty of Medicine, and murder trials in which Orfila was involved as expert during the 1820s and 1830s. These contingent features provided, however, the necessary assets for developing a continued program of research on poisons during three decades, which transformed Orfila's textbook on toxicology into the most famous reference work for that subject in many European countries. In spite of his careful management of the uncertainty surrounding issues such as "normal arsenic", Orfila's research was far from being "junk science in courtrooms". Neither did it provide definitive and completely reliable tools for putting poisoners in prison. While offering new resources for both toxicological research and criminal investigations, the new chemical tests introduced additional challenges and prompted controversies, which proved to be very damaging for Orfila's authority in courts.

Orfila's research on poisons would have been impossible without the data provided by trials such as those of Soufflard, Mercier, Cumon, Rigal, or Lafarge. When chemical analysis and animal experimentation were insufficient or inadequate, the corpses of the victims turned out to be unique sources of information on poisoning. The trials also provided challenging questions on unexpected issues, which encouraged the search for more reliable chemical tests and refined animal experiments. Among the achievements were not only more sophisticated technologies for detecting poisons in criminal investigations, but also substantial data and important conclusions concerning the absorption and effects of poisons. As his Scottish colleague Robert Christison remarked, the research conducted by Orfila during the 1830s was "pregnant alike with interesting physiological deductions and valuable medico-legal applications".[55]

Perhaps the impressive sensibility of the Marsh test produced a sort of "CSI-effect" in the minds of jurors, lawyers, and judges during its first appearances in court. But was it experts like Liebig or Orfila, rather than mass media, who launched this overoptimistic image in their academic publications? The first papers presented by Orfila at the Academy of Medicine in 1839 aroused great expectations concerning the power of new technologies to "hunt crime down to its last refuge". These high hopes were soon lowered by the ensuing chaos of impurities emerging from reagents, graveyard soils, and the insidious normal arsenic. The Marsh test provided in court new forms of material evidence, namely black arsenic-like stains, which seemed to "speak for themselves" without the mediation of experts. However, with the help of skeptical experts like Raspail, defense lawyers questioned the arsenic-like stains as the actual *corpus delicti*. This review has also shown that even jurors could be aware of the uncertainties surrounding the new methods, so they could ask experts about the nature and origins of the black stains obtained by means of the Marsh test.

Thanks to the public interest in poisoning trials, the controversy largely contributed to popularize the new high-sensitivity technologies to a broad audience, moving from courts to classrooms, academies, and salons. The verbatim reports of the oral hearings acquainted lay people with substantial details concerning the new methods. Many of them, like the novelist George Sand, were unimpressed by the alleged virtues of the new high-sensitivity chemical tests. By exposing to the public the shortcomings of traditional methods and introducing new sources of fallibility, the new technologies raised more fundamental doubts about the usefulness of chemical tests in judicial fact-finding. Many observers and stakeholders worried about the reliability of expert reports, particularly when they were destined to inspire guilty verdicts sometimes involving the death penalty. In that way, the controversy expanded to more general issues such as the appropriate chains of custody in a world full of impurities; the rightness of the free evaluation of scientific evidence; the overlapping roles of jurors, judges, and experts; and the nature and extension of the group of experts who could employ the new high-sensitivity technologies in a reliable way. The above review shows that Orfila was a leading protagonist in these debates, which so decisively shaped the activities of forensic doctors and the development of toxicology during the nineteenth century.

Notes

1 See, for instance, the few sentences on Orfila included in J.R. Partington, *A History of Chemistry* (London: McMillan, 1961–1970), vol. IV, p. 478; W.F. Bynum and R. Porter (eds.), *Companion Encyclopedia of the History of Medicine* (London and New York: Routledge, 1993), vol. II, p. 919. Surprisingly enough, Orfila is not included in the biographical dictionary edited by A. Roca,

Ciència i tècnica als Països Catalans: una aproximació biogràfica (Barcelona: FCR, 1995).

2   See S. Jasanoff, *Science at the Bar: Law, Science, and Technology in America* (Cambridge: Harvard University Press, 1995); F. Chauvaud, *Les experts du crime. La médecine légale en France au XIXè siècle* (Paris: Aubier, 2000); T. Golan, *Laws of Man and Laws of Nature: A History of Scientific Expert Testimony* (Cambridge: Harvard University Press, 2004); K. Watson, *Forensic Medicine in Western Society: A History* (London: Routledge, 2011); S. Arapostathis and G. Gooday, *Patently Contestable* (Cambridge: MIT Press, 2013). C. Hamlin, "Forensic Cultures in Historical Perspective: Technologies of Witness, Testimony, Judgement (and Justice)", *Studies in History and Philosophy of Biological and Biomedical Sciences* 44 (2013): 4–15; I. Burney and N. Pemberton, *Murder and the Making of English CSI* (Baltimore: Johns Hopkins University Press, 2016). For a review on current literature on history of poisons, see J.R. Bertomeu-Sánchez and Ximo Guillem-Llobat, "Following Poisons in Society and Culture (1800–2000): A Review of Current Literature", *Actes d'Història de la Ciència i de la Tècnica* 9 (2016): 9–36.

3   This approach can be found in P.W. Huber, *Galileo's Revenge: Junk Science in the Courtroom* (New York: Basic Books, 1991). Of course, another important problem in this approach is the received image of academic science. On this point, see, for instance, the discussion of S. Cole, "Forensic Culture as Epistemic Culture: The Sociology of Forensic Science", *Studies in History and Philosophy of Biological and Biomedical Sciences* 44 (2013): 36–46.

4   See J.R. Bertomeu-Sánchez, "Animal Experiments, Vital Forces and Courtrooms: Mateu Orfila, François Magendie and the Study of Poisons in Nineteenth-century France", *Annals of Science* 69 (2012): 1–26.

5   For a recent critical review, see S.A. Cole, "A Surfeit of Science: The 'CSI Effect' and the Media Appropriation of the Public Understanding of Science", *Public Understanding of Science* 24 (2015): 130–146.

6   See J.R. Bertomeu-Sánchez, "Managing Uncertainty in the Academy and the Courtroom: Normal Arsenic and Nineteenth-Century Toxicology", *Isis* 104 (2013): 197–225.

7   I.A. Burney, *Poison, Detection, and the Victorian Imagination* (Manchester: Manchester University Press, 2006); K. Watson, *Dr. Crippen* (Kew: National Archives, 2007); J.R. Bertomeu-Sánchez, *La verdad sobre el caso Lafarge* (Barcelona: El Serbal, 2015). For a social history of poison and poisoners, see K. Watson, *Poisoned Lives: English Poisoners and their Victims* (London: Hambledon, 2004).

8   On Orfila, see J.R. Bertomeu-Sánchez and A. Nieto-Galan (eds.), *Chemistry, Medicine, and Crime: Mateu J. B. Orfila (1787–1851) and His Times* (Sagamore Beach: Science History Publications, 2006), which offers a review of biographical literature. His autobiography and letters have recently been published in J.R. Bertomeu-Sánchez and J.M. Vidal Hernàndez (eds.), *Mateu Orfila (1787–1853). Autobiografia i correspondència,* (Menorca: IEM, 2011); J.R. Bertomeu-Sánchez, *Venenos, Ciencia y Justicia: Mateu Orfila y su Epistolario* (Alicante: PUA, 2015). Most of Orfila's publications and other relevant documents can be read online at: www.bium.univ-paris5.fr/histmed/medica/orfila.htm.

9   The classical study on this issue is E.H. Ackerknecht, *Medicine at the Paris Hospital, 1794–1848,* (Baltimore: The Johns Hopkins Press, 1967). For a renovated view, see C. Hannaway and A. La Berge (eds.), *Constructing Paris Medicine* (Amsterdam: Rodopi, 1998).

10   See A. Queruel, *Vauquelin et son temps (1763–1829)* (Paris: L'Harmattan, 1994). On the other mentioned professors, see W.A. Smeaton, *Fourcroy: chemist and revolutionary, 1755–1809* (Cambridge: Heffer, 1962). On Thenard, see

the chapter by Antonio García Belmar in Bertomeu-Nieto (eds.), *Chemistry, Medicine and Crime*; and A. García Belmar and J.R. Bertomeu-Sánchez, "Louis Jacques Thenard's Chemistry Courses at the Collège de France, 1804–1835", *Ambix* 57 (2010): 48–63.

11 M. Orfila, *Nouvelles recherches sur l'urine des ictériques* (Paris: Didot Jeune, 1811).

12 Orfila, autobiography, in Bertomeu-Vidal, *Mateu Orfila* (p. 135):

> Je fis un mélange de cette boisson et de la dissolution arsenicale: « Vous allez être convaincus de l'exactitude de ce que j'avance, » dis-je à ces messieurs. Pas du tout! L'eau de chaux, qui devait précipiter en blanc, fournit un trouble gris violacé; le sulfate de cuivre ammoniacal donna un précipité olive noirâtre, au lieu d'un précipité vert pré, etc... Que l'on juge de mon embarras! J'attribuai ces résultats à la présence de matières organiques et colorées, sans pouvoir expliquer au juste ce qui était arrivé.

13 On early nineteenth-century analytical chemistry, see E. Homburg, "The Rise of Analytical Chemistry and Its Consequences for the Development of the German Chemical Profession", *Ambix* 46 (1999): 1–32. On colored test and its problems, see Burney, *Poison, Detection, and the Victorian Imagination*, chapter III. On the difficulties of handling visual colored data in chemistry, see the study on nineteenth-century spectroscopy by K. Hentschel, *Mapping the Spectrum: Techniques of Visual Representation in Research and Teaching* (Oxford: Oxford University Press, 2002).

14 For instance, a postmortem examination performed by Jules Cloquet in March 1813. See M. Orfila, *Traité des poisons* (Paris: Crochard, 1814–1815), vol. I, pp. 219–221.

15 *Procès-verbaux des séances de l'Académie Hendaye*, 1910–1922, vol. 5, p. 263. Letter to Antoni Orfila, Paris, 25 November 1815. Printed in Bertomeu-Vidal, *Mateu Orfila*, pp. 379–381. For details about the different editions and translations, see José Ramón Bertomeu-Sánchez, "Livres et brochures de Mateu Orfila i Rotger (1787–1853)". www.bium.univ-paris5.fr/histmed/medica/orfila/orfila03.htm.

16 Orfila, *Traité des Poisons*, vol. III, p. xvi.

17 See M.P. Earles, "Experiments with Drugs and Poisons in the Seventeenth and Eighteenth Centuries", *Annals of Science* 19 (1963): 241–254; A.H. Maehle, *Drugs on Trial: Experimental Pharmacology and Therapeutic Innovation in the Eighteenth-Century* (Amsterdam: Rodopi, 1999). See also J. Schickore, *About Method: Experimenters, Snake Venom, and the History of Writing Scientifically* (Chicago: University of Chicago Press, 2017).

18 John Cross, *Sketches of the Medical Schools of Paris* (London: Callow, 1815), pp. 55–56.

19 For an overview, see N. Rupke (ed.), *Vivisection in Historical Perspective* (New York: Croom Helm Ltd., 1987); A. Guerrini, *Experimenting with Humans and Animals: From Galen to Animal Rights* (Baltimore: John Hopkins University Press, 2003).

20 *British and Foreign Medico Chirurgical Review* 27 (April 1861): 285–318, quoted on p. 308.

21 M. Orfila, "Note sur l'empoisonnement par l'oxyde blanc d'arsenic", *Archives générales de médecine* 1 (1823): 147–152, quoted on pp. 147–148. "funeste à l'avancement de la science". On early antivivisection movements in France, see Paul Elliot, "Vivisection and the Emergence of Experimental Physiology in Nineteenth-century France", in Rupke (ed.), *Vivisection in Historical Perspective*, pp. 48–77.

22 A. Portal, *Mémoires sur la nature et le traitement de plusieurs maladies* (Paris: Bertrand, 1800–1825), vol. 4, pp. 300–316.

23 George Macilwain, *Memoirs of John Abernethy, F.R.S.* ... (London: Hurst and Blackett, 1853), pp. 194–200, quoted on p. 200. For more details about these debates, see Bertomeu-Sánchez, "Animal Experiments".

24 Orfila, *Traité des poisons*, vol. II, pp. 228–235. Orfila reviewed and answered the criticisms in the subsequent editions of his textbook. See M. Orfila, *Traité de Toxicologie*, 5th edition (Paris: Labé, 1851), vol. I, pp. 45–51.

25 A. Tardieu, *Étude médico-légale et clinique sur l'empoisonnement par* ... (Paris: Baillière, 1867), pp. 10–11 and 112.

26 The sentence was written by the American physician Peter Solomon Townsend in his diary, in 1828. See G. Rosen, "An American Doctor in Paris in 1828: Selections from the Diary of Peter Solomon Townsend, M.D.", *Journal of the History of Medicine and Allied Sciences* 6 (1) (1951): 64–115, on p. 81.

27 *Medical Times* 3 (1840–1841): 106.

28 P.H.M. Bérard, *Eloge d'Orfila prononcé dans la séance de rentrée de la Faculté de médecine* (Paris: Labé, 1854), p. 50: "J'ai obtenu plus de décisions avantageuses pour la Faculté, j'ai mené à bonne fin plus d'entreprises relatives aux études, dans les salons que dans les bureaux des administrations". See also A. Fayol, *La vie et l'œuvre d'Orfila* (Paris: Albin Michel, 1930), pp. 130–143.

29 For more details, see J.R. Bertomeu-Sánchez, "Classrooms, Salons, Academies, and Courts: Mateu Orfila (1787–1853) and Nineteenth-Century French Toxicology", *Ambix* 61 (2014): 162–186.

30 *Journal des débats*, 13 November 1823.

31 J.R. Bertomeu-Sánchez, "El esqueleto de la viuda Houet: Frenología y medicina legal en Francia durante la década de 1830", *Criminocorpus* [online since 10 February 2015]. http://criminocorpus.revues.org/2927; doi:10.4000/criminocorpus.2927.

32 R. Christison, *A Treatise on Poisons*, 4th edition (Edinburgh: Black, 1845), p. 261. See also I.A. Burney, "Languages of the Lab: Toxicological Testing and Medico-legal Proof", *Studies in History and Philosophy of Science* 33 (2002): 289–314 for a larger discussion.

33 *Annalen der Pharmazie und Chemie* 23 (1837): 217–227. Quotation from Liebig in p. 223. J. Marsh, "An Account of a Method of Separating Small Quantities of Arsenic from Substances with Which It May Be Mixed", *Edinburgh New Philosophical Journal* 21 (1836): 229–236. See K. Watson, "Criminal Poisoning in England and the Origins of the Marsh Test for Arsenic". In Bertomeu-Nieto (eds.), *Chemistry, Medicine and Crime*, pp. 183–207.

34 M. Orfila, "De l'empoisonnement par l'acide arsénieux", *Bulletin de l'Académie Royale de Médecine* 3 (1839): 676–683.

35 *L'Expérience*, 91, 28 March 1839, p. 208.

36 M. Orfila and O. Lesueur, *Traité des exhumations juridiques* (Paris: Béchet, 1831).

37 M. Orfila, "Mémoire sur l'empoisonnement par l'acide arsénieux", *Bulletin de l'Académie Royale de Médecine* 3 (1839): 426–464. Quoted on p. 464. See also Archives of the Académie de Médecine de Paris, *Procès-verbaux – Séances générales*, Session 29 janvier 1839.

38 M. Orfila, "Empoisonnement par l'arsenic", *Annales d'hygiène publique et de médecine légale* 24 (1840): 298–313. Quoted on pp. 312–313.

39 *L'Esculape*, 22 December 1839, 1 (29), p. 166. Italics are mine.

40 M. Orfila, "De l'arsenic naturellement contenu dans le corps de l'homme", *Bulletin de l'Académie Royale de Médecine* 4 (1839): 178–203. Quoted on p. 181.

41 M. Orfila, "Mémoire sur plusieurs affaires d'empoisonnement par l'arsenic...", *Bulletin de l'Académie Royale de Médecine* 5 (1840): 465–475. Quoted on p. 474.
42 *Le Droit*, 10 June 1840, 5 (138), p. 561.
43 See the main documents of the trial in *Procès de Mme Lafarge* (Paris: Pagnerre, 1840). Quotation from p. 114. For more details, see Bertomeu-Sánchez, *La verdad sobre el caso Lafarge.*
44 *Procès de Mme Lafarge*, pp. 352–353 and p. 356.
45 *Le Moniteur*, 26 October 1840, p. 2159; *L'Esculape*, 5 November 1840, pp. 109–112. For further information, see Bertomeu-Sánchez, "Managing Uncertainty".
46 Quotations from A.M. Fugier, *La vie élégante ou la formation de Tout-Paris, 1815–1848* (Paris: Fayard, 1990), pp. 170–171, and M. de Bassanville, *Les Salons d'Autrefois* (Paris: Brunet, 1862–1866), vol. 3, pp. 181–187. For more details, see Bertomeu-Sánchez, *La verdad sobre el caso Lafarge.*
47 See J.C. Whorton, *The Arsenic Century: How Victorian Britain was Poisoned at Home, Work, and Play* (Oxford: Oxford University Press, 2010), chapter 4, "The chief terror of poisoners".
48 J. Barse, *Manuel de la cour d'assises* (Paris: Labé, 1845). Quoted on p. 151.
49 Quotes from Lynch et al., "Truth Machine", p. 66. See also pp. 113–141 and 228–254.
50 *Gazette des Hôpitaux*, 31 December 1839, p. 609.
51 Letter to Eugène Delacroix, 22 September 1840, quoted by C. Sobieniak, *Rebondissements dans l'affaire Lafarge* (Paris: Lucien Souny, 2010), pp. 219–220.
52 A. Tardieu, "Médecine légale théorique et pratique par A. Dévergie", *Annales d'Hygiène Publique et de Médecine Légale* 27 (1842): 225–232. Quoted on pp. 226–227:

> A propos de cet empoisonnement par l'arsenic, il semble que l'on ait tout-à-coup et complètement oublié les procédés les plus vulgaires de la philosophie des sciences, et bien plus, les faits les plus communs de leur histoire. D'où vient tout le bruit, si ce n'est que l'on a voulu exiger la certitude absolue là où la vérité ne sera toujours que relative. La preuve en est facile: c'est un perfectionnement bien réel de ces moyens employés qui est venu faire douteur de la valeur de ces moyens mêmes! C'est l'appareil de Marsh qui a rendu suspectes les analyses dès longtemps acceptées pour les matières arsenicales. Il y a dans ce seul fait, quelque chose d'assez étrange pour mettre en saillie sur-le-champ le peu de raison de ces exigences inusitées.

53 See Bertomeu-Sánchez, "Managing uncertainty", for more details.
54 The previous quotation was taken from the study on DNA fingerprints by M. Lynch et al., *Truth Machine*, 340.
55 Christison, *A Treatise on Poisons*, 289.

10 Mercury

"One of the Most Valuable Drugs We Have" (1937)

Andrew Cunningham

1. Original uses of mercury in Western medicine

The title of my chapter here cites the judgement of a very important pharmaceutical guide in its 23rd edition, published in 1937, on the continuing importance of mercury in the treatment of syphilis, Sir William Hale-White's *Materia medica*:

> Mercury in any form is powerfully antisyphilitic. The perchloride is often used for adults, and grey powder for children. This action is so important that it makes mercury one of the most valuable drugs we have... it can completely cure the patient.[1]

No one in the West would make such a claim today, so radically has the position of mercury in the *materia medica* been changed.

Mercury is extremely poisonous to humans in almost every one of its many forms. Yet it has been in widespread use in European medicine, in many forms and for many illnesses and conditions, from at least the late 1490s until the late 1950s, that is, for the best part of 500 years. It is still in regular use in many non-Western medical systems today.[2]

The toxicity of mercury has been known from ancient times, by Greek, Roman and Chinese physicians. It appears in Dioscorides' book on *materia medica* from the 1st century AD.[3] In fact, mercury is not the only toxic metal that has customarily been used in the Western *materia medica*. For instance, *The London Pharmacopoeia* of 1824 has a section on 'The metals and their salts', in which it deals with the preparation and uses of antimony, silver nitrate, arsenic, bismuth, copper, iron, lead and zinc, as well as mercury.[4] All of these minerals, or preparations from them, are poisonous to man. But mercury is probably the most dangerous because it has always been known that contact with or proximity to mercury or even to its vapour, from the moment of first mining it onwards, leads to disruption of breathing, of digestion, of the nerves, skin and the major organs, and it can lead to insanity. Its use in certain industrial applications could make one 'mad as a hatter'. And all this before considering its use in medicine!

Mercury in ointment form was a familiar skin treatment from the medieval period. 'Raw', or liquid, mercury is mixed with animal fat and other ingredients; left for a few days, the fat becomes black, and the medicinal effect of the mercury is thought to become stronger the longer it is left. This ointment had first been used by Arab practitioners to counter the extremely irritating itch of scabies or that of crabs, and it had then been used quite widely in Latin Europe too. Both these skin irritations are now known to be caused by little parasites (scabies by the scab mite and crabs by the pubic louse), but as they are too small to be seen with the naked eye, it was thought that the skin problems – rashes, pimples, pustules, sores, irritations, etc. – were a result of eruptions from within the body, presumably from corrupted blood. The application of mercury ointment does, in fact, kill these parasites after only a couple of applications – it is after all poisonous to most living things, to men, to beasts to insects and to funguses, though not to plants – so the doctors clearly had an effective medicine for diseases seemingly erupting through the skin and causing rashes and irritations.

Mercury has been used against the pox (syphilis) from the 1490s until the mid-20th century. The gradual decline in its use in syphilis came through 'the laboratory revolution in medicine', as it has been called, towards the end of the 19th century, when the laboratory became the arena in which drugs were tested, analysed and developed.[5] The causative microorganism of syphilis was isolated in the laboratory in 1905 by Fritz Schaudinn and Erich Hoffmann at the Charité hospital in Berlin, and thereafter mercury was progressively replaced first by the 'magic bullet', Salvarsan, discovered by Ehrlich in 1910,[6] and then by penicillin, discovered by Fleming and in widespread use from 1943. From the introduction of the Wassermann test in 1906, medical men could detect the presence or absence of the causal microorganism of syphilis in the blood and thus (hopefully) speak authoritatively on the presence or absence of syphilis in a patient. A negative finding in the Wassermann test was good, indicating the absence of the spirochetes in the blood; a positive finding was bad. Much faith was put in this test initially, but it was actually very contested.[7] Nevertheless, it could be claimed as late as the 1930s, as we have seen, that mercury was still 'one of the most valuable drugs we have' for the treatment of syphilis. It is a strange case of a poison known to be a poison – that is, mercury – having been used for centuries as a medicine against another poison – that is, the *virus* of pox, in whatever form that *virus* was imagined to exist and operate. One poison was thought to be the antidote to another poison.

Several other forms of mercury remained in use in the hospital and the sickroom well into the 20th century. It was still in use into the 1950s in various preparations as an antiseptic or germicide, and as a purgative – 'children take mercury very well' as a mild purge[8] – and as a treatment for teething problems in infancy.

It is only really in the last half-century that mercury has been progressively eliminated from the Western *materia medica*, as its dangers to the patient have come to be recognised, and as substitutes for it have been discovered – substitutes that, this time, really work against syphilis.

2. Mercury and the pox

The French pox, or syphilis, first appeared in Europe in the French army besieging Naples in 1494.[9] It was described as a pox because of the pocks it produced on the skin (like smallpox, but larger), and it was French because the soldiers of the French army besieging Naples were the first to suffer from it. An early sufferer, a German soldier called Ulrich von Hutten, recalled that 'there were boils, sharp and standing out, having the similitude and size of acorns, from which came so foul humours and so great stench, that whosoever once smelled it, though himself infect. The colour of these boils was dark green'.[10] Running sores appeared all over the body, and holes appeared in the flesh. These symptoms clearly suggested to physicians and surgeons that the French pox was primarily a skin disease – and our earliest visual representations of it confirm this (Figure 10.1).[11]

Having thus identified the pox as a skin disease, this is how early practitioners set out to treat it. Figure 10.2 shows medical people: the doctor inspecting the urine flask, probably a surgeon applying ointment to the pocks on the skin.[12]

But this new disease also affected the bones and especially the joints, causing almost unbearable pain, which was even worse at night. The first attempts to deal with this disease involved repeatedly covering the body with mercury ointment and then shutting the patient up in a 'stew' or overheated room for weeks on end. 'At length the matter must come to this point, that they should lose their teeth, for they were loosened, their mouth was all in a sore, and through coldness of the stomach and filthy stench they lost appetite'.[13]

A development from this treatment was to heat mercury in a bowl and have the patient breathe in the vapours. To a modern mind, this is simply the worst treatment one could have used. The effect was to make the teeth loose and fall out, and to promote extraordinary amounts of saliva. Our early sufferer, Ulrich von Hutten, reported that 'the disease voided both by the nose and the mouth', and 'all their throats, their tongues, the roofs of their mouths, were full of sores'. If – as one hoped – these were signs of the poison coming out, then they were to be welcomed, however unpleasant they were. Under such treatment, patients also often went mad.

How did the mercury treatment work, if indeed you believed that it did? Your answer would depend on your understanding of the operations of the body in health and disease at the level beyond the visible. So, there was no consistent explanation over the centuries in which it was used, as understandings of physiology and pathology underwent many changes. One important set of explanations was given in 1530 by Girolamo Fracastoro (Hieronymus Fracastorius), the medical professor who first named the disease 'syphilis'. He wrote his account in the form of a Latin poem, 'Syphilis, or the French disease' (*Syphilis, sive Morbus Gallicus*).

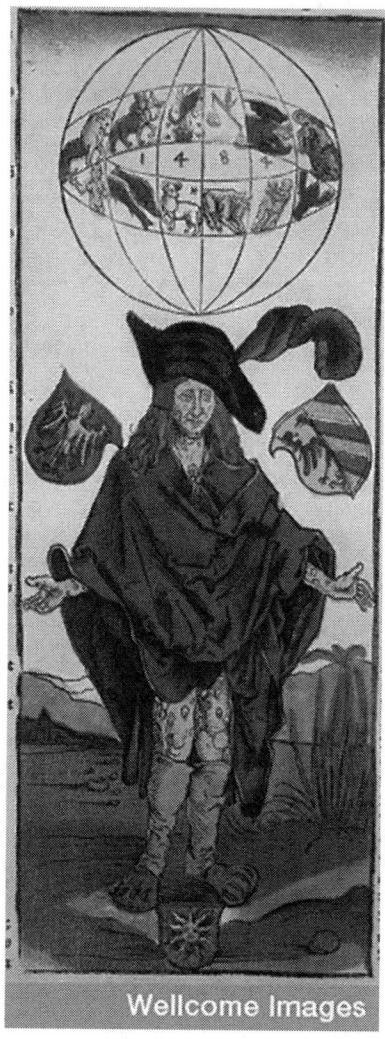

Figure 10.1 Albrecht Dürer, *Soldier with the pox*, Nurnberg broadsheet, 1496. Wellcome Library, London.

His explanation of the cause of syphilis and its cure by mercury was built
on his view that infectious diseases were caused by invisible 'seeds' of disease in the air and that the mercury, in the form of tiny particles, dried up
these seeds in the human body and rendered them innocuous. The poem
opened by asking: 'what seeds conveyed this strange disease, unknown
of any through long centuries?' Conjunctions of planets corrupt the air,
which leads to new diseases. 'The seat of the evil must exist in the air
itself... The air, indeed, is the Father of all things and the Author of their

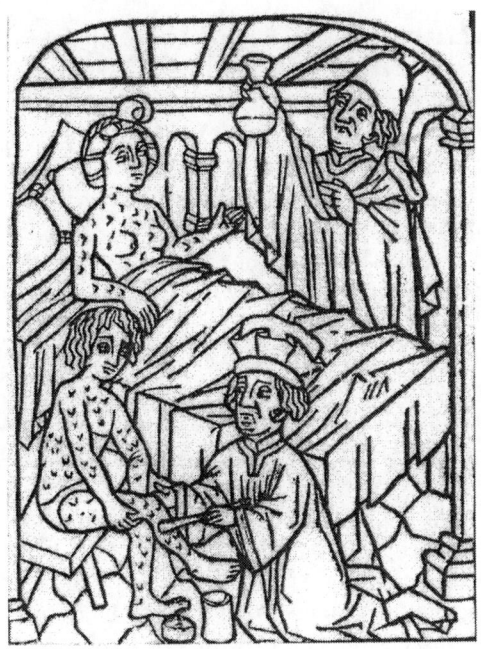

Figure 10.2 Treatment of pox sufferers, 1498. Anon. from B. Steber, *A Mala Franzos Morbo Gallorum, Praeservatio ac Cura*, as reprinted in *The earliest printed literature on syphilis: being ten tractates from the years 1495–1498, in complete facsimile, with an introduction and other accessory material by Karl Sudhoff; adapted by Charles Singer.* Wellcome Library, London.

being. Often, too, it brings grievous maladies to mortals; born in many ways, it starts corruption in the tender body, easily receiving the taint and passing it on' (1.123–9). Of the customary treatments, Fracastoro preferred mercury:

> Most people do better by dissolving everything in quicksilver, since the power inherent in this is wonderful. Whether because it is destined by nature to relieve both chills and fever, by drawing swiftly to itself our bodily heat, or because, being of great density, it dissolves humours and acts more powerfully, just as a glowing flame more keenly consumes iron: or whether the particles of which it is wonderfully compacted, when they lose their internal links and bonds and are carried separately into the body, dissolve away the concretions and dry up the seeds of the pestilence.[14]

A multitude of other accounts of the hidden workings of mercury in the body were given by other practitioners over the centuries.

3. Long-term use of mercury against the pox

One of the difficulties about the history of the French pox is that it is a disease which is now known to return, in up to three different forms, over a period of years, and while this was long suspected, it was not known for certain until the early 19th century. Modern authorities characterise four stages, including a period of latent syphilis between the second and the final stage, which can last from two to fifty years. The development over time of syphilis was first formally distinguished as three distinct stages by the Parisian surgeon and syphilis specialist Phillipe Ricord in his *Traité pratique des maladies vénériennes ou recherches critiques et expérimentales sur l'inoculation appliquée à l'étude de ces maladies*, published in Paris in 1838.[15] There is first the appearance of the initial lesion, a chancre usually on the genitals, but often also on the face and mouth; the second stage appears from four to twelve weeks later and is marked by the appearance of a rash, with mucous patches and condylomata (wart-like lesions on the genitals), and then after a latent period of any period from a few weeks to ten or more years, the tertiary phase, with nodes, tubercles, extreme pain in the bones and even the loss of the nose.

Given this view of the three (or four) stages, one can see that for a patient or a practitioner, mercury would seem to be an effective medicine if the symptoms and pains seemed to have gone away after treatment with mercury. That the disease later returns in a different form cannot, in itself, be taken to indicate that the mercury treatment was ineffective, and this presumably is why this kind of treatment continued for centuries, and why patients submitted to it, loathsome as it was. Charles Rinear, author of *The sexually transmitted diseases*, writes: 'Even without treatment, the chancre [of the first stage] heals completely within 4 to 6 weeks'; of the second, very painful, stage, he writes, 'As with the chancre, secondary syphilitic symptomology becomes asymptomatic even without treatment in approximately 2 to 6 weeks (sometimes longer) of their appearance'. Then comes the latent period. 'The latent period is dangerously deceptive because symptomology is absent. It was during this stage of the disease in the great syphilitic epidemic of the fifteenth century that the condition was thought to be cured'.[16]

Mercury was the treatment of choice in cases of the pox for most practitioners, and indeed for most patients, for hundreds of years. Yet there was never any real evidence that any of the mercury treatments worked against syphilis – that is to say, cured it, or even alleviated the symptoms. The theory and the practice were passed on from master to pupil or from quack to quack. There were no systematic investigations of its efficacy at any time – who would have performed them? who would have paid for them? – and the best we have in this regard are surveys of their own practice made by the occasional practitioner. The very best such compilation was made by Dr Philippe Ricord, the surgeon in the Venereal Hospital of Paris. His *Traité complet des maladies vénériennes*, published in 1851, crowns his many years of specialist work on the pox. In this, he deals with many cases, each extending over time, with details of dates and every particular about the patients and their sex lives, except for their names. In this large atlas, this *Clinique iconographique de l'Hopital des vénériens*, as he calls it, M. Ricord records in detail how he made his exhaustive inspections of patients and their diseased genitals, with the eyes, fingers and speculum. He says these cases have all been witnessed by his coterie of students who followed his rounds. He includes the courses of treatment he proposed in each case including, of course, mercury in various forms, for instance as pills or calomel. If anyone was ever in a position to assess the pros and cons of the mercury treatment, it would have been Ricord.[17] But he didn't, instead just favouring the historic view of the efficacy of mercury in treating syphilis, still treating the disease as the poison and mercury as the antidote.

But there were attackers of the mercury treatment from virtually the beginning of its use to treat the pox, and such fierce arguments continued in print well into the 19th century. Those opposed to the use of mercury argued either that it was useless compared to other treatments, such as bleeding and a low diet, or – much worse – that the mercury caused most of the symptoms it was supposedly being used to cure!

For instance, in London in 1709, Dr Sintelaer published a book called *The scourge of Venus and Mercury*, whose full title promised that it would deal not only with 'the nature, causes, signs, degrees, and symptoms of that dreadful distemper', but would also argue vehemently that mercury, far from curing the patient, actually produced a disease that Sintelaer called 'the mercurial pox, found to be more dangerous than the pox itself'.[18] He used what has become one of the more celebrated images of the treatment of pox with mercury to make his point, calling it 'The martyrdom of mercury' (Figure 10.3).

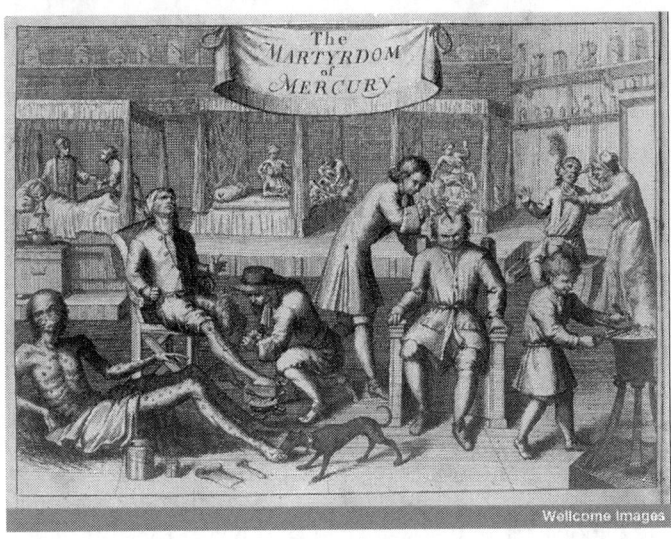

Figure 10.3 The martyrdom of mercury. From J. Sintelaer, *The scourge of Venus and Mercury, represented in a treatise of the venereal disease; giving a succinct, but most exact account of the nature, causes... and symptoms of that dreadful distemper...*, London, 1709. Wellcome Library, London.

The image portrays 'men and women with demolished noses, rotten tibiae, exfoliated skulls, empty alveolae, panther-like skins, fallen palates, and other attributes', which Sintelaer and others blamed on mercury.[19] The patients are being treated in various ways: with hot irons to cauterize sores on the skin of the legs and the head, and in the mouth. A dog is portrayed licking such sores. The patient at the front left of the picture has a bandage around his nose: presumably, his nose is in the course of rotting away, which was one of the final indignities of the pox. All these, according to Sintelaer, are caused by the mercury treatment. And in the bed at the back left of the picture, and also in the bed at the back right, one form of treatment by mercury is portrayed: the patient in his bed breathes in the fumes of mercury from a warm pot full of the mineral in order to promote salivation. This promotion of salivation Sintelaer called 'suffimigation' or fumigating from below, and he considered it an evil practice.

Sintelaer himself believed, from his fifty years of experience as a practitioner in physic, that true pox could be cured primarily by sweating. Together with purging, a 'low' diet and administration of a special decoction, the poison is sweated out. And Sintelaer also promoted the same system to sweat out the mercury a patient had absorbed if he or she had previously undergone the supposed mercury cure.

This sweating treatment, in its essentials, had been first promoted by the Dutch physician Stephen Blankaart, who published on the theme in Amsterdam in 1685, in the book *Venus belegert en ontset oft Verhandelingean de Pokken en des Selfs Toevallen*, and which came complete with practical illustrations. One could be treated lying in a bed or sitting on a chair, either with the vapour of brandy or a simple hot water vapour. Here, in Table V of the book, Blankaart describes the equipment and technique needed for one form of brandy or spirit of wine vapour treatment (Figure 10.4).

> But in addition to sweating, one must burden the patient even more if he wants to be cured: because he has to sweat pure brandy every day once or at least every other day as much as the sufferer can bear. To this end are different methods: The first one is that the patient lies in the bed naked, without wearing a vest, across his body you must arrange four half hoops so that the sheets and blankets can lie across: It being like this, construct another instrument out of tin, the height of the box bed, see the *fifth table* the *first figure* [that is the instrument at the bottom of the picture] in which A.A. is a hollow ascending pipe, which you can attach in pieces to one another, so that it is adjusted to the height of the box bed, E. is the elbow of the pipe AA which moves into pipes E.D., B is hollow like a big funnel, with a small door at the bottom, marked C. The *second figure* of the same table shows the use [that is, the bed with the same instrument set up beside it], while the patient is lying in the bed, and the instrument and hoops have been set: When everything is

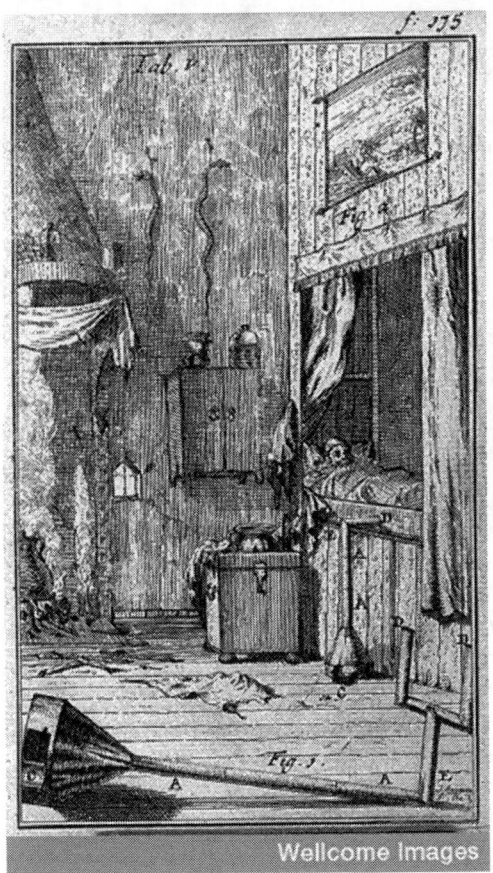

Figure 10.4 Administration of mercury treatment. From Stephen Blankaart, *Venus belegert en ontset oft Verhandelingean de Pokken en des Selfs Toeval-len*, Amsterdam, 1685. Wellcome Library, London.

ready, you open the doors of the tin sweat instrument, and you put a pot of brandy underneath, meanwhile you lay the sufferer down under the hoops, covered with sheets and blankets, so that his head is outside, and the holes are tucked in. Then you light the brandy with a sulphur-stick, so the vapour goes through the pipe A.E.D. up underneath the blankets, so that the sufferer will immediately sweat copiously, so long as he can bear it: When the brandy extinguishes during the procedure, you must pour new brandy in the pot and light it again, every time small amounts, otherwise the sweating is too hasty: At the end of the sweating you give the patient a full mug of hot *Pokkendrank* [that is the 'poxdrink', consisting of a drachm of theriac with a scruple of mercury *dulcis*, and a bolus, given in the evening], and you advise him to remain in bed like this.[20]

The topic of whether mercury was cure or cause of the symptoms of pox treatment remained controversial, with medics repeatedly putting their cases before the public of the merits or the dangers of mercury. In the mid-19th century, Dr Charles Drysdale of London put forward his view 'that mercury is a cause of disease, not a remedy', basing much of his case on the experience of the British army in Portugal in 1812, where the soldiers were treated with mercury and suffered, while the men in the Portuguese army used no mercury, suffered little, and recovered.[21]

One of the original forms of treatment was inunction, which is the rubbing of the skin with mercury ointment. It was still in regular use in the late 19th century. According to a recent history of venereology, *The scars of Venus*, a Viennese doctor, Karl von Sigmund promoted it strongly:

> His obituarist Doyon saw groups of patients sitting in the middle of Sigmund's clinic, all industriously performing their "frictions" under the vigilant eye of a male nurse. "Grey ointment", a trituration [thorough mixing] of metallic mercury in animal fat, was widely used. The inunction was usually performed once a day for at least twenty minutes; those who could afford them employed professional "rubbers".[22]

Even in the early 20th century, children who had been born with syphilis, acquired from their infected mother (or possibly from their infected father) – what is known as congenital syphilis – were treated with mercury. Abraham Jacobi, often credited with creating the speciality of paediatrics, insisted on this in his *Therapeutics of infancy and childhood*, first published in 1896:

> The treatment can be carried out slowly and systematically [on the infant]. It consists in the internal administration of calomel; doses of from one-twentieth to one-sixth of a grain can safely be given three times a day for months in succession... [There are] cases in which the systematic calomel treatment is insufficient. In them it is of the utmost importance to get the system immediately under the influence of mercury. With or without the internal treatment, subcutaneous injections of mercury must be made at once.[23]

Other specialists on the treatment of children born with syphilis recommended rubbing with mercury ointment. Leonard Findlay, doctor at the Sick Children's Hospital in Glasgow, wrote in 1919 that for infants,

> mercury in some form remains the usual and favourite remedy... there is no doubt that in a proportion of the patients complete cures, as evidenced by a persistent negative Wassermann reaction, can be obtained... I always advise the inunction of a piece of Ung. Hydrag. [i.e. rubbing with mercury ointment] about the size of a pea for 10 to 15 minutes daily – one day into the abdomen, the next day into the back, the following day

into one axilla and then on the succeeding day into the other axilla, then into one groin, next the other groin, and then back to the abdomen and so on as before... This daily inunction should be kept up for months.[24]

Towards the end of its use in treating syphilis, and while it was still seen by many practitioners as a specific for the disease, mercury was also now recognised as being 'extremely poisonous in its curative dose, so that small doses have to be used over a long period'.[25]

4. Other uses of mercury in Western medicine

With the development in the 16th century of Paracelsian/Helmontian medicine – 'chemical medicine', as it was sometimes called – mercury, as a metal, came to play a larger role than in traditional *materia medica*, which were largely plant-based.[26] In France and England, this movement was strong in the mid-17th century, and the works of chemists developing new medicines, such as Nicasius Le Febure (le Fèvre), promoted the use of mercury and announced how to make its various forms and how to administer it.[27] Le Febure counselled patience 'in the preparation of those *Arcana's* which are extracted from Mercury, so often recommended by our incomparable *Paracelsus*'. Le Febure's favourite preparation of mercury was 'the red and diaphoretical spirit of mercury', which was not only a true specific against the pox if taken internally, but which had also been used in France for some outstanding cures. An eminent person was born blind but now could see:

> there was no other Remedy us'd but of one grain and half of this pre-pared red Mercury blown with a Quill in the Nostrils, which in a very short time did produce surprising effects! for his Head swell'd in an extraordinary manner; then did he spit, drivel, shed tears, blow his Nose, sneeze, vomit, pisse, had copious and large stools, and sweated likewise, and all this in less than eight hours.

In a few days, he could see perfectly.

Outside of the Paracelsian/Helmontian circle of doctors, the resort to mercury in the pox meant that significant quantities of mercury were now needed by the physician and surgeon. And once mercury had arrived as an important tool in the physician's arsenal for pox, then it rapidly came to be used in other diseases – even though it was known from the beginning that it was highly poisonous. It was used according to the same kind of rationales that underlay the administration of most medicines. For instance, it could be administered with the aim of promoting purging, which in turn could be believed to be an effective means of expelling the poison of particular diseases. So, 'blue pills', which are mercury-based, could be described as aperients (laxatives, 'opening the passages'), and calomel, similarly mercury-based, could be prescribed as both an aperient and a purgative. 'Blue pills' were still being used in the late 19th century.[28] According to one recipe from 1884, they usually consisted of 'mercury in a finely divided state, mixed with confection of roses and liquorice root; the mercury should be in the proportion of 33.33 per cent'.[29]

Here are the different preparations of mercury in the *London Pharmacopoeia* of 1824 and their medical uses.[30] An alterative, according to Dunglisson's *Medical Dictionary* of 1874, is 'An agent considered to be capable of producing a salutary change in a disease, but without exciting any sensible evacuation. As medicine improves, this uncertain class of remedies becomes, of necessity, diminished in number'.

- Mercury with chalk (alterative), 'grey powder' (used as a purgative);
- Nitric oxide of mercury (used externally, stimulant, escharotic, i.e. caustic, as for warts);
- Grey oxide of mercury (alterative, deobstruent, i.e. for opening the pores of the skin);
- Red oxide of mercury (alterative; diaphoretic, i.e. sweat-inducing);
- Oxymuriate of mercury (alterative, must be used with caution);
- Liquor of the oxymuriate of mercury (alterative, antisyphilitic);
- White precipitated mercury (used externally, detergent);
- Purified mercury (acts by its weight, i.e. thought to scour the digestive system);
- Submuriate of mercury [= calomel] (alterative, antisyphilitic, cathartic);
- Black sulphuret of mercury (alterative, vermifuge, i.e. expels worms and other parasites from the intestines);
- Red sulphurate of mercury (alterative).
    In addition to these, there was the ubiquitous 'blue pill'. Mercury-based preparations were also, of course, prominent in 'quack' medicines offered into the 20th century as propriety cures by nostrum makers, such as eye ointments, skin ointments and teething powders.[31]

5. Heroic uses of mercury

When mercury was administered to the patient as a medicine, it was still highly poisonous in almost every form. The cure was almost as bad as the diseases it supposedly treated, and everybody knew this, including those who favoured its use in the pox. In one sense, the only safe way is to take lots of 'raw' mercury: to simply swallow it – daily if you like – and even over a long period.[32] In post-mortems of such patients, globules of mercury are found sticking to the intestines, but actually it seems that almost all of it just goes straight through. There are accounts of people who separated the mercury from their faeces and measured it against how much they had consumed. For instance, there was the case of

an old gentleman who took an ounce of quicksilver for nine months, daily, without doing him either good or harm; and out of the sixteen pounds he had taken in the whole, on washing it from the faeces, when it was weighed, there wanted only one ounce and a half, which he thinks was lost in the washing.[33]

If you were so minded, it was possible to wash it and take it again! But the advocates of oral mercury sometimes insisted that that tiny little bit that doesn't appear again in the stools was the active bit which did all the amazing cures.

There have been crazes in which raw mercury, taken straight, daily, was thought to be a cure-all, such as in the 1720s in France, where it was promoted by Dr Augustin Belloste. He wrote that 'Mercury, whose Virtues I here publish, is a Miracle of Nature, and the greatest Gift of Providence in the whole *materia medica*'. He had come upon the virtues of mercury by chance but found many supposedly incurable cases 'entirely gave way to crude mercury'.[34]

As with so many French crazes over the centuries, this addiction to raw mercury as a cure-all and as warding off diseases was rapidly taken up in England. In the early 1730s, one advocate wrote of it:

> Quicksilver is now much in use, and seems to be growing every day into greater reputation... Formerly people were afraid to take it; the common apprehension of its dire effects, its poisonous qualities, had rendered it a terror to all. Now, strange alteration! These fears are fled; its taken in every little disorder, by children too, without disguise, without mixture, crude in substance; and 'tis as usual to meet with it in families, as snuff or tobacco... This is so far from being disagreeable, that it is inviting, it looks like a finer jelly, is tasteless on the tongue, and hardly felt in going down, or in the stomach.[35]

The primary mode of action attributed to mercury taken in this way was by its weight (*pondus*). It is self-evidently heavy, and it was thought that this heaviness meant that it scoured the intestines: it is 'the greatest deobstruent, by its weight bearing down all obstructions before it'.[36] Equally, in some illnesses, it was thought to work through the break-up of the mineral into tiny globules, which were then taken up into the blood, and acted through their 'roundness' to dull and render harmless the disease-causing sharp, acrid particles in the blood. It 'thins, refines, and subtilizes those heterogeneous mixtures, reducing them to a proper fluidity, and having done his errand, passes out the way he was determined'.[37] And it was all perfectly safe taken this way: 'Some have swallowed in this manner to the weight of twenty, thirty, forty pounds of it. In substance it cannot possibly do the least harm, being as innocent as anything in nature taken this way'.[38]

Calomel (mercurous chloride in modern nomenclature, but known as submuriate of mercury or mercurius dulcis in the early 19th century), is a white medicine which can be administered in the form of a powder or a pill, and has been the most used of the mercurial drugs over the last few centuries.[39] One celebrated episode of using calomel as a 'heroic' medicine was when Benjamin Rush used it against an outbreak of yellow fever in Philadelphia in 1793. Rush regarded himself as a follower of Thomas Sydenham, and his account of his own actions in trying to treat yellow fever does indeed show him in the 'try this, and if no improvement, try that' style of therapeutic proceeding as promoted by Sydenham.[40] 'Baffled in every attempt to stop the ravages of this fever... I did not abandon a hope that the disease might yet be cured',[41] wrote Rush. Reading a manuscript by Dr Mitchell about a previous outbreak of yellow fever, the light dawned for Rush: 'I had been accustomed to raising a weak and low pulse in pneumonia and apoplexy, by means of blood-letting, but I had attended less to the effects of purging in producing this change in the pulse'. But how to find a suitable purge? Rush turned to calomel, and the experience of military physicians, and adopted 'ten and ten', that is ten grains of calomel with ten grains of julep (a sweet drink usually with mint and alcohol), twice a day, 'until it procured large evacuations from the bowels'. Rush slightly modified this dosage and found that it perfectly cured four out of the first five patients he gave it to. It was administered to a patient who was almost on his deathbed. 'At length, it operated and produced two copious, foetid stools... In a few days he was out of danger, and he now lives in good health as the first fruits of the efficacy of mercurial purges in the yellow fever'. Many other medics immediately adopted it. With some added blood-letting, Rush had found the perfect cure: 'Never before did I experience such sublime joy as I now felt in contemplating the success of my remedies'. Rush spread the recipe for the purging powders – the mercurial purges – to all available apothecaries. Rush was opposed by other doctors, and the argument was all about the wisdom or otherwise of administering mercury.[42]

6. Mercury falling out of medical use

It can be seen that mercury was increasingly used in Western medicine for various purposes and with varying rationales, from the 1490s well into the 20th century, despite its evident poisonous nature. But it did eventually fall out of use in the course of the 20th century. The pharmaceutical handbook with which we began, Hale-White's *Materia medica*, is a convenient resource in which we can trace some of the moments when mercury came to be gradually dropped as a medicine first for syphilis and then for anything else, and came to be seen simply as a poison and in no way a beneficial medicine. The handbook was regularly updated, its 32nd edition (and last) being published in 1963, some fifteen years after the death of the original author.

The arsenicals were first presented in the 16th edition (1918) as effective against syphilis, though it was a belts-and-braces approach, with mercury still being recommended too: 'It is believed that full doses of atoxyl or arsacetin drive the trypanosomes out of the blood and that then the subsequent administration of mercury kills them, but both [arsenical] drugs are still on their trial' (p. 232). The new arsenicals Arsenobenzol (= 606, Salvarsan and other trade names) and Novaresenobenzol are presented: 'Sufficient time has not yet elapsed for us to be sure that syphilis is permanently cured by these drugs, and it is wise after the injection of either to give a two or three years' course of mercury' (p. 234). Mercury was still being used with the arsenicals in the 19th (1927) and 20th (1931) editions: 'Usually four to eight arsenical doses are given at intervals of a week; some give weekly intramuscular injections of mercury at the same time, others do not begin the mercury till the completion of the first arsenical course... and arsenic and mercury are thus given for a year or even for two years' (p. 234 in both editions). The situation continues the same in the 28th edition (1949), though penicillin is now also introduced as curing gonorrhoea and syphilis (pp. 503–504), being 'the first instance of a powerful bacteriostatic which has no toxic effect on the host' (p. 113).[43] By the 30th edition (1957), widespread resistance to penicillin is registered, while mercury in various forms is still being used as an antiseptic, antiparasitic and purgative. Its efficacy as a diuretic had improved since 'the introduction of organic double salts of mercury', while 'the metal could not be used freely for its diuretic effect on account of its toxicity' (p. 373). And with respect to syphilis, in the 1957 edition, mercury remained 'powerfully antisyphilitic', yet 'it is no longer used because bismuth has largely replaced it in the treatment of syphilis, just as penicillin has replaced arsphenamine' (p. 372).

Finally, by the 30th edition (1957), 'Grey powder (mercury and chalk) as a purgative for children has been abandoned because it is claimed that mercury produces pink disease'. Josef Warkany and Ann Dally have traced the career of this condition, which was first remarked on in the late 19th century, and then appeared with greater frequency in the early 20th century.[44] Doctors saw 'miserable babies and toddlers, bright pink or red in colour and photophobic, with "raw beef" hands and feet, anorexia, peeling skin and, occasionally, gangrenous extremities'.[45] It was estimated that up to 10% of infants died from the disease. For about half a century, the consensus among the medics was that it was some kind of infection, probably a virus, while some among them subscribed to the view that it was a condition arising from nutritional deficiency – both these causes being currently recognised in other diseases. Only in the mid-1940s did an American doctor discover mercury in the urine of a child with pink disease, and paediatricians began to suspect calomel. In particular, it seems, it was the use of calomel in readily available teething powders, which was the main culprit. One English pharmaceutical firm claimed that it sold 30 million such powders a year.[46]

It was again an instance of a poison – mercury – being given as a medicine, in this case to relieve the pains of infant teething, and its effects turning out to be those of a poison, thus creating a much more dangerous condition than what it was given to cure. Both Warkany and Dally point out the irony that it would have probably readily been seen as a case of mercury poisoning back in the 19th century but, with the decline in the use of mercury for medical purposes, the modern medic was not familiar with the effects that mercury poisoning could create!

Notes

1 Sir William Hale-White, *Materia Medica: Pharmacy, pharmacology and therapeutics*, 23rd edition (1st edition 1892), London, 1937, p. 472.
2 See *Asiatische Studien, special issue: Histories of mercury in medicine across Asia and beyond*, vol. 69, 2015.
3 John M. Riddle, in his *Dioscorides on pharmacy and medicine*, Austin: University of Texas Press, 1985, pp. 154–156, has sorted out Dioscorides' confusions over mercury.
4 I have used the version published as *The pupil's pharmacopoeia; being a literal translation of the London Pharmacopoeia*, translated by W. Maugham, 3rd edition, London, 1824. It should be noted that just about every new edition of the Pharmacopoeia published by the Royal College of Physicians in Latin was rapidly turned into English by some surgeon or apothecary or other. On the poisonous actions of these metals and/or preparations of them, see the exhaustive accounts from doctors and from the law courts in Alfred Swaine Taylor, *On poisons in relation to medical jurisprudence and medicine*, 1st edition, London, 1848. The heavy metals and metalloids are still in Hale-White's *Materia medica* in the 20th century.
5 See Andrew Cunningham and Perry Williams, eds., *The laboratory revolution in medicine*, Cambridge, 1992.
6 'All the organic arsenicals [such as Salvarsan] which find important therapeutic application in certain blood diseases and syphilis are synthetic products and are only feebly poisonous', Reece H. Vallance, *A text-book of inorganic chemistry, vol. 6, part 4, Arsenic*, London, 1938, p. 290.
7 See Ludwig Fleck, *Genesis and development of a scientific fact*, Chicago, 1979; first published in German in 1935.
8 Sir William Hale-White, *Materia Medica: pharmacy, pharmacology and therapeutics*, 18th edition (1st edition 1892), London, 1924, pp. 214–222, see esp. 220–221. I have consulted several editions of this important work. The passages quoted above appear as early as the 2nd edition (1897), pp. 201–202; the same is the case in the 16th (1918), 19th (1927), 20th (1931), 21st (1932) and 23rd (1937) editions.
9 On the pox and its history, see Claude Quétel, *History of syphilis*, first published in French as *Le mal de Naples: histoire de la syphilis*, Paris, 1986; translated by Judith Braddock and Brian Pike, Cambridge, 1990; Jon Arrizabalga, John Henderson and Roger French, *The great pox: the French disease in Renaissance Europe*, London, 1997; J. D. Oriel, *The scars of Venus: a history of venereology*, London, 1994; Charles E. Rinear, *The sexually transmitted diseases*, Jefferson, North Carolina, 1986; Kevin Brown, *The pox: The life and near death of a very social disease*, Stroud, Gloucestershire, 2006.
10 Ulrich von Hutten, *Of the Wood Called Guaiacum, that Healeth the Frenche Pockes, and also helpeth the goute in the feete, the stone, palsey, lepree, dropsy, fallynge evyll, and other diseases*. Translated into English by Thomas Paynel, London, 1536 (first published in Latin in Mainz in 1519, and first issued in English in 1533), 2r.
11 From Wellcome Images.
12 From Bartholmaeus Steber, *A Malafranzos, morbo Gallorum, praeservatio et cura*, Vienna, 1498; as reproduced on p. 263 of *The earliest printed literature on syphilis: Being ten tractates from the years 1495–1498, in complete facsimile: With an introduction and other accessory material by Karl Sudhoff; adapted by Charles Singer*, Florence, 1925, in the series *Monumenta Medica*, ed. Henry E. Sigerist (vol. 3).
13 Hutten, *Of the wood called guaiacum*, f. 8r.

14 Fracastor, *Syphilis or the French disease. A poem in Latin hexameters by Girolamo Fracastoro, with a translation, notes and appendix by Heneage Wynne-Finch*, London, 1935, Book II, lines 270–279. Fracastoro coined this name for the disease, though it did not come into general use until the 19th century.

15 Translated by Henry Pilkington Drummond as *A practical treatise on venereal diseases; or, critical and experimental researches on inoculation, applied to the study of these affections*, London, 1842, see pp. 73 and 159–160.

16 Rinear, *The sexually transmitted diseases*, 1986; the citations are from pages 168, 169 and 170, respectively. Presumably he means the 16th century rather than the fifteenth.

17 *Traité complet des maladies vénériennes. Clinique iconographique de l'Hopital des vénériens. recueil d'observations, suivies de considérations pratiques, sur les maladies qui ont été traitées dans cet hopital*, Paris, 1851. I think this is the most revolting book I have ever seen, and which could put one off sex for life.

18 Sintelaer's book is *The scourge of Venus and Mercury, represented in a treatise of the venereal disease; giving a succinct, but most exact account of the nature, causes ... and symptoms of that dreadful distemper ...*, London, 1709.

19 From the analytical review of various works on syphilis and mercury, by Anonymous, appearing in *The medical-chirurgical review, and journal of medical science (Quarterly)*, vol. 2 for 1821–1822, pp. 597–626; see p. 599 for the description of the plate.

20 Translated for me from pages 175–176 of Blankaart's book by Dr Rina Knoeff, for which many thanks.

21 Charles R. Drysdale, *On the treatment of syphilis and other diseases without mercury; being a collection of evidence to prove that mercury is a cause of disease, not a remedy*, London, 1863.

22 J. D. Oriel, *The scars of Venus. A history of venereology*, London, 1994, p. 86.

23 I use the 3rd edition: Abraham Jacobi, *Therapeutics of infancy and childhood*, Philadelphia, 1903; see pages 176 and 178.

24 Leonard Findlay, *Syphilis in childhood*, London, 1919, p. 131.

25 J. E. R. McDonagh, *Salvarsan in syphilis and allied diseases*, London, 1912, p. 3.

26 On which see the chapter by Georgiana Hedesdan in the present volume.

27 Nicasius le Febure, *A compleat body of chymistry ... teaching the most exact preparation of animals, vegetables and minerals, so as to preserve their essential Vertues ... dedicated to the use of all Apothecaries &c.*, London, 1664, first published in French in 1660. The quotations are from pages 209 (Paracelsus) and 215–216.

28 Not to be confused with today's 'blue pill', which is Viagra and which is not mercury-based at all.

29 Alexander Wynter Blyth, *Poisons: Their effects and detection*, London, 1784, p. 598.

30 From *The pupil's pharmacopoeia*. The preparations are given on pages 61–70; I have added the uses of each from the Table at the end of the book.

31 See *Secret remedies, what they cost and what they contain. Based on analyses made for the British Medical Association*, London, 1909.

32 The case is quite different from other forms of mercury, such as mercury (II) salts (or mercury chloride), which is readily absorbed from the intestinal tract.

33 George G. Sigmond *Mercury, blue pill, and calomel; their use and abuse*, London, 1840, p. 16, quoting a 'Mr Bradley', whom I have not been able to identify. (The Bradley is not Thomas who wrote the *Treatise on worms*, 1813.)

34 Augustine Belloste, *An essay on mercury*, translated by J.B., M.D., Dublin, 1733, first published in French in 1725, pp. 4–5.

35 *Encomium argenti vivi: A treatise upon the use and properties of Quicksilver;
    or, the natural, chymical, and physical history of that surprising MINERAL,
    extracted from the writings of the best naturalists, chymists, and physicians ...
    By a Gentleman of Trinity College, Cambridge* [London, 1733], p. i.
36 *Encomium Argenti vivi*, p. iii.
37 *Encomium Argenti vivi*, p. iv.
38 *Encomium Argenti vivi*, p. vii.
39 On the preparation of calomel, see A. and C. R. Aikin, *A dictionary of
    chemistry and mineralogy*, 2 vols., London, 1807, vol. 2, pp. 82–83. The
    chemical language used here is both pre- and post-Lavoisier's reforms in
    nomenclature.
40 On Sydenham, see my 'Thomas Sydenham: epidemics, and the "Good Old
    Cause"', in Roger French and Andrew Wear, eds., *The medical revolution of
    the seventeenth century*, Cambridge, 1989, 164–190.
41 Benjamin Rush, *An account of the bilious remitting yellow fever, as it appeared
    in the city of Philadelphia in the year 1793*, Philadelphia, 1794; the quotations
    are from pages 196–204.
42 On the controversies, see J. H. Powell, *Bring out your dead. The great plague
    of yellow fever in Philadelphia in 1793*, Philadelphia, 1949, esp. 114–139. On
    Rush's reasoning, see Carl Binger, *Revolutionary doctor: Benjamin Rush,
    1746–1813*, New York, 1966, pp. 207–234.
43 On the early adoption of penicillin, see Joseph Earle Noore, *Penicillin in syphilis*,
    Oxford, 1947.
44 It was sometimes known as *acrodynia*, a coinage from Latin and Greek, mean-
    ing 'painful condition of the extremities', referring to the hands, feet and nose.
45 Josef Warkany, 'Acrodynia – Postmortem of a disease', *American Journal of
    Diseases of Children*, 1966 (112), 146–156; Ann Dally, 'The rise and fall of
    pink disease', *Social history of medicine*, 1997, 291–304. The quotation is from
    Dally, p. 29.
46 Warkany, p. 150. The firm is not named here.

11 Collateral benefits

Ergot, botulism, *Salmonella* and their therapeutic applications since 1800

Anne Hardy

The culture of poison and antidote, which so dominated European culture from the Antiquity to the seventeenth century, had faded long before the new medical science of the post-Enlightenment world began to realise the concept of food poisoning – of accidental poisoning caused by the ingestion of naturally occurring toxins in apparently wholesome foodstuffs. Although the attribution of stomach trouble to food, especially to, for example, unripe fruit, decayed foods or meats derived from sick animals, is probably of historic standing, it was only in the early nineteenth century that these beliefs coalesced in the denomination 'ptomaine poisoning', relating to the toxins of decay present in visibly or invisibly rotting foodstuffs. While these beliefs were under scientific scrutiny and doubt by the 1850s, the popular attribution of food poisoning to ptomaines persisted into the twentieth century.[1] Diseased and decayed meat were among the first concerns of early public health reformers.[2] With the development of toxicology as a science after 1800 and the emergence of public health professionals from the 1850s, medical attention began to focus on food rendered unwholesome by adulteration, and in England occasioned the passing of the Food and Drugs Act 1875, the first such legislation to be implemented.[3]

The realisation of the modern concept of food poisoning and its emergence as a recognised problem in public health took place only after 1880. While the work of William Budd and John Snow had shown that the 'poisons' of typhoid and cholera could be transmitted in contaminated liquids, it was only in the 1880s that epidemic outbreaks related to solid foods were placed on the public health agenda.[4] By 1923, when food poisoning was a well-established health concern, Gerald Leighton, investigator of one of Britain's most notorious food poisoning incidents, set out a simple classification of the condition that took the source of the poisoning material as a basis.[5] According to this, three types of food poisoning exist: from the ingestion of poisonous plants, such as laburnum seeds; from the deliberate, accidental or inadvertent presence of metallic poisons such as arsenic or lead introduced from some outside source, as can happen in murders, or as happened in the English brewing industry in the later nineteenth century;[6] and finally from bacterial or viral poisons, where food or drink has been infected by a living organism at some stage in its growth or production.[7] Among the plethora of potential food poisoning threats to human (and animal) health encompassed by these three categories, a handful of poisoning agents have been identified with the potential to deliver therapeutic applications. For the most part, they do not include practical defensive applications that can protect against episodes of food-related illness, while some poisonous plants with medical uses, such as foxglove, would not commonly be regarded as a possible food resource.[8]

Four agents stand out from the crowd in this respect. In order of historical realisation, they are as follows: ergot, a fungal parasite of rye and other cereals, responsible for Holy Fire, St Anthony's Fire and other convulsive manifestations, as in, for example, the medieval dancing epidemics; the bacterium *Clostridium botulinum*, the cause of botulism; and the cholera and the *Salmonella* families of bacteria, among the latter of which *S. typhosa*, the agent of typhoid, is the most virulent for humans. This group of one fungus and three (in the case of the *Salmonella*, in fact, over 2,600 types) bacteria may be sliced differently: ergot and botulinum have therapeutic applications unrelated to their prevention, whereas the cholera and the *Salmonella* can only provide defences against themselves.[9] The potential of ergot and botulinum was recognised through clinical observation and deduction well before medical science was capable of identifying the specific poisons concerned; the potential of cholera and the *Salmonella* was realised only after the bacteria had been identified, after immunology had emerged as a science and as increasingly sophisticated bacteriological techniques were developed in the years after 1890. None the less, the therapeutic potential of the cholera vibrio and the typhoid bacillus was realised relatively early, in the ferment of bacteriological-related research that engulfed Western medical science around the turn of the nineteenth century.[10] The potential of ergot and botulinum toxin waited on twentieth-century developments in physiology and pharmacology.

The pharmacological richness and complexity of ergot and the unexpected applications of botulinum have created a curious disjunction in the historiography surrounding these two substances, compared with that on the bacteria and the immunology of cholera and the *Salmonella*. The literature on ergot and botulinum is far richer than that on cholera and *Salmonella*, and almost all of it has been written by scientists engaged in elucidating the pharmacological properties and medical applications of the two agents. In the case of ergot, two major historical monographs were published in 1931 and 1970.[11] Its history relating to obstetrics has attracted both participant and historical attention, while its association with one of the twentieth century's most notorious recreational drugs, LSD (lysergic acid diethylamide), generated a number of scholarly articles, as well a first-hand account by its discoverer, Albert Hofmann.[12] Ergot's wider scientific history – the elucidation of its active principles and their therapeutic applications – has been set out in masterly fashion by another engaged scientist, Barbara Clark.[13] The account of ergot as poisoner and therapeutic, presented here, is heavily dependent on this existing corpus, and especially on the work of Barbara Clark. The historiography of botulism is even more skewed. While the first recorded observations of its role as a food poisoner date from the late eighteenth century, it was not until its therapeutic, and in a lesser degree its cosmetic, applications, began to achieve recognition between 1970 and 2000, that participant history began to emerge.[14] The wider history of botulism was set out in Elliott Dewberry's *History of Food Poisoning* in the 1950s.[15] The cholera and typhoid vaccines meanwhile have generated little detailed attention from either historians or practitioners.[16]

As a food poisoner, ergot has perhaps the highest historical profile among these disparate agents, for its association with the medieval dancing epidemics, with witch trials, werewolves, the 1951 outbreak at Pont-Saint-Esprit which it was proposed had been generated by the CIA, and of course, LSD.[17] Ergot is found in the sclerotium of *Claviceps purpurea*, a parasitic fungus of rye (and sometimes of other grasses). It was described by its first recorder, the German botanist Adam Lonicer (1528–1586) in 1582 as 'the long, black, hard, narrow corn pegs ... often protruding like long nails from between the grains in the ear'.[18] Lonicer also recorded the consumption of just three of these kernels by some women to increase contractions of the uterus in childbirth.[19] Ergot poisoning occurred during or after wet summers, which favoured the fungus, when infected rye flour was eaten as bread. It took two different forms. In France, it occurred in a gangrenous form, where tissue on the legs and arms blackened like charcoal until eventually the affected limb fell off. In Germany, however, it took a convulsive form, which was recorded from the late sixteenth century. The difference between these two manifestations of the poison derived from deficiency of vitamin A in the diets of German peasant populations in areas where dairy products were not part of the local agricultural economy.[20] The geographical distribution of ergot is reflected in the differing numbers of national synonyms for the fungus. The word ergot is French; in German, the principal term is 'mutterkorn'. The French have twenty-five synonyms for ergot; the Germans sixty-two (although all but five of these are mythological or descriptive). All other people use versions of either the French or the German; the Dutch have twenty-one synonyms for it, and the English a mere nine.[21]

The popular use of ergot in childbirth was probably well established in Germany by the time Lonicer recorded it, but its use by medical professionals seems only to have begun discreetly sometime after 1750.[22] Ergot emerged into the public medical eye only in 1808, when the American physician John Stearns learned of its use from an émigré German patient, tested it himself and communicated his discovery to colleagues.[23] By 1820, ergot was listed as an official drug in the American Pharmacopoeia and had become an accepted therapeutic agent.[24] Already by 1822, however, it was recorded that its introduction had been accompanied by a greatly increased number of still births, so that its use began increasingly to be limited to the control of post-partum haemorrhage.[25] Because of its obstetric interest, however, the new science of analytical chemistry found ergot an attractive subject, and already in the 1830s, attempts were being made to isolate its active principles. By the early 1900s, several chemically impure fractions had been obtained which seemed to owe their activity to a single alkaloid, isolated in the form of crystalline salts by the English researchers George Barger and F. H. Carr in 1906.[26] Named ergotoxine, the alkaloid itself was isolated twenty years later (1926), but it proved chemically and pharmacologically erratic. Much work was done on and with ergot by Barger, Carr and Henry Dale in the years that followed, while John Chassar Moir, a clinician at University College Hospital, working with the chemist H. W. Dudley, was instrumental in bringing ergot back into obstetric practice.[27] Moir and Dudley's discovery of the alkaloid ergometrine early in 1935, again for use in post-partum haemorrhage, was claimed to have played a part in sharply falling maternal deaths from the mid-1930s, although the more or less simultaneous introduction of the sulphonamide drugs, and soon after of greatly improved blood transfusion services and of penicillin, largely obscured the role played by ergometrine.[28]

The therapeutic applications of ergot derivatives have not, however, been limited to post-partum haemorrhage. By 1900, ergot was widely viewed as a problematic entity with pharmacological effects that merited investigation. Thus, when the young Henry Dale took up a research post at the Wellcome Physiological Research Laboratories in 1904, he was asked to try to 'clear up the problem of ergot'.[29] Although not initially enthused by the problem, Dale's career was to be intimately linked to ergot, and the work he did on it with his colleagues F. H. Carr and the chemist George Barger would revolutionise pharmacological thinking.[30] Dale's initial observation that ergometrine had a marked sympatholytic effect on the autonomous nervous system, which manifested itself as antagonism to adrenaline, had become the basis for the extensive use of ergot preparations in internal medicine and neurology by the 1960s.[31]

Wellcome was not the only drug company with an interest in ergot, however. The Swiss company Sandoz (now Novartis) recruited the chemist Arthur Stoll in 1917, with instructions to set up and manage a pharmaceutical research department.[32] Stoll's brief was to isolate and investigate natural products, in their original state, with a view to utilising them in medicine and pharmacy.[33] Starter projects included ergot, squill, digitalis, strophanthus and senna. Ergot was one of the first drugs Stoll tackled, on the grounds that there was still 'great uncertainty' surrounding its active principles. Stoll was well aware of the inadequacy of existing galenical ergot preparations in treating post-partum haemorrhage, and he set himself the task of isolating its active principle in pure form. His aim was to find a substance that could be administered as a weighed dose with a consistent, utterly reliable, effect.[34] Within a few weeks, he had obtained the preparation known as ergotamine (1918) which could be used to control post-partum haemorrhage. Stoll's research team at Sandoz went on to isolate various ergot alkaloids in subsequent decades and played a very significant part in the development of their therapeutic applications beyond the field of obstetrics. The Swiss laboratory, along with others in Chicago and Baltimore, isolated ergometrine almost simultaneously with Moir and Dudley in 1934.[35]

Among the non-obstetric applications for ergot is its use in aborting migraine attacks, which Ernest Rothlin, one of Stoll's team, elucidated in the mid-1920s.[36] Rothlin ran an extensive series of experiments with ergotamine and found (as had Dale and Spiro) that its actions were identical to those of the ergotoxine complex.[37] Taking into account ergotoxine's adrenalin-blocking properties, and in line with contemporary discussions around the discovery of the neurohumoral transmitter mechanism within the autonomic nervous system, Rothlin decided to test the effects of ergotamine on patients with severe, intractable migraine. Although experience showed that ergotamine was not suited to long-term daily treatment, it was being used across Europe for the treatment of migraine attacks by the late 1920s, with America following suit in the 1930s.[38] Research on ergot alkaloids continued at Sandoz through the 1940s and 1950s, and provided the basis for the development of further therapeutic applications in the treatment of hypertension, angina pectoris and peripheral circulatory disorders.[39] Ergot alkaloids continue to be used today in the treatment of deep vein thrombosis and orthostatic hypertension.[40]

Ergotoxine also proved useful in treating disorders of the human reproductive system. Ergot had been used in the early nineteenth century not only to prevent and control uterine bleeding but also to stimulate it in cases of amenorrhoea.[41] In the early 1950s, ergotoxine was found by Israeli researchers to be effective in disrupting the process of egg implantation in the rat uterus, and although the finding was not applicable to humans, it was indicative of new lines of research being pursued at that time.[42] At Sandoz, meanwhile, Ernest Flückiger had begun to look for a natural ergot alkaloid derivative with a specific effect on prolactin (luteotropin, the hormone which enables mammals to produce milk) secretion which would be better tolerated, succeeding in 1965 with the synthesis of bromocriptine.[43] Although its development was a commercially risky venture, since it was uncertain that it would have any clinical applications, Sandoz took the decision to follow up research to the point where the drug could be tested in humans.

By the early 1970s, however, the signs were promising. Bromocriptine was found to inhibit lactation in new mothers, and trials were begun on non-puerperal galactorrhoea, a condition usually associated with amenorrhoea in women and impotence in men. In fact, bromocriptine led to the discovery of a previously unsuspected group of neuroendocrine abnormalities, for which it offered a treatment. Within days or weeks of beginning on bromocriptine, 'normal menses and fertility were restored in women, and potency and libido returned in men'.[44] Bromocriptine heralded a new class of drugs useful in treating a range of disorders, including infertility, amenorrhoea, galactorrhoea and Parkinson's disease.[45] Research into ergot alkaloid derivatives continued at Sandoz and elsewhere into the 1980s and beyond.[46]

In 1965, in his Hanbury Memorial Lecture before the Pharmaceutical Society of London, Arthur Stoll described ergot as 'a veritable treasure house for drugs'.[47] Over and above the applications described earlier, the active constituent of ergot also played a part in the discovery of histamines and antihistamines,[48] and indeed of perhaps the twentieth century's most infamous drug, (d)-lysergic acid diethylamide, or hallucinogenic LSD.[49] Although the early history of LSD was characterised by high hopes for its potential therapeutic applications, this was one part of the ergot story where the apparent treasure proved to be fool's gold.[50] None the less, as Barbara Clark pointed out in 1984, LSD for the first time introduced the idea that mental disease might reflect biochemical abnormalities in the brain.[51] LSD notwithstanding, Stoll was right to describe ergot as a treasure house for drugs, a judgement that came after a career working with the fungus that spanned nearly fifty years.

Ergot was not the only organism to receive such an accolade. Four decades later, an enthusiast for the new cosmetic uses of another historical poison, botulinum toxin, described it as 'the most exciting new drug from the (twentieth) century' – a judgement that Stoll might have disputed.[52] Botulinum toxin A, commonly known today as Botox (or BTX or BoNT in clinical circles), is (as is well recognised) the most modern, most highly hyped, and now increasingly questioned, treatment in cosmetic surgery, or aesthetic surgery as its advocates prefer to call it. In 2006, Botox was claimed to be fast becoming 'the world's most frequently administered aesthetic procedure'.[53] Behind this enthusiasm, which has resulted in what is probably the world's largest ever medical vanity project, and a lucrative and self-perpetuating medical industry, lies some very serious science and valuable therapeutic applications that are a far cry from lip-filling and the removal of wrinkles – procedures for which the drug is not even licenced. Yet botulinum toxin was once described as 'the most poisonous poison', and in its natural state retains the power to be just that.[54]

The historical record for botulism is much shorter than that for ergot, dating back only to the late eighteenth century. It is caused by ingestion of an anaerobic neurotoxin producing bacterium, *C. botulinum*, which is widely found in soil and water, and its emergence into public prominence seems to have been an unexpected consequence of the French Revolutionary Wars, which left Southwest Germany in near famine conditions in the 1790s.[55] Recorded cases of fatal food poisoning increased in the Württemberg region in that decade, and in 1815, the medical officers of two small towns in the region reported on lethal outbreaks associated with blood sausages which had occurred in their localities. One of these medical officers, the young Justinius Kerner, followed up on these reports, collecting more cases and publishing monographs on the topic in 1820 and 1822.[56] Kerner accurately described all the intestinal, autonomic and neuromuscular symptoms of infection, and mentioned such clinical details as the disappearance of tear fluid, saliva, ear wax, mucus and sperm; difficulty in urination and extreme drying out of the palms of the hands, soles of the feet and eyelids.[57] Not content just to describe the symptoms, Kerner experimented with aqueous sausage extracts and observed symptoms comparable to those in human infection in both birds and animals. He concluded that the toxin developed in bad sausages under anaerobic conditions, that the toxin was a biological substance, which was strong and potentially lethal even in small doses, and that it acted on the motor and autonomic nervous systems. He suggested methods of treatment and prevention, and in his second monograph on the topic discussed the potential therapeutic use of the toxin in minimal dose for a variety of disorders, including hyperactivity or hyperexcitability of the motor and autonomic nervous systems. Other conditions suggested by Kerner for treatment included hypersecretion of sweat or mucus, ulcers from malignant disease, delusions, rabies, pulmonary tuberculosis and yellow fever.[58]

As with ergot, botulism has attracted little attention from professional historians, and its history has largely been written by the scientists who have worked with it. The most substantial contribution to the older history of botulism is that by Elliott Dewberry, published in his book *Food Poisoning* in 1959.[59] In particular, Dewberry recorded that most of the earlier outbreaks of sausage poisoning in Central Europe were caused by blood sausages, popular foods among the poorer classes and often eaten raw or partly cooked, and occasionally semi-decayed, and by hams.[60] Poisoning from the consumption of fish was first recorded in Russia in the mid-1830s and was proved by Thorvald Madsen, who investigated an outbreak caused by pickled mackerel on the tiny Danish island of Orø in the early 1900s, isolating a bacillus identical with *C. botulinum*.[61] In the history of the causal organism, a long pause had followed Kerner's observations, until in December 1895 a significant outbreak of botulism occurred in the small Belgian village of Ellezelles. The members of a local music club had played at a funeral, and afterwards shared a meal of raw ham.[62] Almost all were taken ill, and within a week, three were dead and ten nearly died. Symptoms included digestive and visual disturbances, burning thirst, problems in secreting saliva and increasing paralysis. Survivors did not fully recover for months afterwards.[63] Medical science being well into the age of bacteriology, Emile van Ermengem, Professor of Bacteriology at the University of Ghent, was called in to investigate. Van Ermengem was well aware of food poisonings due to *Salmonella* (then known as Gärtner's bacillus and varieties), as well as the possibility of botulism, given the symptoms.[64] His team conducted extensive animal feeding experiments with the suspect hams and subjected their remains, urine samples from two patients, organs from several autopsied corpses and the large number of dead experimental animals to bacteriological investigation.[65] They identified an anaerobic bacterium which they named Bacillus botulinus in honour of Kerner's sausages (botulus being the Latin for sausage).[66]

For much of the twentieth century, the history of C. *botulinum* and its toxin pursued a quiet way. Outbreaks were generally small and aroused little public health interest, except in the United States, where cases associated with the traditional home canning of fruit and vegetables led the authorities in the 1920s and 1930s to regard it as the national food poisoner.[67] (In Europe, by contrast, *Salmonella* infections were held to predominate.[68]) The science of botulism moved slowly forwards. A 1904 outbreak in Germany due to tinned white beans demonstrated that meat and fish were not the only sources of infection and also led to the discovery that the organism involved was serologically different from that at Ellezelles.[69] By 2002, a further four different strains had been identified, named on an alphabetical system as toxins A–G, following a suggestion made by Georgina Burke of Stanford University in 1919.[70] The potential of botulinum as a bacteriological weapon was recognised during the First World War.[71] During the Second World War, the United States conducted extensive research into biological weapons, including botulinum, at the US Army Laboratory at Fort Dettrick, Maryland.[72] In the course of this work, Carl Lamanna and James Duff developed concentration and crystallisation techniques (1946) that were later applied to the production of toxin for clinical use by their colleague Edward J. Schantz.[73] Schantz, whose career had hitherto been with the US Chemical Warfare Service, transferred to the Food Research Institute, Wisconsin, with the closure of Fort Dettrick in 1972.[74] From there, he continued to produce botulinum toxin in concentrated form for experimental purposes and kept the academic research community generously supplied – yet another example of wartime research benefitting peacetime medicine. Without the concept of bacteriological warfare and the war-related research at Fort Dettrick, botulinum toxin would not have been available to civilians in usable form.[75]

Among those who contacted Schantz was Alan B. Scott, a surgeon at the Smith-Kettlewell Eye Institute in San Francisco who, inspired by the animal experiments of D. B. Drachman, was in search of a toxic substance that could be injected into hyperactive eye muscle as an alternative to surgery for strabismus (cross-eyes), for which re-operative rates were high.[76] Scott began human experiments with strabismus in 1977, and by 1982 was treating strabismus, nystagmus (continuous to and fro movement of eyes), retraction of the eyelid, hemi facial spasm, and blepharospasm (involuntary contraction or twitch of eyelid), as well as dystonia (involuntary muscle contraction) of the limbs and neck.[77] But Scott also perceived a wider use of the treatment for muscle contractures and was frustrated by the reluctance of his Californian colleagues to experiment – a reluctance which he attributed to reservations about using a known poison in human therapeutics. The first botulinum treatments for torticollis (twisted neck) were carried out in Vancouver in the mid-1980s, after which use of the toxin in motility disorders gradually extended.[78]

Official sanction for the first of these clinical uses of botulinum came in December 1989, when the Food and Drug Administration (FDA) approved the use of botulinum toxin for use in the treatment of strabismus, blepharospasm and hemi facial spasm in patients over 12 years of age.[79] The experimental use of the toxin in a wide range of neuromuscular and other disorders in the years that followed proved its usefulness in many trying conditions, some of which had originally been foreseen by Kerner. Within a decade, botulinum (or BoNT as it came to be known) had shown itself to be 'safe, effective, specific in effect, and reversible' and had come to be considered a 'powerful and versatile tool' for a wide range of disorders, including overactive bladder/urinary incontinence, hyperhidrosis (excessive sweating), migraine and obesity.[80] In the 1990s, it became a globally popular adjunctive treatment for adult spasticity and juvenile cerebral palsy.[81] By 2000, it had also proved itself useful in yet other distressing conditions, including anal fissure.[82] FDA approval for many of these treatments took time in coming – for primary axillary hyperhidrosis, for example, it was only forthcoming in 2004 – and for some, it has not yet come. Many treatments in use today, including all but one cosmetic treatment, remain unapproved.

Despite its many and various uses for painful and embarrassing medical conditions, botulinum remains most famous – or notorious – for its cosmetic or, as many practitioners prefer to call it, its aesthetic applications. The cosmetic use of botulinum was created by the wife-and-husband team Jean and Alastair Carruthers.[83] Jean Carruthers was working with Alan Scott's team in the 1980s, when he was treating patients for blepharospasm, injecting the toxin around the eyes and upper face every three or four months, since the effects of the toxin waned in that time.[84] Carruthers noticed that many of these patients would joke on return that they had come back 'to get the wrinkles out'. As Alan Scott recorded, it took the Carruthers' joint specialisms of aesthetic dermatology and ophthalmology to realise the potential for this application of the toxin. Noting with cautious praise the couple's 'thoughtful and rational application of toxin to selective agonist-antagonist muscles in the face, to lift the brow, flatten folds', Scott further observed that their practice 'is probably now overtaken by less discriminate use'.[85] That was in 2004, two years after the FDA had given approval (12 April 2002) for the use of BTX-A specifically for the treatment of severe glabellar (vertical frown) lines between the eyebrows, with corrugator and/or procerus muscle activity, causing emotional stress to the patient, in patients aged 65 and under.[86] This was the first and still remains the only area of the face for which the FDA approved a cosmetic application of botulinum.[87]

Jean Carruthers and her husband were quick to develop the commercial potential of the new treatment, extending its applications and tapping into the growing culture of youth, beauty and celebrity that swept global societies from the later 1990s.[88] In 1999, Botox treatment was virtually unheard of; within five years, it had become a household name.[89] Already in 2002, the American Society of Plastic Surgeons recorded 1,123,510 persons as treated with the toxin, making it the top-ranking non-surgical procedure performed by certified plastic surgeons.[90] In the following year, the Carruthers' published the first clinical guidebook, *Using Botulinum Toxins Cosmetically*, in which they discussed the practical aspects of 'common facial and neck neurotoxin treatments' to provide 'a stimulus to physicians to advance the understanding and use of this important cosmetic modality'.

The drivers behind this publication are clearly manifest in the Carruthers' text. Both the 'Foreword' and the section headed 'Aesthetic Philosophy' drove home the social and cultural importance of retaining a youthful face: 'Society does not welcome a tired and aged appearance', they wrote; 'today ... people ... seek to appear rested, relaxed and at peace'.[91] Cultural references emphasised the point: African masks, they noted, show vertical lines in the face to convey negative emotion – 'anger, depression, fatigue, bitterness, disappointment and envy'. Horizontal lines across the brow and radiating from the corners of the eyes, they declared, 'may be masculinising features'; vertical lip lines 'are seen as the hallmark of the aged female lower face'; vertical neck bands 'give the impression of age and weakness', and when seen in younger people are 'suggestive of obesity'.[92] The Carruthers' plainly perceived an immensely lucrative market: 'Self-rejuvenation', they wrote, 'has become a huge industry because of the power of beauty to modify perception and behaviour in our colleagues and peers, friends and family'. And the demographic trend was in favour of the new aesthetic practitioners: seventy-eight million baby boomers born in the United States between 1946 and 1964 'wish to present their best to the world but with little or no downtime'.[93] These people needed and wanted botulinum; it was up to the Carruthers and their colleagues to supply their needs.

This is not the place to detail the rapid descent from triumphalism which took place, but the 'wildly unsafe' use of non-approved botulinum toxin in Florida in late 2004 presaged an explosion of 'aesthetic surgical practice' among persons with minimal, irrelevant or no qualifications.[94] There was in parallel the speedy development of an unregulated market in toxin products of varying strengths, with different units of biological activity, whose units were not equivalent.[95] Whereas the first edition of Anthony V. Benedetto's compendium *Botulinum Toxins in Clinical Aesthetic Practice*, published in 2006, carried a foreword by Jean Carruthers and no warnings at all about drawbacks to these procedures, the second, 2011, edition was punctuated throughout with hazard warnings, notably an entirely new contribution by David J. Goldberg, Clinical Professor of Dermatology at Mount Sinai School of Medicine and Adjunct Professor of Law at Fordham University School of Law, on the legal pitfalls of aesthetic practice.[96] Perhaps also significantly, there was no contribution from Jean Carruthers in this edition. The most poisonous of poisons was beginning to revenge its co-option into aesthetic practice.

Both ergot and *C. botulinum* are natural phenomena containing power-ful agents that can be isolated and recreated for use in clinical settings. By contrast, bacteria of the *Salmonella* family can be reinvented as vaccines to protect vulnerable populations against infection but remain about 75 per cent effective only.[97] The development of vaccines for typhoid and cholera was among the first concerns of late-nineteenth-century bacteriology, and vaccines for the both were developed around 1900, for cholera much less successfully than for typhoid.[98] Across the spectrum of food poisoning or-ganisms, however, a range of other pathogenic organisms continue to be of far more significance in terms of human misery than ergot or botulism, cholera or typhoid. The 2,600 or so lesser *Salmonellas* all have the poten-tial to cause human infection, and since their identification from the late 1970s, *Campylobacter*, norovirus and cryptosporidium have joined *Salmo-nella* as major agents of human infection. Despite the human and economic costs of these infections, developing vaccines against all the food poison-ing *Salmonella* is neither necessary nor desirable. In certain circumstances, however, a vaccine may provide a solution, or a remedy, for particular pub-lic health problems. Such was the case with *Salmonella enteritidis* phage Type 4 (or PT4 as it is commonly known), an environmentally highly adapt-able variant, which in the 1980s and early 1990s emerged as a major global pandemic, for reasons which have never been satisfactorily explained.[99] Although this was a global pandemic, it was related to the consumption of hen eggs. The incidence of egg-associated *Salmonella* is much higher in Europe than in the United States,[100] and using the English experience as a case study here is not unduly parochial.

Food poisoning, broadly speaking, has been a core concern of the English Ministry of Health and its successors since 1920.[101] Throughout the twen-tieth century, *Salmonella* infections were a major preoccupation. Until the early 1980s, when they were joined by *Campylobacter* (identified 1977), the *Salmonellas* were considered as by far the dominant bacterial food poi-soner in Great Britain.[102] Before 1988, *Salmonella typhimurium* remained the most frequently isolated serotype. In 1985, however, the Chief Medical Officer reported that *S. enteritidis* phage Type 4 infections were increas-ingly being reported in tourists returning from the Iberian Peninsula.[103] By 1988, *S. enteritidis* infections 'far exceeded' those for *S. typhimurium*; the trend continued into 1989, and increasingly these isolations were of PT4.[104] By now, these were not just imported cases. In fact, PT4 turned out to be an unusually environmentally adaptable organism, which could be communi-cated directly from humans to chickens, and which has been shown to have adapted to survival in hen houses, mice, chickens, eggs and humans.[105] By the summer/autumn of 1988, evidence had accumulated to link PT4 with *Salmonella* outbreaks due to the consumption of raw eggs and raw-egg dishes, such as mayonnaise, and of lightly cooked egg. In December, the Ministry therefore advised vulnerable groups only to eat eggs cooked until both whites and yolks were solid, and took out full-page advertisements in the national press to ensure that the message reached as many people as possible.[106] Already in June, the Department of Health had called a meeting of interested parties – the Ministry of Agriculture, Farming and Fisheries (MAFF), the National Farmers' Union, the British Poultry Federation and the British Egg Industry Council – to declare that eggs were a health risk. The industry's veterinarians began checking thousands of eggs for infection.[107] The MAFF meanwhile organised a consumer survey to determine consumer opinions and habits relating to food poisoning and food hygiene – an exercise that revealed depressingly low levels of engagement with hygienic principles.[108] The Department of Health began issuing public warnings from the end of June. It was against this background that the junior Agriculture Minister, Edwina Currie, made her now-infamous announcement to ITN News on 3 December that 'most of the egg production in this country is infected with *Salmonella*'.[109]

The upshot of the devastating (to the egg industry) food scare that followed this pronouncement was, inevitably, the search for a remedy. The Microbiological Committee on the Safety of Foods was set up in February 1989, and a new Food Safety Act aimed at tightening up procedures for regulation, inspection and enforcement of safety standards was passed in 1990, effective from 1 January 1991.[110]

The Act established the 'statutory role' of Food Examiner to carry out the microbiological examination of foodstuffs, just as the much older post of Public Analyst (Food and Drugs Act 1872) performed chemical analyses to detect adulteration. Powers regarding the withdrawal of hazardous foods were reinforced, and a new defence of 'due diligence' was introduced in prosecutions for inadequate food safety procedure.[111] At much the same time (March 1989), the Zoonoses Order 1989 made compulsory the slaughter of *Salmonella*-infected poultry and the reporting of positive test results for *Salmonella* in poultry mandatory.[112] The *Salmonella* problem was one of the factors that led to the establishment of the Food Standards Agency in 1998.[113]

As a result of the food scare, no doubt, 1990 was the first year since 1986 in which total food poisoning notifications were down; on the other hand, the number of PT4 notifications saw a significant increase. Although MAFF had initiated the *Salmonella* control measures for poultry in March 1989, not all were in place before April 1990.[114] Despite the new precautions, human *Salmonella* notifications peaked in 1993, and although they then stabilised, PT4 continued to increase its market share.[115] In parallel to this pattern, a 1991 Department of Health survey found that *Salmonella* were present in eggs from high street retail outlets at a rate of one in 650, and by 1995/1996, the rate had increased to one in 560.[116] In the absence of 'any obvious explanation' for this scenario, the Advisory Committee on the Safety of Food decided in 1998 to set up a second working party to try to establish the factors determining *Salmonella* contamination in or on eggs.[117]

By the mid-1990s, it was clear that administrative and educational measures were not effective, and it was increasingly obvious that PT4 had caused widespread environmental contamination, which it was proving 'remarkably difficult' to eradicate.[118] While the British have proved signally reluctant to protect their domestic livestock by immunisation – witness the 2001 controversy over foot-and-mouth disease – other countries have been less reluctant.[119] Given the established models of typhoid and paratyphoid vaccines, vaccines against the lesser *Salmonella* were a realistic prospect. By the mid-1990s, scientific communities across the world were investigating the possibility of vaccinating hens against PT4.[120] In 1994, a small number of British breeders of broiler chickens began to use vaccination to protect their birds against *S. enteritidis*, with some two million being immunised. By 1997, the number had risen to five million, and in that year, four and a half million commercial laying birds were also vaccinated, although in Northern Ireland vaccination was not begun until the second half of 1998.[121] Nevertheless, human notifications of *S. enteritidis* continued to rise, and in 1997, a survey conducted by the Public Health Laboratory Service indicated that levels of contamination in shell eggs had not changed significantly since 1991, and also that British egg consumption was 'in long-term decline', having fallen by 60 per cent following Currie's 1988 announcement and continuing to fall by 8 per cent a year thereafter.[122]

It was at this point that the British Egg Industry Council intervened, introducing the Lion Code of Practice which required that all pullets destined for Lion Quality egg-producing flocks be vaccinated against *S. enteritidis*. By the end of 1999, it was estimated that 85 per cent of layers in production in the British laying flock had been so protected.[123] Human infections with *S. enteritidis*, which had stood at over 15,000 notifications in 1997, fell by more than half by 1999.[124] While the *Salmonella* problem was one of the factors that led to the establishment of the Food Standards Agency in 1998,[125] the Agency's role in resolving the problem remains doubtful. It was noted in 2012 that the 'temporal relationship between vaccination program and the reduction in human disease is compelling'.[126] As a remedy for controlling PT4 in both poultry and human populations, vaccination had proved more effective than all the hygienic admonitions of health workers and industry advisers put together.

Salmonella, botulinum and ergot each represent a different path by which a food poisoning agent becomes a remedy. *Salmonella* bacteria are themselves translated by laboratory procedures into defensive barriers against the parent infection. The toxin of *C. botulinum* is extracted, processed and utilised to treat conditions relating to the motor and autonomic nervous systems. The different alkaloids contained in ergot are isolated and used to treat a range of conditions from post-partum bleeding to migraine and infertility. Among a host of food poisoning agents, these three stand out for having qualities which, enabled by the laboratory, allow them successfully to be used for therapeutic purposes. If botulism is 'the most poisonous of poisons', it is at least mercifully rare, as now is ergot, given modern knowledge, food habits and farming systems.[127] *Salmonella* food poisoning, by contrast, if less common in Britain and Europe than it was fifteen years ago,[128] remains a continuing hazard of modern life across the world.[129]

Notes

1   W. H. Michael, 'Case of fatal poisoning by German sausages', *Edinburgh Medical Journal*, 2 (1856), pp. 176–77; William Osler, *The Principles and Practice of Medicine*, Edinburgh and London, 1892, pp. 1012–15; Gerald Leighton, *Botulism and Food Preservation (The Loch Maree Tragedy)*, London, 1923, p. 6.

2   Editorial, 'Sale of bad meat in London', *Journal of Public Health and Sanitary Review*, 2 (1856), p. 311; see also Keir Waddington, *The Bovine Scourge, Meat, Tuberculosis and Public Health, 1850–1914*, Woodbridge, 2006, chapter 2.

3   Michael French and Jim Philips, *Cheated Not Poisoned. Food Regulation in the United Kingdom, 1875–1938*, Manchester, 2000.

4   Anne Hardy, *Salmonella Infections, Networks of Knowledge, and Public Health in Britain, 1880–1975*, Oxford, 2015, p. 88.

5   Leighton, *Botulism* (n. 1), p. 4.

6   See Jim Phillips and Michael French, 'The pure beer campaign and arsenic poisoning, 1896–1903', *Rural History*, 9 (1998), pp. 195–209.

7   Leighton, *Botulism* (n. 1), pp. 4–5. Leighton was unaware of the role of viruses; it was only in the latter part of the twentieth century that the role of viruses in food poisoning was realized.

8   For foxglove and digitalis, see Jeffrey Aronson, *An Account of the Foxglove and Its Medical Use, 1785–1985*, Oxford, 1985. It was noted in 1992 that in recent years, a great multitude of poisonous substances from plants and microorganisms had been found of use in studies on animal physiology and that 'some are used medicinally on humans': Edward J. Schantz and Eric A. Johnson, 'Properties and use of botulinum toxin and other microbial neurotoxins in medicine', *Microbiological Reviews*, 56 (1992), p. 80.

9   On the cholera family, see Christopher Hamlin, *Cholera. The Biography*, Oxford, 2009, pp. 253–65, 273–74. For the *Salmonella* family, see T. A. Cogan and T. J. Humphrey, 'The rise and fall of *Salmonella* Enteritidis in the UK', *Journal of Applied Microbiology*, 94 (2003), p. 114S.

10 E. H. Hankin, 'Remarks on Haffkine's method of protective inoculation against cholera', *British Medical Journal*, 1892, ii, pp. 569–71; W. M. Haffkine, 'A lecture on vaccination against cholera', *B.M.J.*, (1895), ii, pp. 1541–44; A. E. Wright and W. B. Leishman, 'Remarks on the results which have been obtained by the antityphoid inoculations', *B.M.J.*, (1900), i, pp. 122–29.

11 George Barger, *Ergot and Ergotism. A Monograph*, London, 1931; Frank James Bové, *The Story of Ergot*, Basel and New York, 1970.

12 John Chassar Moir, 'The history and present day use of ergot', *The Canadian Medical Association Journal*, 72 (1955), pp. 727–34; E. M. Tansey, 'Ergot to ergometrine: An obstetric renaissance', in Anne Hardy and Larry Conrad (eds), *Women and Modern Medicine*, Amsterdam, 2001, chapter 9; Albert Hofmann, *LSD: My Problem Child*, New York, 1980; John S. Haller, 'Smut's dark poison: Ergot in history and medicine', *Transactions of the College of Physicians of Philadelphia*, series V, vol. III, no. 1 (1981), pp. 62–78.

13 Barbara Clark, 'The versatile ergot of rye', in M. J. Parnham and J. Bruinvels (eds), *Discoveries in Pharmacology*, 2, Philadelphia, 1984, chapter 1.

14 The first such study appears to be Frank J. Erbguth and Markus Naumann, 'Historical aspects of botulinum toxin. Justinus Kerner (1786–1862) and the "sausage poison"', *Neurology*, **53** (1999): pp. 1850–53. But see Barger, *Ergot* (n. 11), chapter 1; Leighton, *Botulism* (n. 1), Chapter 2. Leighton was the Medical Officer in charge of the investigation into the 1922 Loch Maree incident – Britain's first and worst botulism outbreak, with eight cases and eight deaths. There have been a further ten incidents between 1932 and 1998; see Surveillance Report, *Botulism in the United Kingdom*: www.eurosurveillance.org/ViewArticle.aspx?ArticleId=45, accessed 6 July 2014.

15 Elliott B. Dewberry, *Food Poisoning, Food-Borne Infections and Intoxications*, 4th edition, London, 1959, chapters xvi–xviii.

16 But see George H. Bornside, 'Waldemar Haffkine's cholera vaccine and the Ferran-Haffkine priority dispute', *Journal of the History of Medicine and Allied Sciences*, **37** (1982): pp. 399–422; Anne Hardy, ' "Straight back to barbarism": Anti-typhoid inoculation and the Great War, 1914', *Bulletin of the History of Medicine*, **74** (2000), pp. 265–90.

17 John G. Fuller, *The Day of St Anthony's Fire*, London, 1969; Mary K. Matossian, *Poisons of the Past: Molds, Epidemics, and History*, New Haven, 1989; J. W. Bennett and Ronald Bentley, 'Pride and prejudice: The story of ergot', *Perspectives in Biology and Medicine*, **42** (1999), pp. 333–55. For Pont-Saint-Esprit and the CIA, see Hank P. Albarelli Jr., 'CIA: What really happened in the quiet French village of Pont-Saint-Esprit', at www.voltairenet.org/article 164447.html.

18 Clark, 'Ergot' (n. 13), p. 4.

19 Bové, *Story* (n. 11), p. 26. The dosage so contained, circa half a gram, repeated several times, was that still used in midwifery practice in the mid-twentieth century.

20 Edward Mellanby, 'The relation of diet to health and disease. Some recent investigations', *B.M.J.*, (1930), ii: 577–81, p. 679; Clark, *Ergot* (n. 13), pp. 5–7.

21 Bové, *Story* (n. 11), pp. 3–9.

22 Clark, 'Ergot' (n. 13), p. 7.

23 Barger, *Ergot* (n. 11), pp. 13–19; Bové, *Story* (n. 11), p. 273.

24 Bové, *Story* (n. 11), p. 276.

25 Barger, *Ergot* (n. 11), p. 18.

26 G. Barger and F. H. Carr, 'Note on ergot alkaloids', *Chemical News*, **94** (1906), p. 89.

27 See W. S. Goldberg, 'Henry Hallett Dale', *Biographical Memoirs of Fellows of the Royal Society*, **16** (1970), pp. 127–31, 135–37; H. W. Dudley and J. Chassar Moir, 'The substance responsible for the traditional effect of ergot', *B.M.J.*, (1935), i, pp. 529–32; JCMB, 'J. Chassar Moir', *B.M.J.*, (1977), ii, p. 1551; J. Chassar Moir, 'The history and present day use of ergot', *Canadian Medical Association Journal*, **72** (1955), pp. 727–34. See also Tansey, 'Ergot to ergometrine' (n. 12).

28 Moir, 'History' (n. 12), p. 733. Dudley and Moir, 'Substance' (n. 27), p. 523, state ergometrine to be 'without doubt the constituent to which ergot owes its introduction into medicine'.

29 Clark, 'Ergot' (n. 13), p. 11.

30 Ibid. For the role of ergot in Dale's career, see Goldberg, 'Dale' (n. 27).

31 Arthur Stoll, 'Ergot – A treasure house for drugs', *The Pharmaceutical Journal*, **194** (1965), p. 605.

32 For Stoll, see L. Ruzicka, 'Arthur Stoll', *Biographical Memoirs of Fellows of the Royal Society*, **18** (1972), pp. 566–93.

33 Stoll, 'Ergot' (n. 31), p. 605.

34 Ibid, pp. 605–6.

35 Ibid, p. 606.
36 Rothlin is described by Barbara Clark as the man who dominated the field of ergot pharmacology in the years 1925–1950: Clark, 'Ergot' (n. 13), p. 18.
37 Ibid, p. 18.
38 Ibid, pp. 18–19.
39 Ibid. pp. 20–25.
40 Roger F. J. Shepherd, 'Ergotism', in Rodney A. White and Larry H. Hollier (eds), *Vascular Surgery: Basic Science and Clinical Correlations*, Oxford, 2005, p. 103.
41 Clark, 'Ergot' (n. 13), p. 28.
42 Ibid, pp. 25–26.
43 Ibid, p. 26.
44 Ibid, pp. 27–28.
45 Ibid, pp. 28–29.
46 Ibid, pp. 30–31; J. Mukherjee and M. Menge, 'Progress and prospects of ergot alkaloid research', *Advanced Biochemical Engineering Technology*, **68** (2000), pp. 1–20; H. Hulvova et al., 'Parasitic fungus Claviceps as a source for biotechnological production of ergot alkaloids', *Biotechnological Advances*, **31** (2013), pp. 79–89, Epub. 2012 January 12.
47 Stoll, 'Treasure house' (n. 31), pp. 612–13.
48 Haller, 'Smut's dark poison' (n. 12), p. 79.
49 See Clark, 'Ergot' (n. 13), pp. 13–18; Hofmann, *My Problem Child* (n. 12). For Hofmann, see www.telegraph.co.uk/news/obituaries/2004/1912485/Obituary_Albert-Hofmann-LSD-inventor, accessed 15 July 2014.
50 Robert F. Ulrich and Bernard M. Patten, 'The rise, decline, and fall of LSD', *Perspectives in Biology and Medicine*, **34** (1991), pp. 561–78.
51 Clark, 'Ergot' (n. 13), p. 16.
52 Jean Carruthers, 'Foreword', in Anthony V. Benedetto (ed), *Botulism Toxin in Clinical Dermatology*, Abingdon, 2006, p. xi.
53 Ibid.
54 Carl Lamanna, 'The most poisonous poison: What do we know about the toxin of botulism? What are the problems to be solved?' *Science*, **130** (1959), pp. 763–72.
55 Ebgurth and Naumann, 'Historical aspects' (n. 14), p. 1850.
56 Frank J. Ebgurth, 'Historical notes on botulism, *Clostridium botulinum*, botulinum toxin, and the idea of the therapeutic use of the toxin', *Movement Disorders*, **19**, Supplement 8 (2004), pp. S2–S6, at p. S3. See also Ebgurth and Naumann, 'Historical aspects' (n. 55), pp. 1850–53.
57 Ebgurth, 'Notes' (n. 56), pp. S4–S5.
58 Ibid, p. S5.
59 Dewberry, *Food Poisoning* (n. 15), pp. 294–344. Dewberry appears to have been a Royal Army Medical Corps officer, 1914–1920s (RAMC/803, Wellcome Library), but is coy about his qualifications, except MBE, and public health society Fellowships, on the cover page of the book.
60 Ibid, p. 296.
61 Ibid. Madsen's account is given in Kraus and Levaditis (eds), *Handbuch der Technik und Methodik der Immunitätsforschung* (1908), Bd 1 u. 2. I have been unable to trace a copy in Britain.
62 Many accounts describe the ham variously as smoked, or as 'pickled and smoked hams'. Van Ermengem himself described it as raw (salted), but also mentions bacon (n. 63, below), pp. 701, 702.
63 See E. van Ermengem, 'A new anaerobic bacillus and its relation to botulism', (Classics in Infectious Diseases), *Reviews of Infectious Diseases*, **1** (1970), pp. 701–19 at p. 702.
64 Ibid, pp. 703–4.

65 Ibid, pp. 706–11.
66 J. K. Torrens, 'Clostridium botulinum was named because of association with "sausage poisoning"', *B.M.J.*, (1998), **316**, p. 151.
67 Editorial, 'The problem of food poisoning', *American Journal of Public Health*, **15** (1925), p. 896; J. Geiger and J. P. Gray, 'Food poisoning – a public health problem', *A.J.P.H.*, 23 (1933), pp. 1039–44. See also James Harvey Young, 'Botulism and the ripe olive scare of 1919–20', *Bulletin of the History of Medicine*, **50** (1976), pp. 372–91.
68 Editorial, 'Problem' (n. 67), p. 896.
69 F. J. Ebgurth, 'From poison to remedy: The chequered history of botulinum toxin', *Journal of Neural Transmission*, **115** (2008), pp. 555–70 at p. 562.
70 G. S. Burke, 'Production of anti-toxin: Technique for isolating B. botulinus', *Journal of Bacteriology*, 4 (1919), pp. 557–64 at p. 564. On strains, see also Dewberrry, *Food Poisoning*, (n. 15), pp. 314–17.
71 A. Lamb, 'Biological weapons: The facts not the fiction', *Clinical Medicine*, 1 (2001), pp. 502–4.
72 Roland Böni, 'Botulinum toxin in warfare', in O. P. Kreydon, R. Böni and G. Burg (eds), "Hyperhydrosis and Botulinum Toxin in Dermatology", *Current Problems in Dermatology*, 30 (2002), pp. 101–6.
73 Schantz and Johnson, 'Botulinum toxin' (n. 8), p. 319.
74 Ibid, p. 321. See also Jeremy Pearce, 'Edward J. Schantz, pioneering researcher of toxins, including botox, dies at 96', *New York Times*, 4 May 2005 at www.nytimes,com/2005/05/04/national/04schantz.html?_r=O.
75 Alan B. Scott, 'Development of botulinum toxin therapy', in Arnold W. Klein (ed), "The Clinical Use of Botulinum", *Dermatologic Clinics*, 22 (2004), pp. 131–33 at p. 132.
76 Ibid, p. 132.
77 Ibid.
78 Ibid.
79 Schantz and Johnson, 'Botulinum toxin' (n. 8), p. 317.
80 Vishwanath S. Hanchanale et al., 'The unusual history and urological applications of botulism neurotoxin', *Urologia Internationalis*, **85** (2010), pp. 125–30 at p. 128 (quotation); Rod J. Rohrich et al., 'Botulinum toxin: Expanding role in medicine', *Plastic and Reconstructive Surgery*, **112**, Supplement 5 (2003), p. 51.
81 K. Roger Aoki, 'Pharmacology, immunology, and current developments', in Anthony V. Benedetto (ed), *Botulinum Toxins in Clinical and Aesthetic Practice*, 2nd edition, London, 2011, p. 16.
82 Ernst Stein, 'Botulinum toxin and anal fissure', in Kredon et al., (eds), "Hyperhydrosis" (n. 72), pp. 218–26.
83 Scott, 'Development' (n. 75), p. 132.
84 Aoki, 'Pharmacology' (n. 81), p. 17.
85 Scott, 'Development' (n. 52), p. 132. The Carruthers' first publication of the frown line treatment was in 1992: Jan D. Carruthers and J. Alastair Carruthers, 'Treatment of glabellar frown lines with C. Botulinum-A exotoxin', *Journal of Dermatological Surgery and Oncology*, 18 (1992), pp. 17–21.
86 Aoki, ''Pharmacology' (n. 81), p. 17.
87 Benedetto, *Botulinum Toxins* (n. 81), p. x.
88 See Anthony Elliott, *Making the Cut: How Cosmetic Surgery is Transforming Our Lives*, London, 2008; also Elizabeth Haiken, *Venus Envy: A History of Cosmetic Surgery*, Baltimore and London, 1998.
89 Arnold W. Klein, 'Preface', in Arnold W. Klein and Bruce H. Thiers (eds), "The Clinical Use of Botulinum Toxin", *Dermatologic Clinics*, 22 (2004), p. ix.
90 Rod J. Rohrich, 'Botulinum toxin: Expanding role in medicine', in Klein and Thiers (eds), "Clinical Use", p. 15.

91 Jean and Alastair Carruthers, *Using Botulinum Toxin Cosmetically*, London and New York, 2003, pp. 1, 3.
92 Ibid, p. 3.
93 Ibid. Printed inside front hardcover.
94 Benedetto (ed), *Botulinum Toxins* (n. 81), p. xi.
95 Aoki, 'Pharmacology', in Benedetto (ed), *Botulinum Toxins* (n. 81), p. 7.
96 David J. Goldberg, 'Medicolegal considerations of cosmetic treatment with botulinum toxin injection', in Benedetto (ed), *Botulinum Toxins* (n. 81), pp. 263–66. For the 1st edition, see note 52.
97 Kenneth F. Kiple (ed), *The Cambridge World History of Human Disease*, Cambridge and New York, 1993, pp. 643–44, 1074.
98 Hamlin, *Cholera* (n. 9), p. 285.
99 Jean Guard-Petter, 'Minireview. The chicken, the egg and *Salmonella enteritidis*', *Environmental Microbiology*, 3 (2001), pp. 421–30 at www.black-wellspubliching.com/products/journals/freepdf/emi213.pdf, accessed 17 July 2014; Advisory Committee on the Microbiological Safety of Foods, *Second Report on Salmonella in Eggs*, London (2001), p. 1. For *Salmonella* control in the EU, see Richard Ducatelle, 'An update on *Salmonella* prevention and control in poultry by vaccination, including emerging monophasic *S. Typhimurium*', *Salmonella 360' Newsletter* at www.Salmonella360.com/cms3/assets//fullsize/582, accessed 16 July 2014.
100 Guard-Petter, 'Minireview' (n. 99), p. 423.
101 See Chief Medical Officer's Annual Report, Ministry of Health [CMOAR], 1920, p. 134.
102 Ibid, 1984, p. 3.
103 Ibid, 1985, p. 52. For naming practice of the *Salmonella*, see Hardy, *Salmonella Infections* (n. 10), pp. 156–57.
104 CMOAR, 1988, p. 8.
105 Guard-Petter, 'Minireview' (n. 99), pp. 424, 426.
106 CMOAR, 1988, p. 9.
107 Christopher G. Forshner, 'The British Government, mad cows and rotten eggs: Decision-making, uncertainty and risk as it occurs in the real world', unpublished MPhil dissertation, Oxford University, 1993, p. 67.
108 CMOAR, 1988, p. 132.
109 Forshner, 'Decision-making' (n. 107), p. 67.
110 Food Safety Act 1990, at www.legislation.gov.uk/ukpga/1990/16/contents. See also CMOAR, 1989, p. 9; 1990, p. 16.
111 CMOAR, 1990, pp. 16–7.
112 www.safe-poultry.com/SalmonellacontrolUK.asp?print=col, accessed 13 June 2014; www.legislation.gov.uk/uks/1989/285/made?view=plan, accessed 18 July 2014.
113 CMOAR, 1997, p. 21.
114 Ibid, p. 132.
115 Ibid, 1993, p. 159; 1996, p. 213; 1997, p. 21.
116 Advisory Committee, *Second Report* (n. 99), p. 1.
117 Ibid, pp. 1–2.
118 Ibid, p. 1.
119 Among EU countries, Sweden and Finland forbade the use of vaccines against *Salmonella* in poultry; Northern Ireland forbade the import of eggs from vaccinated flocks: Ibid, p. 43.
120 See, for example, N. Nagamine et al., 'Evaluation of the efficacy of a bacterin against Salmonella enteritidis infection and the effect of stress after vaccination', *Avian Diseases*, 35 (1994), pp. 717–24; G. L. Cooper et al.,

'Vaccination of chickens with strain CVL30, a genetically defined Salmonella enteritidis aroA live oral vaccine candidate', *Infection and Immunity*, 62 (1994), pp. 4747–54; T. J. Nassar et al., 'Use of live and inactivated Salmonella enteritidis phage type 4 vaccines to immunise laying hens against experimental infection', *Reviews of Science and Technology*, 13 (1994), pp. 855–67 at www.oie.int/doc/ged/D8924.PDF, accessed 30 June 2014.

121 Advisory Committee, *Second Report* (n. 99), p. 42.

122 CMOAR, 1997, p, 21; Laurence Gibbons, 'British Lion Scheme helps "eradicate salmonella" in eggs: Report', at www.foodmanufacture.co.uk/content/view/print/708593, accessed 13 June 2014.

123 Advisory Committee, *Second Report* (n. 99), p. 42.

124 Ibid, p. 9, Table 2.1.

125 Ibid, 1997, p. 21.

126 S. J. O'Brien, 'The decline and fall of non-typhoidal salmonella in the United Kingdom', *Clinical Infectious Diseases*, 56 (2013), pp. 705–10, Epub. 2012 November 19.

127 The last documented outbreak was that at Pont-Saint-Esprit, France, in 1951.

128 Salmonella control programmes in poultry were implemented in all EU member states from 2003: European Food Standards Authority, 'Topic: Salmonella' at www.efsa.europa.eu/en/topics/ropic/salmonella.html, accessed 20 July 2014.

129 August 2014 saw an outbreak in England linked to imported eggs from a single source outside the United Kingdom, with cases also occurring in France and Austria: see Public Health England, Salmonella Outbreak Investigation Update at www.gov.uk/goverment/news/salmonella-outbreak-investigation-update (22 August 2014), accessed 19 October 2014; Public Health England, Bulletin no. 2014301 (29 August 2014). Recent outbreaks in the United States, some of them interstate, have been linked to nut butter, organic chia powder, backyard poultry, pet bearded dragons and raw cashew cheese; see www.cdc-gov/salmonella/, accessed 19 October 2014.

12 It *does* all depend on the dose. Understanding beneficial and adverse drug effects since 1864

Clinical and experimental attitudes to the Law of Mass Action and concentration–effect curves

Jeffrey K. Aronson and Robin E. Ferner

Introduction

Just over 150 years ago, on 15 March 1864, the Norwegian chemist Peter Waage (1833–1900) and his brother-in-law, the mathematician and chemist Cato Maximilian Guldberg (1836–1902) (Figure 12.1), published a paper in which they propounded what has come to be known as the Law of Mass Action [1, 2]. Coincidentally, their paper appeared just 300 years after the posthumous publication of the *Septem Defensiones* by Paracelsus (Philippus Aureolus Theophrastus Bombastus von Hohenheim, 1493–1541) in 1564.

Since then, the Law of Mass Action has come to inform our understanding of many biological functions, including control of cellular pH, the catalytic actions of enzymes and their inhibitors, the transmembrane transport of anions and cations, the binding of drugs to proteins, and the actions of drugs at receptors and other pharmacological targets. It is the basis of the Henderson–Hasselbalch, Michaelis–Menten, Hill, Adair, Schild, and other eponymous equations; the Langmuir adsorption isotherm; and comparable equations used in physiology and pharmacology.

In pharmacology, application of the Law of Mass Action has led to the concept of dose-responsiveness. Here, we describe the genesis of this idea, its clinical relevance, and how attitudes to it have changed in recent years.

Terminology

A concentration–effect curve is a visual representation of the relation between the concentration at the site of action of a drug in a biological system and the magnitude of a selected measurable effect that it has on that system. This relation can be drawn on a graph using Cartesian (i.e. linear–linear)

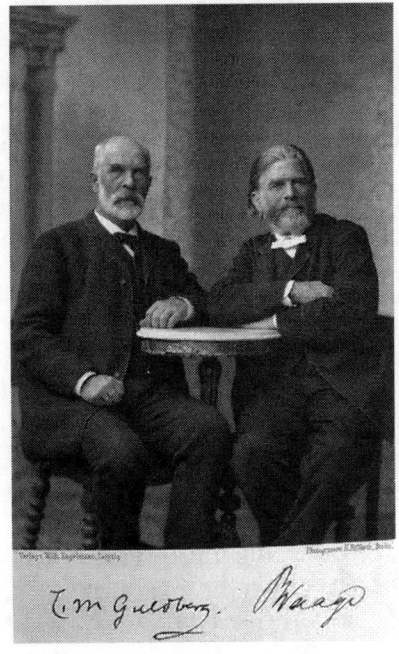

Figure 12.1 Cato Guldberg and Peter Waage.
Photogravure by H. Riffart, Berlin, Zeitschrift für Physikalische Chemie, Band 8, 1891. Image scanned, processed, and uploaded by Kuebi = Armin Kübelbeck [Public domain], via Wikimedia Commons.

coordinates, when, in the simplest case, it generally takes the form of a rectangular hyperbola. It is nowadays more usual to draw it with the concentration of the drug on a horizontal logarithmic axis and the effect on a linear vertical axis, when the curve becomes sigmoid and approximately linear at values of the effect between 20% and 80% of the maximal possible effect. Before 1926, such curves were not drawn. Equations that describe concentration–effect curves, which can be fitted to experimental data, can also be derived theoretically from the Law of Mass Action, using structural models and under certain assumptions.

The term "dose–response curve" should properly be reserved for an analogous representation of the relation between the administered dose of a drug and its observed effect in a whole animal or human. Since there is expected to be a predictable relation between the administered dose of a drug and the consequent drug concentration at the site of action that causes the measured effect, the *in vivo* dose–response curve is often taken to be a surrogate for the concentration–effect curve, which generally cannot be measured in the intact animal. The two terms are often used interchangeably.

Examples of both of these types of curve are given in the following discussion.

Benefits and harms, poisons and toxicity

Benefits are favourable outcomes in individuals or populations.

Drug harms (adverse drug effects and reactions) are unwanted outcomes from medicines: symptomatic hurt (e.g. pain, breathlessness); organ damage, either symptomatic (e.g. rash, stroke) or asymptomatic (e.g. agranulocytosis, QT interval prolongation); or combinations of these.

Diseases and medicines both provide hazards, which are potential sources of harm. Risk describes the probability of such harms during or after exposure to the hazard. Risks can also describe probabilities of benefits (a good risk, a desirable risk, a preferred risk), even though we are not used to thinking of the chance of benefit as a risk.

The balance of benefit to harm of a therapeutic intervention can be assessed by weighing up three probabilities (or risks) [3]:

• The probability of benefit from the treatment.
• The probability of harm from the treatment.
• The probability of harm if you don't use the treatment.

"Poison" is defined in the *Oxford English Dictionary* (OED) as "Material that causes illness or death when introduced into or absorbed by a living organism, esp. when able to kill by rapid action and when taken in small quantity...", the earliest citation being from the early 13th century [4]. However, the dictionary does not specify what it means by "in small quantity". In answer to the question "how small?" one might well say "large enough". Many animal and plant toxins, for example, are toxic to human in very small quantities. In humans, the average estimated lethal dose of ricin, a toxin found in the beans of the castor plant *Ricinus communis*, if given by inhalation or by intramuscular or intravenous injection, is 5–10 micrograms/kilogram, that is, 350–700 micrograms in a 70-kilogram adult [5]. [1 microgram = 10^{-6} grams.] Some bacterial toxins, such as botulinum toxin, shiga toxin, and tetanus toxin, are even more toxic, and nanogram amounts can be fatal. [1 nanogram = 10^{-9} grams.] In contrast, other compounds are very safe and require very large doses (milligrams, grams, or even kilograms) before toxic effects occur.

"Toxicity" is defined in the OED as "Toxic or poisonous quality, esp. in relation to its degree or strength", and "toxic" is defined as "caused or produced by a poison". These are vague definitions, and we prefer a definition of toxicity that is based on the pharmacological principles that proceed from the Law of Mass Action, as we shall describe later.

Poisons have been known and used as such for hundreds of years. For example, it is not known for sure what Socrates was given to procure his death in 399 BC, hemlock or otherwise [6], but it was certainly a poison. Fear of poisoning led the Greeks to search for theriacs (antidotes). Mithridates, King of Pontus (120–63 BC), advised by his physician Krateuas, tried to develop an antidote to poisoning (hence called a mithridate) by combining many substances in a single formulation, which he then took in increasing doses in an attempt to achieve immunity to their toxic effects [7]. This approach was imitated for many years (one 17th-century recipe listed 48 different ingredients), until William Heberden debunked it in his *Essay on Mithridatium and Theriaca* of 1745. A mithridate, he wrote, is "made up of a dissonant crowd collected from different countries, mighty in appearance, but in reality an ineffective multitude, that only hinder one another".

Even at times when medical practitioners—doctors, apothecaries, and quacks—had access to few effective drugs, some of the compounds they used were pharmacologically effective, albeit not necessarily specific, and could cause toxicity. Other compounds had no therapeutic efficacy but were toxic nevertheless. It is much easier to poison someone than to treat them effectively—you just have to give a large enough dose.

As an instance, poisons feature in several of Shakespeare's plays, often without mention of their provenance. Hamlet's father is, we are told, poisoned, as is Gonzago in the play within a play, and by the end, all the main characters have been poisoned too, in one way or another. On three of the four occasions when Shakespeare mentions apothecaries, who would have been expected to purvey beneficial medicines, it is in the context of poisons. Romeo, for example, obtains a poison from a Mantuan apothecary, who sells it to him illegally, risking the punishment of death, but persuaded to do so by virtue of poverty. The misanthropic Timon says "Trust not the physician / His antidotes are poison", although Shakespeare, in contrast to his Elizabethan and Jacobean contemporaries, never actually portrayed physicians as poisoners.

Paracelsus and dose

In the year of Shakespeare's birth, 1564, the *Septem Defensiones* by Paracelsus (Philippus Aureolus Theophrastus Bombastus von Hohenheim, 1493–1541) was published posthumously. In the third defence in that work, Paracelsus wrote his now much quoted text: "Was ist das nit gifft ist? alle ding sind gifft/und nichts ohn gifft/Allein die dosis macht das ein ding kein gifft ist". In English, "What is there that is not a poison? Every thing is a poison and nothing is not a poison. Only the dose determines that a thing is not a poison". A Latin translation appears in the margin of the first edition of the text: "Nil sine veneno praesertim dosi non servari" or "nothing lacks poison[ous effects] especially if the dose is not heeded".

The word "ding", as used by Paracelsus, is potentially ambiguous. Instead of the traditional medical philosophy, based on the four humours, the four elements, and Aristotle's four qualities, he proposed a tripartite system, reflecting the Trinity and threefold human nature, consisting of soul, spirit, and body [8]. The three educational pillars on which he thought his system should be built were astronomy, natural philosophy, and alchemy, reflecting the heavens, the earth, and human biology. Seeking a name for the elements of his new philosophy and wanting to avoid the word "elements" itself, he rejected words such as the Latin terms corpora (bodies), essentiae (essentials or essences), and species (classes), and the German words ersten (first things) and stücke (pieces), and finally settled on "dingen".

Paracelsus's tripartite scheme involved the use of mercury, sulphur, and salt as therapeutic principles, or arcana (secret remedies), which he called "drei dingen" and which he considered to be the prime sources of all the matter in the universe, the causes of diseases and at the same time possible cures. By "salt", he meant what we would nowadays call metallic salts, such as those of antimony, arsenic, copper, iron, lead, magnesium, mercury, and potassium, particularly potassium nitrate (sal nitri, nitre, or saltpetre).

Paracelsus wrote *The Third Defence* in response to criticism of his treatment of syphilis with these "things". Thus, "alle ding sind gifft", read in isolation, as it is usually quoted, cannot be clearly interpreted: he might have been specifically referring to the drei dingen, the therapies that he had used, mercury, sulphur, and salt[s]. The implication would be that while he recognized that the use of large doses of such substances could be harmful, the doses that he was accustomed to using were purely beneficial.

Nevertheless, elsewhere in *The Third Defence*, Paracelsus spells out his view that all therapeutic substances are indeed potential poisons. His reply to those who criticized him for using poisons in his therapeutic practice takes the line that there are poisons in nature, but that God put them there, and when used properly, they do not have to be poisonous. "Why should a poison be denounced?" he writes. "He who denounces a poison does not understand its composition". Take purgatives, for example. "Wa[s] ist ein Purgatio?" he asks, and the answer, in the marginal Latin translation, is "Omnis purgatio venenum, si non servetur dosis"; "Every purgative is a poison if the dose is not heeded". Theriac, he points out, used as an antidote to poison, was itself obtained from the venom of poisonous vipers. Even food and drink is poisonous, he suggests, if taken in too great quantities.

From this, we cannot tell whether Paracelsus had any conception of the graded effects of medicines, in which for each outcome that a medicine produces, there is a no-effect level, an increasing effect as the dose increases, and no further effect as the dose is increased beyond the maximum effective. Indeed, since he espoused a kind of dualism in which good and evil coexisted as natural forces, it is possible that he thought that there was a dose or range of doses that was beneficial and a separate dose or range of doses that was poisonous. This opinion would have been reinforced by his knowledge that different salts of the same metal could have different actions, beneficial and harmful.

However, others have argued that Paracelsus did at least understand the principle of the no-effect dose [9], citing five reasons:

1 He does not ask "What is a poison?" but "What is not a poison?"
2 He uses the word "thing" instead of drug, medicine, remedy (or others), and thus advances a much broader approach.
3 He also refers to food and drink.
4 In saying "only the dose determines that a thing is not a poison" (the negative definition), he is looking at the dose–response relationship downwards.
5 Elsewhere in *The Third Defence*, he states that "while a thing may be a poison, it may not cause poisoning".

These arguments are only partly convincing. Paracelsus certainly asks, "What is there that is not a poison?" (the negative formulation), but then says that "every thing is a poison and nothing is not a poison" (both positive and negative). Here and elsewhere, he stresses that although the remedies that he uses are poisons (i.e. defending himself), so are those that others use (i.e. attacking others), and that there is a beneficial dose and a harmful dose. None of this necessarily implies that he understood the concept of gradation.

Immediately after telling his critics that purgatives are poisons, he adds: "The main point is that the dose should not be too large or too small. He who uses a middling dose will not cause poisoning". It would be surprising if Paracelsus had not recognized that too little of anything, or at least any thing, would be ineffective. His view that the same things, mercury, sulphur, and salt[s], could both cause and cure diseases was not Hahnemann's homoeopathic view that the cure could be diluted away to nothing and remain effective. Given that Paracelsus appreciated that a dose might be too small to be effective and that too large a dose would be poisonous, it seems likely that he would have thought it logical that there must be a dose in between that would be both effective and not poisonous. This description may even have been seen as according with his more general tripartite theory. However, even this does not convincingly demonstrate that he fully understood the complete nature of the graded dose–response curve.

The nature of the concentration–effect curve

In order to understand the history of the concentration–effect relation, it is necessary to understand the nature of the curve. The major principles are demonstrated in Figure 12.2, from the work of R P (Steve) Stephenson (1925–2004), published in a paper [10] that some have considered the most important pharmacological paper to have been published in the 20th century [11].

Stephenson generated concentration–effect relationships by exposing guinea pig ileum (part of the small bowel) *in vitro* to a series of alkylated trimethylammonium salts, which caused the ileum to contract. His data, plotted as log concentration on the horizontal axis and effect as a percentage of maximum on the vertical, illustrate three different features of concentration–effect curves: different potencies, different maximum efficacies, and, in one case, hormesis.

Consider the curve generated by exposure to the ethyl salt. The curve is sigmoid in shape. At a concentration of about 10^{-6} molar (i.e. 10^{-6} mol/L), there is no contraction; as the concentration rises to just above 10^{-4} molar, there is increasing contraction, and at higher concentrations, no further contraction is achieved. The curves for the butyl and hexyl salts are similar; they have the same sigmoid shape and plateau at the same maximum contractile effect. However, these three curves are set apart—the same effects are produced by different concentrations; the butyl salt is more potent than the hexyl salt, producing its effects at lower concentrations, and in turn, the hexyl salt is more potent than the ethyl salt.

The curves for the heptyl, octyl, and nonyl salts are different. They too have different potencies, but in each case, the maximum contractile effect (the so-called maximal efficacy) is less than the maximum possible. These compounds have lower efficacy—a concept that Stephenson introduced—than the butyl, hexyl, and ethyl salts.

Note that had Stephenson plotted the data on Cartesian coordinates, the curves would have been rectangular hyperbolas, as we shall see later.

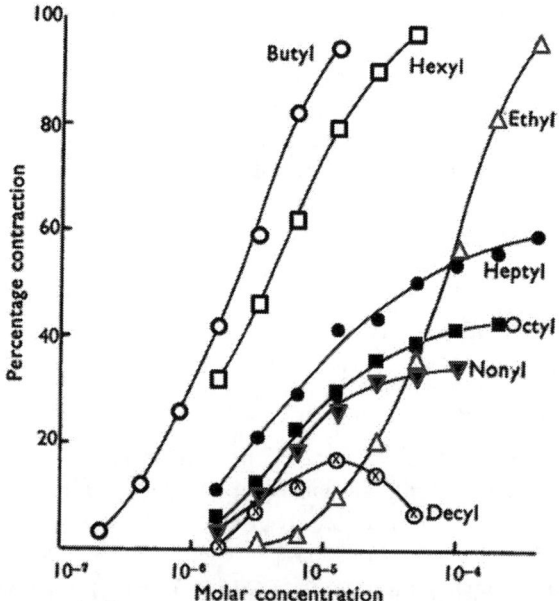

Figure 12.2 Concentration–effect relationships for a series of alkylated trimethylammonium salts causing contraction in guinea pig ileum *in vitro*.

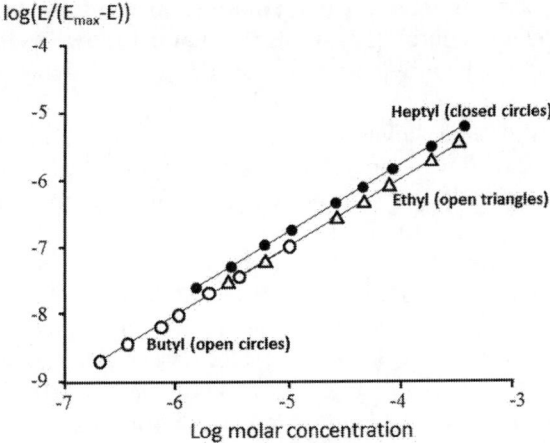

Figure 12.3 Hill plots for the data shown in Figure 12.2 for the butyl, ethyl, and heptyl salts.

Analysing these curves using the Hill equation shows that they all have the same slope of 1 (Figure 12.3), implying that one molecule of the compound interacts with one molecule of the effector responsible for contraction.

The mathematical derivations of these equations are given in the Appendix.

The decyl salt is a case apart. It has a biphasic effect, increasing contraction at concentrations between 10^{-6} and 10^{-5} molar and reducing it at higher concentrations. This is the phenomenon known as hormesis, which has been discussed in detail by Calabrese [12, 13].

The Law of Mass Action: defining dose-responsiveness

The concept of "affinity" as the chemical force that holds together dissimilar substances was ascribed to Herman Boerhaave (1668–1738), the influential Leiden physician and the author of *Elementa chemiae* [14], by William Whewell (1794–1866) in 1840 [15]. In Whewell's words, "When we make a chemical solution, not only are the particles of the dissolved body separated from each other, but they are closely united to the particles of the solvent".

The French chemist Claude Louis Berthollet (1748–1822), in considering the driving force behind chemical reactions, then established the relation between the mass of a substance and the rate at which it undergoes a chemical reaction. He set this idea down in his 1801 treatise *Recherches sur les lois de l'affinité*, which described "the laws of the affinity by which bodies tend to join together or combine" [16]. The relevance of chemical affinity to therapeutics was quickly recognized. For example, Jonathan Pereira in *The Elements of Materia Medica* (1854) wrote that "The action of a medicine on one organ rather than on another is accounted for on the chemical hypothesis, by assuming the existence of unequal affinities of the medicinal agent for different tissues" [17]. Others extended the concept to the idea that there must be specific elements in tissues on which drugs acted, paving the way for the concept of receptors to be developed [18].

It was not until 1864, however, that the Norwegians Cato Guldberg and Peter Waage clearly propounded the Law of Mass Action in a neglected paper in Norwegian [1], at a time when the population of Norway was around 1.7 million and few if any scientists elsewhere would have spoken Norwegian [19]. Greater currency was obtained when Guldberg and Waage published a paper in French in 1867, titled *Etudes sur les affinités chimiques* [20]. Even then, however, the idea had to be rediscovered in 1877 by the Dutch chemist Jacobus van 'tHoff (1852–1911), who classified chemical reactions and defined their orders [21]. Based on van 'tHoff's work, the Swedish chemist Svante Arrhenius deduced a formula for the change in reaction rate constant with temperature.

It was then not long before the term "Law of Mass Action" started to be used to describe the phenomenon that Guldberg and Waage had described. In 1879, for example, Matthew Moncrieff Pattison Muir published an annotation of the 1867 French paper, which had been donated to the library of the Chemical Society [of London] in its year of publication, in which he described its contents in detail. "The law of mass action formulated [by Guldberg & Waage]", he wrote, "was applied in the authors' 'Études' to the cases of chemical action already cited and also to the case of ether formation" [22]. By the next year, Muir was referring to Guldberg and Waage's paper as "their celebrated memoir" [23].

The problem that had occupied Guldberg and Waage was to give a mathematical description of the affinities that drive chemical reactions. This involved both the rates of the reactions, which they described as chemical dynamics, and, for reversible reactions, the final equilibrium between the forward reaction and the backward reaction, which they designated chemical statics. The two separate parts of the problem have sometimes been forgotten, as Mysels [24] and Guggenheim [25] pointed out.

Taking the question of the rate of reaction first, the Norwegians proposed that for a reversible reaction taking place in one phase (their data were derived from reactions in solution), the rate was proportional to the "active mass" of the reactants ("La force est porportionelle au produit des masses actives des deux corps A et B"), where "active mass" is the mass per unit volume—that is, the concentration. Thus,

$$A + B \rightleftharpoons A' + B' \tag{12.1}$$

The rate is therefore related to the number of species involved in the reaction, and so it depends on the precise reaction path. This means that if there is a series of intermediate reactions whose form is not known, it may not be possible to calculate the rate of each reaction, even when the overall reaction is known. As Guggenheim later pointed out, "The point ... that the kinetic behaviour of a particular reaction must be determined experimentally and cannot be predicted from the stoichiometric formula was better appreciated by ... van 'tHoff than by many subsequent writers, especially writers of textbooks" [23].

The simple analysis of the rate of change of the concentration of the reactant and the pharmacokinetic treatment of the disappearance of a drug from the sampling compartment are identical. In particular, if the disappearance of a reactant A follows first-order kinetics, it follows that

$$-d[A]/dt = k[A]. \tag{12.2}$$

In due course, theoretical treatments of reaction kinetics have taken into account the energy required for a species to react, the time for a suitably energized species to react, and the spatial arrangement of the reactant [26].

The law governing reversible chemical reactions at equilibrium does not depend on any intermediate steps, only on the concentrations of the reactants and products. For a simple one-step reaction, in which A + B $\rightleftharpoons$ AB, the ratio of concentrations of reactants to product is a constant, the equilibrium constant, given by:

$$[AB]/[A].[B] = K_{eq} \tag{12.3}$$

where K_{eq} is the ratio of the backward and forward rate constants.

More complex interactions lead to correspondingly more complex equilibrium conditions. Pharmacology has benefited greatly from simple equilibrium considerations, and they form the basis of the description of interactions between receptor and drug.

Receptors

Paul Ehrlich (1854–1915) first set out his view of the specificity of reactions with cellular components in his doctoral thesis on the staining of tissues with aniline dyes, 'Beiträge zur Theorie und Praxis der histologischen Färbung', which he presented at Leipzig University on 18 June 1878 [27]. He argued that the interaction was purely chemical, that the specificity was explained by preferential reactions, and that the structure of the aniline dye determined what cellular components it would stain. He later more explicitly stated that there is a direct relation between chemical structure and function, and that the binding of molecules by receptors mediates most physiological functions [28, 29]. In his 1908 Nobel Lecture, Ehrlich explained why the action of a toxin "can only be caused by the *adhesion of the toxic substance to quite definite cell complexes*" which he called '*receptors*' [30].

Charles Scott Sherrington (1857–1952), Professor of Physiology in Liverpool and subsequently in Oxford, coined the term "chemoreceptors" in 1904, in his Silliman Lectures, delivered at Yale University, published as *The Integrative Action of the Nervous System* in 1906: "Thus, we may take in illustration the two sets of selective chemo-receptors, the gustatory and the olfactory" [31]. Paul Ehrlich seems to have done likewise independently a year later, in his Harben Lectures [32]:

> I have now formed the opinion that in like manner a part of the chemically defined substances is attached to the cell by groups corresponding to these [toxin] receptors; these atom groupings I will distinguish from the toxin-receptors by the name of 'chemo-receptors.'

In the same lectures, he reported that "The existence of receptors can be proved experimentally".

Meanwhile, in 1905, John Newport Langley (1852–1925), Professor of Physiology in Cambridge, suggested that what he called "receptive substances" were responsible for the effects of nicotine and curare on skeletal muscle [33]:

> In all cells two constituents at least must be distinguished, (1) substance [*sic*] concerned with carrying out the chief functions of the cells... and (2) receptive substances especially liable to change and capable of setting the chief substance in action.

The importance that Langley attached to the term "receptive substance(s)", which did not appear in the title of his paper, is demonstrated by its inclusion in the running head "NERVE-ENDINGS AND RECEPTIVE SUBSTANCE".

The Law of Mass Action and the concentration–effect curve

The 19th century

Even before the enunciation of the Law of Mass Action in 1864, pharmacologists had observed graded responses to pharmacological interventions.

In 1854, Rudolf Virchow (1821–1902) observed a concentration-dependent reduction in the beating activity of tracheal epithelial ciliae (hair cells) in post-mortem human mucosa in response to increasing doses of sodium and potassium hydroxide; however, he also observed *increased* beating activity of the ciliae at low concentrations [34]. Then in the 1880s, Hugo Paul Friedrich Schulz (1853–1932), Professor of Pharmacology at the University of Greifswald, showed that in yeasts a range of antiseptics (iodine, bromine, mercuric chlorite, arsenic acid, chromic acid, salicylic acid, and formic acid) affected fermentation, increasing the production of carbon dioxide at low concentrations and inhibiting it completely at higher concentrations [35, 36]. As Schulz wrote in his 1887 paper, "Die physiologische Wirkung eines Medicaments auf ein Organ ist weiter abhängig vonder Quantität des Arzneimittels", "the physiological effect of a drug on an organ depends on the amount of drug present".

These experiments were associated with attempts to find a justification for homoeopathic theory, linking it to the apparent biphasic effects that Chester Southam and John Ehrlich were later to christen hormesis [37]. The work of Schulz and his colleague Arndt gave rise to the now discredited Arndt–Schulz rule, namely that small doses of a substance stimulate, moderate doses inhibit, and large doses kill. However, hormesis is the phenomenon of a biphasic effect of a compound at measurable concentrations (Figure 12.2), and it cannot be used to justify homoeopathic reasoning [38].

In 1875, Robert Koppe studied the effects of oral digitoxin and treated himself with a total of 3.5 milligrams over five days: 0.5 milligram on the first day, 1 milligram on the next, and 2 milligrams four days later [39]. He experienced severe toxicity and attributed the increasing slowing of his pulse and other effects to dose-related actions. However, he did not appreciate that digitoxin has a very long half-life and that the increasing effects he experienced while taking increasing doses were due to accumulation of the drug rather than to individual doses. Others, notably Emil Juckuff [40] and Harnack [41], built on Koppe's misleading experience, taking a mathematical approach and recognizing two main classes of drugs: those in which the lethal dose was much higher than the effective dose and those for whom there was little difference between beneficial and toxic doses. We would nowadays refer to the latter as having a narrow therapeutic window or a low toxic-to-therapeutic ratio.

An unusual set of data can be found in a publication from 1894, in which Spenzer reported the effects of ether on respiratory carbon dioxide production [42]. The relation between dose of ether and the effect on carbon dioxide was linear. This is an uncommon example of a linear response relation, which is occasionally reported [43]. However, again Spenzer did not plot his data, which are shown in Figure 12.4. Perhaps observations of this kind held up the development of ideas about log dose–response curves.

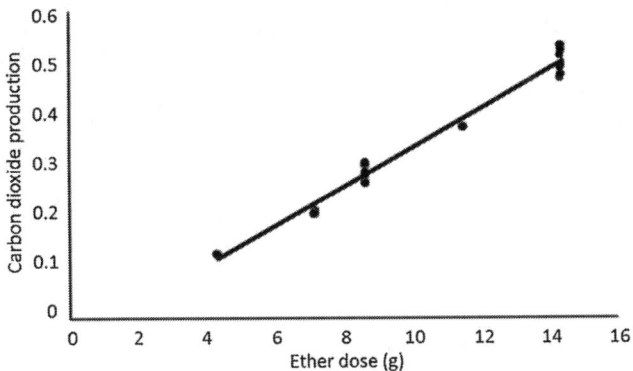

Figure 12.4 The effects of inhaled ether on respiratory carbon dioxide production; note the Cartesian coordinates.

The 20th century

In the early 20th century, the idea of graded doses started to emerge. Experimenters such as Pearce [44] and Bull and Pritchett [45] referred to the "carefully graded doses" that they used in their experiments. Experiments designed to study concentration–effect or dose–response relations were based mainly on two types of research, on the effects of disinfectants on microorganisms and on pharmacological and toxicological effects of various drugs in isolated tissues, animals, and humans.

Claus Ludwig Theodor Bernhard Krönig (1863–1918) and Theodor Paul (1862–1928), following the studies of Kahlenberg and True in plants [46], applied chemical principles to disinfection at the end of the 19th century and observed that the rate at which bacteria are killed by a disinfectant depended on the concentration of the disinfectant and the temperature [47]. In 1908, Harriette Chick (1875–1977) at the Lister Institute extended their results, demonstrating that the rate of bacterial death was proportional to the number of surviving bacteria, n:

$$-dn/dt = K \cdot n \tag{12.4}$$

The form of this equation is identical to that of equation (12.2). "This latter equation", Chick wrote, "is deduced directly from the Law of Guldberg and Waage: that the velocity of any reaction is at any moment proportional to the active mass of reacting substance present at that moment" [48]. She should have added "at equilibrium" after "any reaction". For the number of anthrax spores remaining after the addition of 5% phenol, the value of K calculated by Chick was approximately 0.047 per hour. In the same year, Herbert Watson observed that the rate of disinfection depended on the concentration of the disinfectant [49]. The Chick–Watson equation incorporates measures of concentration and time of exposure in calculating the dose of disinfectant required to kill bacteria, in chlorinated water, for example.

One early investigation of the relation between dose and effect of a drug in the class of compounds for which the lethal dose was much higher than the effective dose was by J Theodore Cash (1854–1936), Regius Professor of Materia Medica at the University of Aberdeen, who studied the effects of indaconitine on temperature in rabbits [50]. He presented his data in tabular form and graphically, and we have redrawn them in Figure 12.5. The main graph shows the raw data plotted on a semi-log plot, and the inset shows the Hill plot derived from the same data; the slope of the latter is 0.9, very close to 1, as would be expected for a simple dose–response curve. Nevertheless, Cash did not attempt to analyse his data mathematically.

Failure to plot data is a common feature of reports detailing the effects of varying doses of drugs on various endpoints at this time. For example, in 1901, Hunt reported changes in blood pressure in response to epinephrine (adrenaline) in dogs whose vagus nerves had been cut [51]. His results were

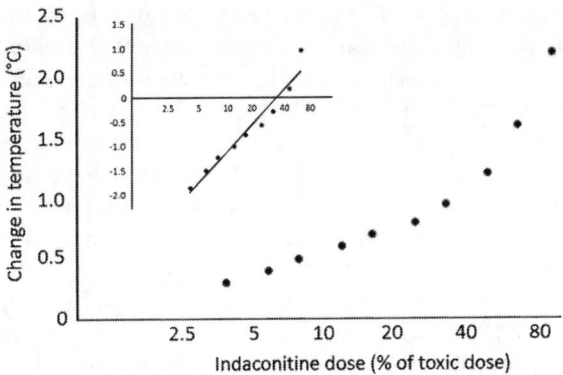

Figure 12.5 The effects of indaconitine on rectal temperature in rabbits.

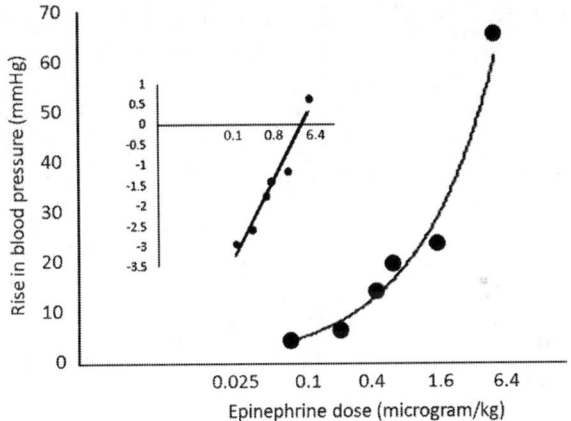

Figure 12.6 The effects of epinephrine on blood pressure in vagotomized dogs, plotted from data given by Hunt in 1901; the inset shows the derived Hill plot, but the estimate of the slope (0.89) at an E_{max} of 100 mmHg has a very large confidence interval, because of the paucity of data at the upper end of the dosage range.

later cited as evidence of a saturable effect of the drug at high doses, but the data were never plotted. They are shown in Figure 12.6. In general, pharmacological data at this time were given in the form of kymograph tracings, and when the resultant data were plotted, it was almost always to show the time courses of events, not their relation to dose or concentration.

The first evidence of a mathematical approach to the problem came from Archibald Vivian Hill (1886–1977). While he was being supervised by Langley, and before he went on to become Professor of Physiology at University College, London, Hill examined the temperature coefficient of the effect of nicotine on muscle contraction. In his first published paper, in 1909, citing Arrhenius's work, he concluded that the effect could not be accounted for by physical diffusion: the "combination between nicotine or curare and the combining constituent of the muscle is of an ordinary chemical nature. This combination is a reversible one between two molecules..." [52]. Hill derived the hyperbolic form of the dose–response curve from the premise of a chemical combination of drug and receptor. The derivation of what has come to be known as the Hill equation, from his analysis of the relation between oxygen tension and the binding of oxygen to haemoglobin (the oxygen saturation curve), is described in the Appendix. In neither case did Hill draw the log concentration–effect curve from the data that he had obtained.

It took another 17 years before anyone thought to publish concentration–effect curves in both Cartesian and semi-logarithmic plots.

In 1923, Lyon investigated the effects of epinephrine (adrenaline) on blood pressure in anaesthetized cats [53]. He plotted the data on Cartesian coordinates (Figure 12.7), but he assumed that Weber's law ("as the stimuli are increased arithmetically, the effects only increase logarithmically") applied, and he fitted the data to a function of the form $E = a\log_e S + b$, and the line that he drew through the data points corresponded to the formula $E = 21.43\log_e S + 91.83$, i.e. a straight line corresponding to the central part of the expected logarithmic dose–response curve, as one would expect from an application of Weber's law (see the Appendix).

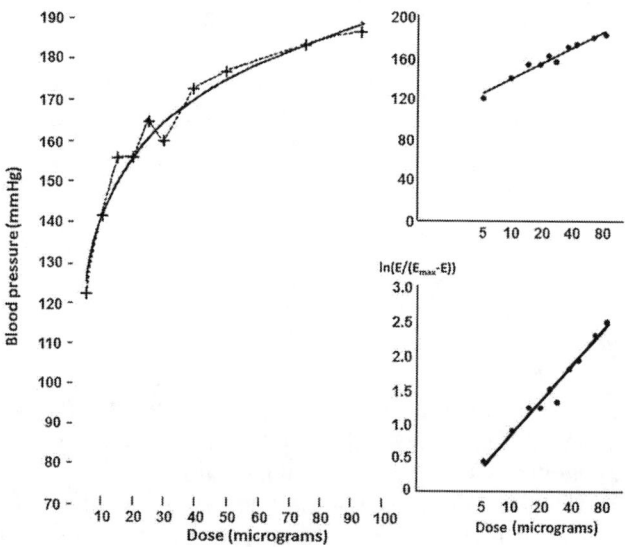

Figure 12.7 The effect of epinephrine (adrenaline) on blood pressure in anaesthetized cats; the main figure is adapted from Lyon 1923; the insets are Hill plots calculated from the published data; in the upper inset the units on the ordinate are in mmHg and in the lower $\ln(E/(E_{max}-E))$.

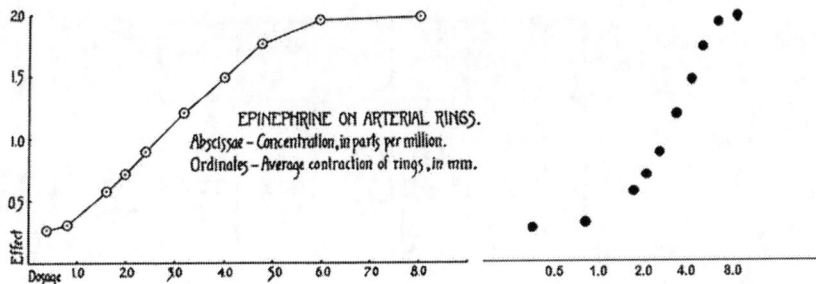

Figure 12.8 The effect of adrenaline (epinephrine) on sheep carotid arterial rings; note the Cartesian coordinates (left-hand panel); plotting the data using logarithmic concentrations yields a sigmoid curve (right-hand panel).

When we replotted the data we found a similar relation: $E = 20.5\log_e S + 93.8$. However, Lyon's conclusion was based on data from an incomplete concentration–effect curve (upper inset in Figure 12.7), which, had data at lower blood pressures been obtained, would probably have been sigmoid. A Hill plot of Lyon's data (lower inset in Figure 12.7) had a slope of 0.68.

Similarly, in 1924, Shackell et al. studied sheep carotid arterial rings and showed increasing contraction with increasing doses of epinephrine (adrenaline), again only on Cartesian coordinates (Figure 12.8) [54].

The first example we have found of a pharmacological plot of response against the logarithm of the dose, that is, the classical log concentration–effect curve, was published in 1926, when Alfred Joseph Clark (1885–1941), at that time Professor of Pharmacology at University College, London, and about to become Professor of Materia Medica at Edinburgh University, used it to demonstrate the action of acetylcholine on frog rectus abdominis muscle [55]. Clark noted that

> the relation between the concentration and action of acetylcholine in most cases follows the formula $K \times x = y/(100 - y)$ and the simplest explanation of this fact is to suppose that a reversible monomolecular reaction occurs between the drug and some receptor in the cells.

His paper contains five figures showing eight log dose–response curves and one figure showing two Hill plots. His Figures 6 and 7 are reproduced as Figure 12.9 here.

Clark assumed that the effect of a drug is directly proportional to the concentration of drug–receptor complex and that the maximum effect occurs when all the receptors are occupied. From this, he derived the apparent dissociation constant of the interaction of a drug with its receptor (K_D in

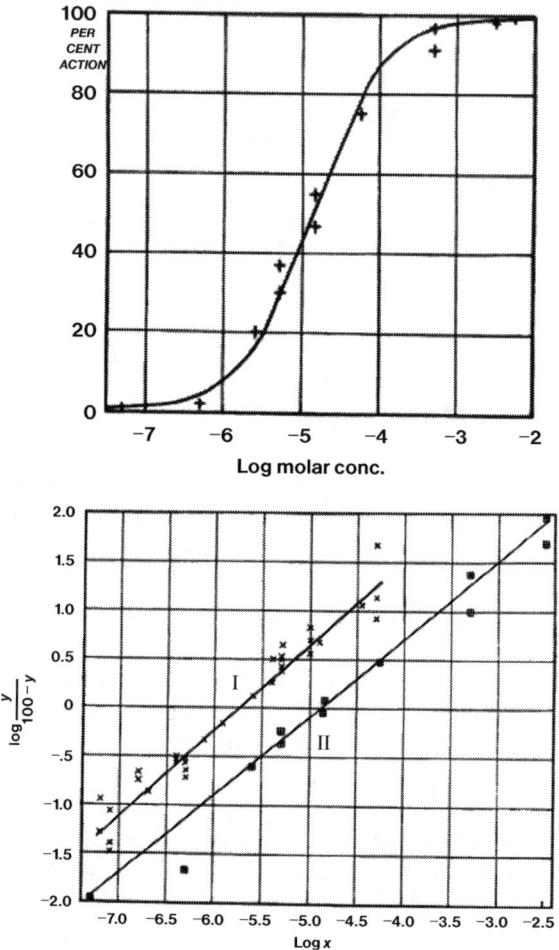

Figure 12.9 Top panel: Figure 6 from Clark's 1926 paper, showing the effect of acetylcholine in producing isotonic contraction of frog rectus abdominis muscle *in vitro*. Bottom panel: Figure 7 from Clark's 1926 paper; line II is the Hill plot derived from the data in his Figure 6.

equation A5 in the Appendix). Clark was also aware of the work of Francis Galton (1822–1911) [56] and Donald MacAlister (1854–1934) [57] on the log normal distribution, which could be used to interpret many data on human attributes, including those attributes explained by Weber's law, later generalized by Fechner, originally applied to psychological stimuli, that the least discernible increment in stimulus was a constant proportion of the initial stimulus [58]. Clark pointed out that the log concentration–effect curve was approximately linear across concentrations that produced

20–80% of the maximum effect. He also stressed that unless concentrations were chosen from across the whole spectrum of effects, from none to maximum, it would not be possible to distinguish the equation he used to fit the data from other possible equations [59].

The quantitative analysis of competitive antagonism by the "dose ratio" method was introduced by John H Gaddum (1900–1965), when he was Professor of Pharmacology at University College London (UCL), later to become Professor of Pharmacology at the University of Edinburgh [60], and was later elaborated by Heinz Otto Schild [61], who was to become one of Gaddum's successors at UCL. Classical theory was later extended by the Dutch pharmacologist Everhardus Jacobus Ariëns (1918–2002), Professor of Pharmacology at the Catholic University of Nijmegen, who used the term "intrinsic activity" to describe the proportionality constant relating effect to the concentration of drug–receptor complex [62].

Modifications to classical receptor theory came when its basic assumptions were questioned, at first by Stephenson (see above), who showed that the assumption of proportionality between occupancy and effect was incorrect and postulated [10] that a maximum effect can be produced without total occupancy of receptors (spare receptors). He coined the term "efficacy" as a measure of the ability of a drug to activate receptors and cause a response. Other later developments, too many and complex to detail here, included Paton's rate theory [63], Changeux's allosteric theory [64], and the elucidation of models to try to explain the difficult concept of efficacy [65]. Add to this the various behaviours of G-protein-coupled receptors, related to spontaneous production of receptor active states, ligand-selective receptor active states, oligomerization with other proteins, and allosteric mechanisms [66], and the increasing complexity of the subject can be readily appreciated. The observation of hormesis, in which there are stimulatory effects at low concentrations and inhibitory effects at high ones [67], adds an extra dimension, which is not vitiated by its uncritical adoption by the homoeopathic lobby. Indeed, it is salutary that A J Clark's contribution to receptor theory was important in debunking homoeopathic theories of the time.

Adverse drug reactions and defining toxicity

It is striking, as one looks through the literature on concentration–effect and dose–response relations since the middle of the 20th century, that the vast majority have been derived from studies in cells or tissues *in vitro* or from experiments in animals. Gaddum's 1954 paper, based on his Walter Ernest Dixon Memorial Lecture delivered at the Royal Society of Medicine in December 1953, included seven figures containing 19 log dose–response curves derived from data obtained in human subjects [68]. However, since then relatively few sets of pharmacodynamic data have been published showing human experiments across wide ranges of concentrations or doses. Notable exceptions include the relation between urinary concentrations of loop diuretics and their effects on the rate of urinary sodium excretion [69, 70] and the relation between plasma propranolol concentrations and the effect of propranolol in reducing exercise-induced tachycardia [71]. Even so, the latter extends only over the linear part of the sigmoid logarithmic concentration–effect curve.

Even rarer are dose–response curves that also incorporate time as a factor. When Hughes looked for such data, hand-searching all issues of four clinical pharmacology journals from 1980 to 2005 for articles that presented pharmacodynamic response versus time curves for four or more different doses, a total of over 18,000 articles in 189 volumes, he found only 33 examples [72].

However, the most striking neglect of the dose–response curve has been in relation to adverse drug reactions, the history of whose classification is summarized in Table 12.1.

From the time when Edward Johnson Wayne (1902–1990), Regius Professor of the Practice of Medicine at the University of Glasgow, classified adverse drug reactions in 1958 as "toxic" and "unpredictable", the latter implying non-dose-relatedness, which Ruth Levine made explicit in 1973, the idea that some adverse reactions are not related to the dose of the drug, and hence to the concentration at the site of action, has dominated the field of pharmacovigilance. The problems with this have been discussed in detail elsewhere [86], but the main objection is that the Law of Mass Action dictates that the magnitude of a pharmacological reaction increases with increasing dose. This is true even of immunological reactions and would be expected to apply to all adverse reactions.

This observation has led to the formulation of a new classification of adverse reactions, called DoTS, which is based on the Dose-relatedness and Time course of the reaction and the Susceptibility of the individual to it. The dose-related aspect of this classification divides reactions into three types (Figure 12.10), depending on whether the adverse reaction occurs at doses below the doses that produce benefit (hypersusceptibility reactions), in the same region as those that produce benefit (collateral reactions), or above those that produce benefit (toxic reactions). Thus, drug toxicity can now be defined more precisely than before, as an adverse effect of a drug that occurs at a range of doses of the drug above the range of doses that are normally expected to produce a beneficial effect.

The implications of this for various aspects of clinical pharmacology, including drug regulation [87], pharmacovigilance planning [88], interpretation of mechanisms of adverse drug reactions [89], prevention of adverse drug reactions [90], adherence to drug therapy [91], and the difference between adverse effects of drugs and the adverse reactions they cause [92], have been discussed elsewhere.

Table 12.1 The history of classifications of adverse drug reactions based on dose-relatedness and time course

Date	Classification based on supposed dose-relatedness	Classification based on time course	References
1958	Distinguishes predictable effects ("toxic effects … related to the main action of the drug or to its side effects") and unpredictable effects ("not related to the main or subsidiary pharmacological action of a drug")	–	[73]
1973	Distinguishes dose-related ("toxic" and "idiosyncratic") reactions from non-dose-related ("allergic") reactions	Distinguishes acute, subacute, and chronic toxic reactions	[74]
1976	Distinguishes dose-related and non-dose-related effects	Distinguishes long-term and teratogenic effects	[75]
1977	Proposes two types of reactions, types A and B	–	[76]
1981	Adds a mnemonic: type A reactions = "augmented"; type B reactions = "bizarre"	–	[77]
1984	Classifies types A and B as dose-related and non-dose-related reactions	Adds two time-related categories, long-term and delayed	[78]
1990	–	Distinguishes acute, subacute, and latent allergic reactions	[79]
1992	–	Labels types C and D long-term and delayed, respectively	[80]
1992	–	Splits type C into two types, type C (continuous) and type E (end of use)	[81]
1997	–	Distinguishes five different patterns of time course that are useful in diagnosing adverse reactions	[82]
2000	Adds a sixth category, F for failure	–	[83]
2002	Adds a seventh category, G for genetic/genomic	–	[84]
2003	DoTS—distinguishes three types of dose-related reactions—toxic, collateral, and hypersusceptibility reactions (see definitions in the text)	Distinguishes time-independent and time-dependent reactions, the latter with six subtypes	[85]

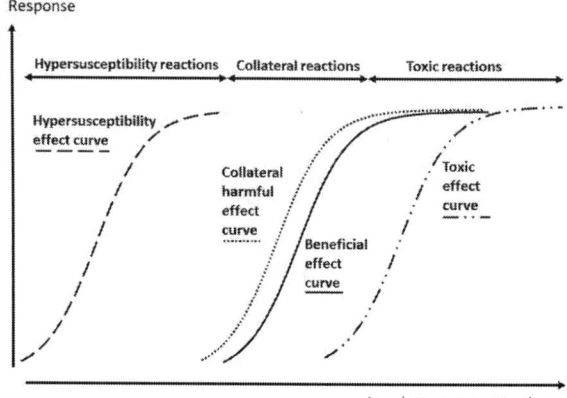

Figure 12.10 Types of adverse drug reactions based on the positions of the dose–response curves of the adverse reactions relative to the dose–response curve for the beneficial effect; a dose–response curve for a hypersusceptibility reaction is shown.

Conclusion

Guldberg and Waage's work on chemical reactions, resulting in what we now call the Law of Mass Action, was the foundation for our quantitative treatment of pharmacological phenomena. Hill postulated a simple reversible combination between two molecules, and A J Clark pioneered the use of log-linear depiction of concentration–effect relations. These approaches have served pharmacologists well. Modern analysis, which allows for more complex interactions and incorporating more recent ideas about chemical kinetics, has been described by Kenakin [93].

Appendix

The ligand-binding equation

We can represent the interaction of a ligand L with its receptor R as follows:

$$L + R \underset{k_{diss}}{\overset{k_{ass}}{\rightleftharpoons}} LR \tag{A1}$$

where k_{ass} and k_{diss} are the rate constants of the relative rates of association and dissociation, respectively, of ligand and receptor. We assume that one molecule of ligand reacts with one receptor. If we let [LR] be the concentration of receptors occupied by the ligand and [R] be the concentration of receptors unoccupied, then, by the Law of Mass Action, at equilibrium the rate at which receptors are being occupied must be the same as the rate at which drug–receptor complexes are dissociating. Thus,

$$[L][R]k_{ass} = [LR]k_{diss} \tag{A2}$$

Rearranging equation (A2), we get

$$[L][R]/[LR] = k_{diss}/k_{ass} \tag{A3}$$

The ratio of the two rate constants, k_{diss}/k_{ass}, is itself a constant and can be replaced by a new constant, K_D, whose interpretation will emerge. If the total concentration of receptors available for binding the drug is $[R_{tot}]$, then

$$[R_{tot}] = [R] + [LR] \tag{A4}$$

Substituting for [R] in equation (A3), we find that

$$[L][R_{tot} - LR]/[LR] = k_{diss}/k_{ass} = K_D \tag{A5}$$

and that therefore,

$$[LR]/[R_{tot}] = [L]/(K_D + [L]) \tag{A6}$$

and therefore,

$$LR = \frac{R_{tot}[L]}{K_D + [L]} \tag{A7}$$

or, put another way

$$b = \frac{B_{max}[L]}{K_D + [L]} \tag{A8}$$

where b is the amount of ligand bound and B_{max} is the total number of binding sites available.

The concentration–effect equation

Assume that the intensity of the effect (E) that a ligand [drug] produces is proportional to the number of receptors the ligand occupies [LR]. Then,

$$E = k'[LR] \tag{A9}$$

where k' is the proportionality constant.
If the maximum possible effect, E_{max}, occurs when all the receptors are occupied, then,

$$E_{max} = k'[R_{tot}] \tag{A10}$$

Dividing (A9) by (A10), we find that

$$\frac{E}{E_{max}} = \frac{[LR]}{[R_{tot}]} \tag{A11}$$

Now substitute (A11) into (A7)

$$\frac{E}{E_{max}} = \frac{[L]}{K_D + [L]} \tag{A12}$$

Rearranging equation (A12) gives

$$E = \frac{E_{max}[L]}{K_D + [L]} \tag{A13}$$

Equation (A13) defines the shape of the classical concentration–effect curve, which has the following properties:

1 When $[L] = 0$, $E = 0$. In other words, when there is no ligand, there is no effect.
2 When the effect is half-maximal, $E = E_{max}/2$. Substituting this into equation (A13), we find that $K_D = [L]$. In other words, K_D is the concentration of ligand required to produce a half-maximal effect.
3 When $[L]$ is very low, $[L] \ll K_D$ and thus,

$$E \approx [L] \times E_{max} / K_D \tag{A14}$$

In other words, at low concentrations of the drug, the response is directly proportional to the drug concentration $[L]$.
4 When $[L]$ is very high, $[L] \gg K_D$ and thus,

$$E \approx E_{max} \tag{A15}$$

In other words, high concentrations of the drug produce effects that are near maximal. This means that further increases in concentration produce only small increases in effect.

The Hill equation

An assumption of this derivation is that one molecule of the ligand interacts with only one molecule of the receptor, or whatever moiety is responsible for the observed effect, and that each interaction has the same affinity. However, that is not always the case. Sometimes more than one molecule interacts, and sometimes the affinity of the interaction changes (increases or decreases) as increasing numbers of molecules bind (so-called positive and negative cooperativity). These phenomena are dealt with by modifying equation (A13) as follows:

$$E = \frac{E_{max}[L]^{n_H}}{(K_D)^{n_H} + [L]^{n_H}} \tag{A16}$$

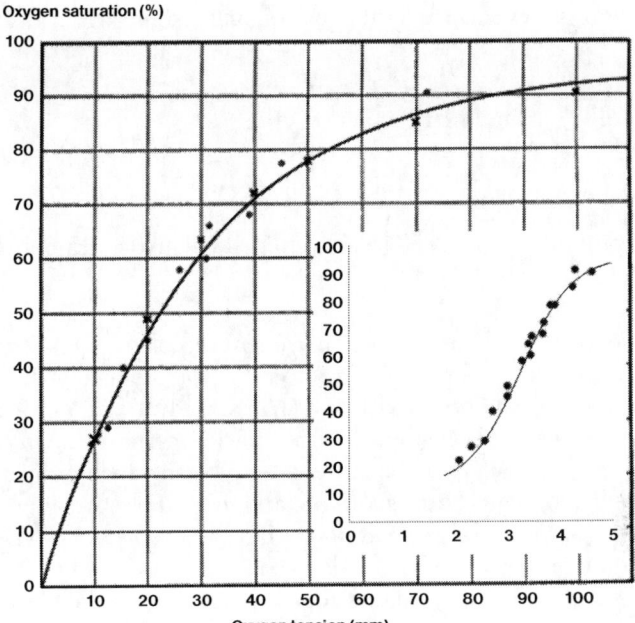

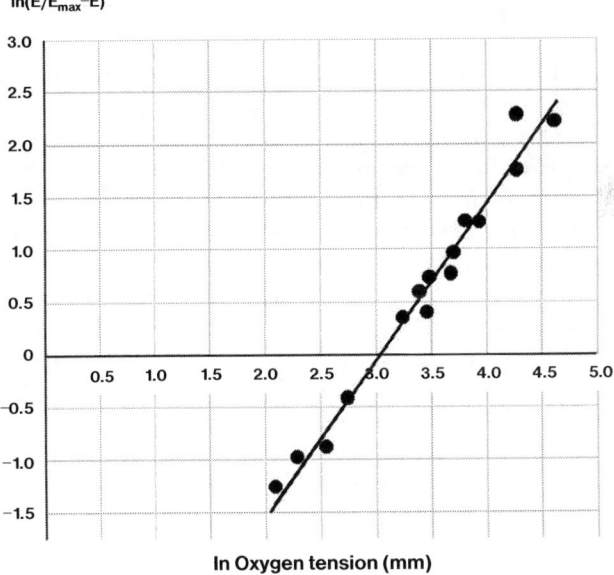

Figure A.1 Upper panel: The effect of oxygen tension on the binding of oxygen to haemoglobin ("oxygen saturation"). The main figure is from Hill's 1910 paper, and the inset is the same data with oxygen tension plotted on a logarithmic scale, a plot that Hill did not draw. Lower panel: The Hill plot drawn from Hill's data, read directly off the main graph in the upper panel and using equation (A17); the slope of the line, n_H, is 1.488; Hill's calculation, using the original data and his equation B, gave a value of 1.405.

This equation, known as the Hill equation, can be linearly transformed as follows:

$$\ln\left(\frac{E}{E_{max}-E}\right) = n_H \ln[L] - n_H \ln[K_D] \qquad (A17)$$

where ln is the natural logarithm.

Thus, a plot of $\ln\left(\frac{E}{E_{max}-E}\right)$ versus ln [L] will give a straight line whose slope is the Hill coefficient n_H.

A Hill coefficient of one implies that one molecule of ligand reacts with one molecule of the moiety that is responsible for producing the measured effect. In that case, equations (A13) and (A16) are identical. A Hill coefficient different from one implies either that the stoichiometry of the interaction is not one to one, or that if it is, then the affinity with which individual molecules of the ligand bind changes as more and more molecules bind (cooperativity). This is what Hill described in relation to the effect of oxygen tension on the binding of oxygen to haemoglobin (Figure A.1) [94]. For more details about non-linear Hill plots, Adair's equation, and other related theories, see Bindslev [95].

The Weber–Fechner law

In 1834, Ernst Heinrich Weber (1795–1878), Professor of Anatomy in Leipzig, published data on people's ability to discriminate weights [96]. Weights of 20 and 21 grams could be discriminated in each hand, but at higher weights, a 1-gram difference could not be discriminated. Weights of 40 and 42 grams, of 60 and 63 grams, of 80 and 84 grams, and of 100 and 105 grams were the limits of discrimination, in each case a 5% difference. Other senses yielded similar findings.

Weber therefore formulated the law that the "just noticeable difference" in the intensity of a stimulus is proportional to the original stimulus. In other words, the just noticeable difference is a function of the logarithm of the stimulus.

Later, Gustav Theodor Fechner (1801–1887), Professor of Physics in Leipzig, further studied this law and named it Weber's law. The generalized form of Weber's law is therefore now referred to as the Weber–Fechner law, as represented by Fechner's equation:

$$S = c \cdot \log R \qquad (A18)$$

where S is the sensation experienced, R is the size of the stimulus, and c is a constant that is different for each type of sensory modality. Plotting S against logR yields a straight line with slope c.

Stevens subsequently refined this by turning it into a power function [97]:

$$\Psi = k \cdot S^n \qquad (A19)$$

Taking logarithms,

$$\ln \Psi = \ln k + n \cdot \ln S \qquad \qquad \qquad (A20)$$

So, plotting ln ψ (S in equation A18) against ln S (R in equation A18) yields a straight line with slope n.

From time to time in the history of the development of ideas about concentration–effect relations, the view has been expressed that such relations obey Weber's law. For example, in a discussion of the effects of diuretics, Marshall wrote that "I am even sanguine that by and by we shall be able to generalize Weber's law, and make it applicable to the stimulation of cells" [98], and Lyon even titled his paper on adrenaline "Does the reaction to adrenalin obey Weber's law?", concluding that it did [53].

However, the problem with Weber's law is that it does not apply at the lower and upper extremes. In other words, it fits at most only the central log-linear portion of the sigmoid log concentration–effect curve, the section that covers, as A J Clark pointed out, 20–80% of the maximum effect possible.

References

1 Waage P, Guldberg CM. Forhandelinger: Videnskabs-Selskabet i Christiana, 1864: 35.
2 Ferner RE, Aronson JK. Cato Guldberg and Peter Waage, the history of the Law of Mass Action, and its relevance to clinical pharmacology. British Journal of Clinical Pharmacology 2016; 81(1): 52–55.
3 Aronson JK. Good prescribing: benefits, hazards, harms, and risks. BMJ 2016; 352: i537.
4 "poison, n.". OED Online. Oxford University Press. http://ezproxy-prd.bodleian.ox.ac.uk:2355/view/Entry/146669?rskey=G5kJ7f&result=1.
5 Bradberry SM, Dickers KJ, Rice P, Griffiths GD, Vale JA. Ricin poisoning. Toxicological Reviews 2003; 22(1): 65–70.
6 Ober WB. Did Socrates die of hemlock poisoning? New York State Journal of Medicine 1977; 77(2): 254–58.
7 Watson G. Theriac and Mithridatium. A Study in Therapeutics. London: Wellcome Historical Medical Library, 1966.
8 Webster C. Paracelsus. Medicine, Magic and Mission at the End of Time. New Haven and London: Yale University Press, 2008; Chapter V: 131–68.
9 Deichmann WB, Henschler D, Holmstedt B, Keil G. What is there that is not poison? A study of the *Third Defense* by Paracelsus. Archives of Toxicology 1986; 58(4): 207–13.
10 Stephenson RP. A modification of receptor theory. British Journal of Pharmacology and Chemotherapy 1956; 11(4): 379–93.
11 Kelly J, Stephenson J. Dr RP Stephenson (1925–2004). *pA$_2$* Online 2004; 2(3). www.pa2online.org/Vol2Issue3Stephenson.html.
12 Calabrese EJ. Hormesis: from mainstream to therapy. Journal of Cell Communication and Signaling 2014; 8(4): 289–91.
13 Calabrese EJ. Historical foundations of hormesis. Homeopathy 2015; 104(2): 83–89.
14 Muir MMMP. A History of Chemical Theories and Laws. New York: John Wiley & Sons, 1907: 381.

15 Whewell W. Chapter II: Establishment and development of the idea of chemical affinity. In: The Philosophy of the Inductive Sciences: Founded Upon Their History.. London: John W Parker, West Strand; Cambridge: J & JJ Deighton, 1840: 374.

16 Berthollet CL. Recherches sur les lois de l'affinité. Paris: Baudouin, 1801.

17 Pereira J. The Elements of Materia Medica. 4th edition. London: Longman, Brown, Green & Longmans, 1854: 1–91.

18 Parascandola J. The development of receptor theory. In Parnham MJ, Bruinvels J, editors. Discoveries in Pharmacology. Volume 3. Pharmacological Methods, Receptors and Chemotherapy. Amsterdam: Elsevier, 1986: 129–56.

19 Drake M. Population and Society in Norway, 1735–1865. Cambridge: Cambridge University Press, 1969.

20 Guldberg CM, Waage P. Etudes sur les affinités chimiques. Christiana, 1867.

21 van 'tHoff JH. Etudes de dynamiques chimiques. Amsterdam: Frederik Muller, 1884.

22 "M.M.P.M." Chemical Affinity. By GULDBERG and WAAGE (J. pr. Chem., [2], 19, 69–114). Journal of the Chemical Society Abstracts 1879; 36: 580–86.

23 Muir MMP. XXVII.—Contributions from the laboratory of Gonville and Caius College, Cambridge. No. V. Note on chemical equilibrium. Chemical Society Abstracts 1880; 37: 424–29.

24 Mysels KJ. Textbook errors. VII: The laws of reaction rates and of equilibrium. Journal of Chemical Education 1956; 33: 178–79.

25 Guggenheim EA. Textbook errors. XI: More about the laws of reaction rates and of equilibrium. Journal of Chemical Education 1956; 33: 544–45.

26 Wright MR. Fundamental chemical kinetics. In: An Exploratory Introduction to the Concepts. Chichester: Horwood Publishing, 1999.

27 Crivellato E, Beltrami CA, Mallardi F, Ribatti D. Paul Ehrlich's doctoral thesis: a milestone in the study of mast cells. British Journal of Haematology 2003; 123(1): 19–21.

28 Prüll C-R. Part of a scientific master plan? Paul Ehrlich and the origins of his receptor concept. Medical History 2003; 47: 332–56.

29 Silverstein AM. Paul Ehrlich's passion: the origins of his receptor immunology. Cellular Immunology 1999; 194: 213–21.

30 Ehrlich P. Partial cell functions. Nobel Lecture, December 11, 1908.

31 Sherrington CS. The Integrative Action of the Nervous System. New Haven: Yale University Press; London: Humphrey Milford, Oxford University Press, 1906.

32 Ehrlich P. Experimental Researches on Specific Therapeutics. The Harben Lectures for 1907 of the Royal Institute of Public Health. New York: Paul B Hoeber, 1909.

33 Langley JN. On the reaction of cells and of nerve-endings to certain poisons, chiefly as regards the reaction of striated muscle to nicotine and to curari. Journal of Physiology 1905; 33(4–5): 374–413.

34 Virchow R. Ueber die Erregbarkeit der Flimmerzellen. [On the irritability of ciliated cells.] Archiv für Pathologische Anatomie, Physiologie und für Klinische Medizin 1854; 6(1): 133–34.

35 Schulz H. Zur Lehre von der Arzneiwirkung. [On the theory of drug effects.] Virchows Archiv für Pathologische Anatomie und Physiologie und für Klinische Medizin 1887; 108(3): 423–45.

36 Schulz H. Ueber Hefegifte. [On toxic yeasts.] Pflügers Archiv für die Gesamte Physiologie des Menschen und der Tiere 1888; 42(1): 517–41.

37 Southam CM, Ehrlich J. Effects of extract of Western red-cedar heartwood on certain wood-decaying fungi in culture. Phytopathology 1943; 33: 517–24.

38 Oberbaum M, Gropp C. Update on hormesis and its relation to homeopathy. Homeopathy 2015; 104(4): 227–33.

39 Koppe R. Untersuchungen über die pharmakologischen Wirkungen des Digitoxins, Digitalins und Digitaleïns. [Investigations into the pharmacological actions of digitoxin, digitalin, and digitalein.] Archiv für Experimentelle Pathologie und Pharmakologie 1875; 3(3–4): 274–301.

40 Juckuff E. Versuche zur auffindung eines Dosirungsgesetzes: eine toxicologisch–mathematische Studie. [Attempts to find a law affecting dosages: a toxicological–mathematical study.] Leipzig: FCW Vogel, 1895.

41 Harnack E. Ueber den Begriff cumulativen Wirkung in ihren Verhältniss zu den Dosirungsgesetzen. [On cumulative effects in relation to the laws regulating dosages.] MMW Münchener Medizinische Wochenschrift 1896; 44: 1065–67.

42 Spenzer JG. Ueber den Grad der Aethernarkose im Verhältniss zur Menge des eingeathmeten Aetherdampfes. [On the extent of ether narcosis in relation to the amount of ether inhaled.] Archiv für Experimentelle Pathologie und Pharmakologie 1894; 33(6): 407–14.

43 Holford NHG, Sheiner LB. Understanding the dose–effect relationship: clinical application of pharmacokinetic–pharmacodynamic models. Clinical Pharmacokinetics 1981; 6(6): 429–53.

44 Pearce RM. An experimental glomerular lesion caused by venom (*Crotalus adamanteus*). Journal of Experimental Medicine 1909; 11(4): 532–40.

45 Bull CG, Pritchett IW. Toxin and antitoxin of and protective inoculation against *Bacillus welchii*. Journal of Experimental Medicine 1917; 26(1): 119–38.

46 Kahlenberg L, True RH. On the toxic action of dissolved salts and their electrolytic dissociation. Botanical Gazette 1896; 22(2): 81–124.

47 Krönig B, Paul Th. Die chemischen Grundlagen der Lehre von der Giftwirkung und Desinfektion. [The chemical foundations of the study of disinfection and of the actions of poisons.] Zeitschrift für Hygiene und Infektionskrankheit 1897; 25(1): 1–112.

48 Chick H. An investigation of the laws of disinfection. Journal of Hygiene 1908; 8(1): 92–158.

49 Watson HE. A note on the variation of the rate of disinfection with change in the concentration of the disinfectant. Journal of Hygiene 1908; 8(4): 536.

50 Cash JT. The relationship of action to dose especially with reference to repeated administration of indaconitine. British Medical Journal 1908; i: 1213–18.

51 Hunt R. On the effects of intravenous injections of minimal doses of epinephrine sulphate upon the arterial blood-pressure. American Journal of Physiology 1901; 5(2): vii.

52 Hill AV. The mode of action of nicotine and curari, determined by the form of the contraction curve and the method of temperature coefficients. Journal of Physiology 1909; 39(5): 361–73.

53 Lyon DM. Does the reaction to adrenalin obey Weber's law? Journal of Pharmacology and Experimental Therapeutics 1923; 21(4): 229–35.

54 Shackell LF, Williamson W, Deitchman MM, Katzman GM, Kleinman BS. The relation of dosage to effect. I. Epinephrine on arterial rings. Journal of Pharmacology and Experimental Therapeutics 1924; 24(1): 53–65.

55 Clark AJ. The reaction between acetyl choline and muscle cells. Journal of Physiology 1926; 61(4): 530–46.

56 Galton F. The geometric mean, in vital and social statistics. Proceedings of the Royal Society of London 1879; 29(196–199): 365–67.

57 McAlister D. The law of the geometric mean. Proceedings of the Royal Society of London 1879; 29(196–199): 367–76.

58 Ferner RE. Harms from medicines: inevitable, in error or intentional. British Journal of Clinical Pharmacology 2014; 77(3): 403–9.

59 Clark AJ. The Mode of Action of Drugs on Cells. London: Edward Arnold & Co, 1933.

238   *Jeffrey K. Aronson and Robin E. Ferner*

60 Gaddum JH. The quantitative effects of antagonistic drugs. Journal of Physiology 1937; 89(Suppl): 7P–9P.
61 Schild HO. pA, a new scale for the measurement of drug antagonism. British Journal of Pharmacology 1947; 2(3): 189–206.
62 Ariëns EJ. Affinity and intrinsic activity in the theory of competitive inhibition. I. Problems and theory. Archives International de Pharmacodynamie et de Thérapie 1954; 99(1): 32–49.
63 Paton WDM. A theory of drug action based on the rate of drug-receptor combination. Proceedings of the Royal Society of London Series B 1961; 154(954): 21–69.
64 Changeux JP, Thiery J, Tung Y, Kittel C. On the cooperativity of biological membranes. Proceedings of the National Academy of Sciences of the United States of America 1967; 57(2): 335–41.
65 Rang HP. The receptor concept: pharmacology's big idea. British Journal of Pharmacology 2006; 147(Suppl): S9–S16.
66 Kenakin T. Principles: receptor theory in pharmacology. Trends in Pharmacological Sciences 2004; 25(4): 186–92.
67 Calabrese EJ, Baldwin LA. Hormesis: U-shaped dose responses and their centrality in toxicology. Trends in Pharmacological Science 2001; 22(6): 285–91.
68 Gaddum JH. Clinical pharmacology. Proceedings of the Royal Society of Medicine 1954; 47(3): 195–204.
69 Chennavasin P, Seiwell R, Brater DC. Pharmacokinetic–dynamic analysis of the indomethacin–furosemide interaction in man. Journal of Pharmacology and Experimental Therapeutics 1980; 215(1): 77–81.
70 Brater DC, Chennavasin P, Day B, Burdette A, Anderson S. Bumetanide and furosemide. Clinical Pharmacology and Therapeutics 1983; 34(2): 207–13.
71 McDevitt DG, Shand DG. Plasma concentrations and the time-course of beta blockade due to propranolol. Clinical Pharmacology and Therapeutics 1975; 18(6): 708–13.
72 Hughes DA, Aronson JK. A systematic review and empirical analysis of the relation between dose and duration of drug action. Journal of Clinical Pharmacology 2010; 50(1): 17–26.
73 Wayne EJ. Problems of toxicity in clinical medicine. In: Walpole AL, Spinks A, editors. The Evaluation of Drug Toxicity. London: J & A Churchill Ltd, 1958: 1–11.
74 Levine RR. Factors modifying the effects of drugs in individuals. In: Pharmacology. Drug Actions and Reactions. Boston: Little, Brown and Co, 1973: 261–91.
75 Wade OL, Beeley L. Adverse Reactions to Drugs. 2nd edition. London: William Heinemann Medical books Ltd, 1976: Chapter II.
76 Rawlins MD, Thompson JW. Pathogenesis of adverse drug reactions. In: Davies DM, editor. Textbook of Adverse Drug Reactions. Oxford: Oxford University Press, 1977: 44.
77 Rawlins MD, Thompson JW. Pathogenesis of adverse drug reactions. In: Davies DM, editor. Textbook of Adverse Drug Reactions. 2nd edition. Oxford: Oxford University Press, 1981: 11.
78 Grahame-Smith DG, Aronson JK. In: The Oxford Textbook of Clinical Pharmacology and Drug Therapy. Oxford: Oxford University Press, 1984: 134.
79 Hoigné R, Jaeger MD, Wymann R, Egli A, Muller U, Hess T, Galeazzi R, Maibach R, Kunzi UP. Time pattern of allergic reactions to drugs. Agents and Actions Supplement 1990; 29: 39–58.
80 Park BK, Pirmohamed M, Kitteringham NR. Idiosyncratic drug reactions: a mechanistic evaluation of risk factors. British Journal of Clinical Pharmacology 1992; 34(5): 377–95.

81 Laurence DR, Bennett PN. Clinical Pharmacology. Edinburgh: Churchill Livingstone, 1992: 121–22.

82 Ferner R, Mann RD. Drug safety and pharmacovigilance. In: Page C, Curtis MJ, Sutter MC, Walker MJA, Hoffman BB, editors. Integrated Pharmacology. 1st edition. London: Mosby, 1997: 83–90.

83 Hartigan-Go KY, Wong JQ. Inclusion of therapeutic failures as adverse drug reactions. In: Aronson JK, editor. Side Effects of Drugs. Annual 23. Amsterdam: Elsevier, 2000: xxvii–xxxiii.

84 Aronson JK. Drug therapy. In: Haslett C, Chilvers ER, Boon NA, Colledge NR, editors, Hunter JAA, international editor. Davidson's Principles and Practice of Medicine. 19th edition. Edinburgh: Elsevier Science Limited, 2002: 147–63.

85 Aronson JK, Ferner RE. Joining the DoTS. Classifying adverse drug reactions by dose responsiveness, time course, and susceptibility. BMJ 2003; 327(7425): 1222–25.

86 Aronson JK. Adverse drug reactions: history, terminology, classification, causality, frequency, preventability. In: Talbot J, Aronson JK, editors. Stephens' Detection and Evaluation of Adverse Drug Reactions: Principles and Practice. 6th edition. Oxford: Wiley-Blackwell, 2011: 1–119.

87 Aronson JK, Price D, Ferner RE. A strategy for regulatory action when new adverse effects of a licensed product emerge. Drug Safety 2009; 32(2): 91–98.

88 Callréus T. Use of the dose, time, susceptibility (DoTS) classification scheme for adverse drug reactions in pharmacovigilance planning. Drug Safety 2006; 29(7): 557–66.

89 Aronson JK, Ferner RE. The Law of Mass Action and the pharmacological concentration–effect curve: resolving the paradox of apparently non-dose-related adverse drug reactions. British Journal of Clinical Pharmacology 2015; 81(1): 56–61.

90 Aronson JK, Ferner RE. Preventability of drug-related harms. Part 2: Proposed criteria, based on frameworks that classify adverse drug reactions. Drug Safety 2010; 33(11): 995–1002.

91 Roughead EE, Pratt NL. Impact on drug safety of variation in adherence: the need for routinely reporting measures of dose intensity in medication safety studies using electronic health data. Drug Safety 2015; 38(12): 1145–52.

92 Aronson JK. Distinguishing hazards and harms, adverse drug effects and adverse drug reactions: implications for clinical trials, biomarkers, monitoring, and surveillance. Drug Safety 2013; 36(3): 147–53.

93 Kenakin T. The mass action equation in pharmacology. British Journal of Clinical Pharmacology 2016; 81(1): 41–51.

94 Hill AV. The possible effects of the aggregation of the molecules of hæmoglobin on its dissociation curves. Journal of Physiology 1910; 40(Supplement): iv–vii.

95 Bindslev N. In: Drug–Acceptor Interactions. Modeling Theoretical Tools to Test and Evaluate Experimental Equilibrium Effects. CRC Press, 2017. https://www.taylorfrancis.com/books/9781351660587.

96 Ross HE, Murray DJ (editors and translators). E.H. Weber on the Tactile Senses. 2nd edition. Erlbaum, UK: Taylor & Francis, 1996. https://books.google.co.uk/books?id=xEd8JglYzFwC&printsec=frontcover&source=gbs_ge_summary_r&cad=0#v=onepage&q&f=false.

97 Stevens SS. On the psychophysical law. Psychological Review 1957; 64(3): 153–81.

98 Barr J, Marshall CR, Atkinson GA, Smith RS. A discussion on diuretics. British Medical Journal 1897; 2(1928): 1697–709.

Index